EAT
THIS
NOT
THAT!

EAT THIS NOT THAT!

THE BEST (& WORST)

FOODS IN AMERICA

BY DAVID ZINCZENKO

Ballantine Books

New York

No book can replace the diagnostic expertise
and medical advice of a trusted physician.
Please be certain to consult with your doctor before
making any decisions that affect your health,
particularly if you suffer from any medical condition or
have any symptom that may require treatment.

Published in the United States by Ballantine Books,
an imprint of Random House,
a division of Penguin Random House LLC, New York.

BALLANTINE and the HOUSE colophon are
registered trademarks of Penguin Random House LLC.

ISBN 978-1-5247-9670-9
ebook ISBN 978-1-5247-9669-3

Printed in China on acid-free paper

246897531

Book design by J. HEROUN and LAURA WHITE

To the 8 million men and women who have made *EAT THIS, NOT THAT!* a publishing phenomenon and who have spread the word to friends and relatives about the importance of knowing what's really in our food. Because of your passionate efforts, food manufacturers and restaurant chains are waking up to the fact that more and more of us demand good, solid information about our food, and healthy choices that will let us drop pounds and stay lean for life.

And to the men and women working in America's fields, farms, and supermarkets, waiting tables, and toiling in kitchens everywhere: It is because of your hard work that Americans have so many options. This book is designed to help us choose the best of what you've created.

—*DAVE ZINCZENKO*

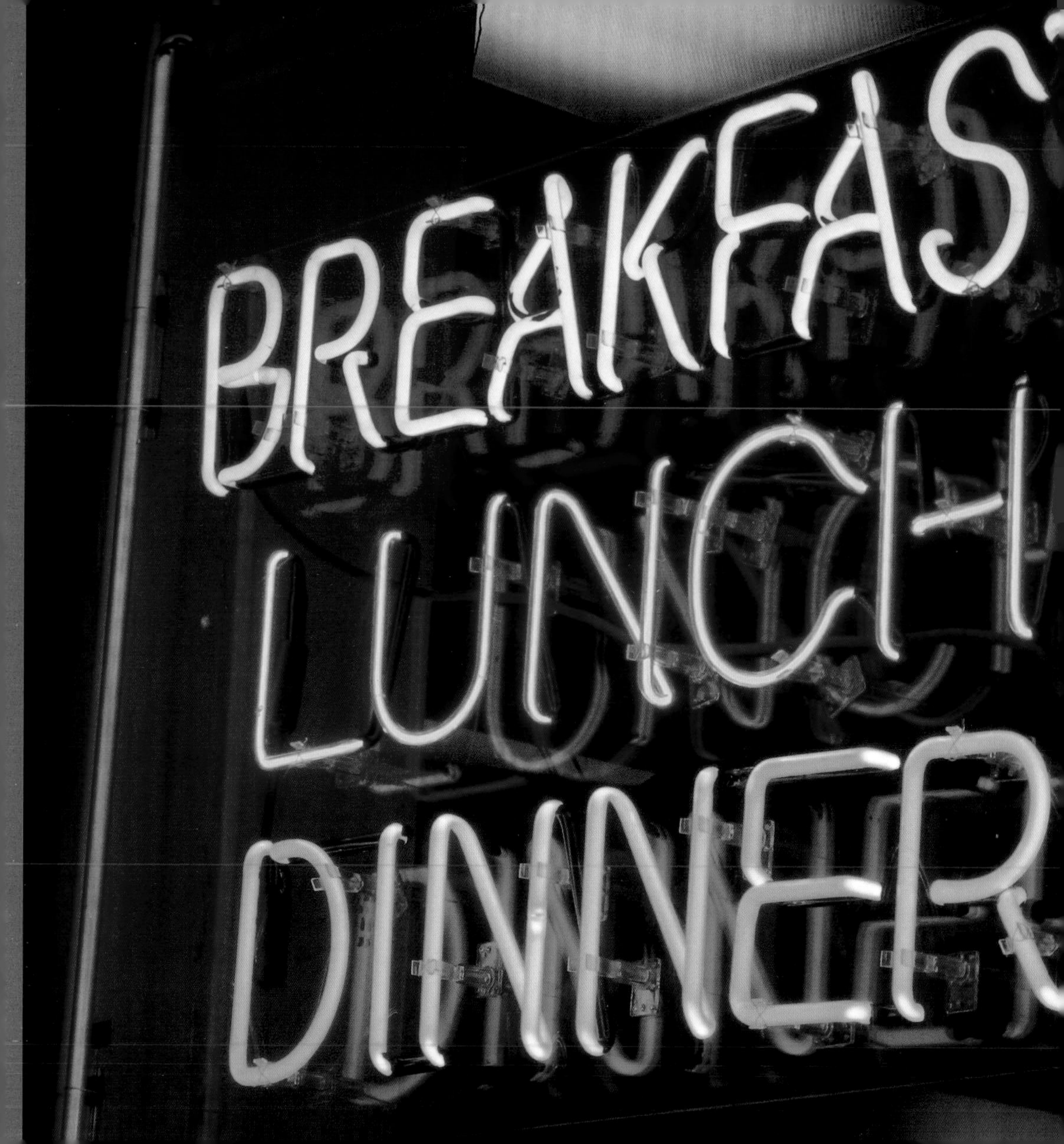
BREAKFAS
LUNCH
DINNER

CONTENTS

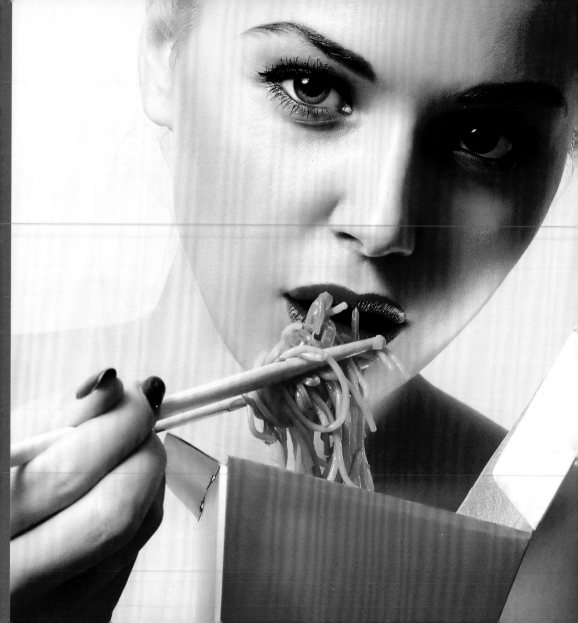

WELCOME TO THE

FUTURE OF FOOD

IF A COTERIE of science fiction writers had gotten into a room 40 years ago and imagined what 2020 would look like, what would they have thought up?

Flying cars? We're not there yet. Teleportation? Still waiting. Cure for the common cold? They're working on it. Food appearing out of nowhere at the touch of a button?

Ah. Bingo. The time it takes to go from "I'd like a hamburger" to "That was a delicious hamburger" has shrunk exponentially from the time of our great-grandparents, who had to tramp through snow to the butcher shop, lug home a pound of chuck, grind it, and fry it up themselves. Even our own parents, back in the dark ages of the last millennium, had to rummage around for a menu, make a phone call (from their house!), and then wait 40 minutes for dinner to show up. Today, you can accidentally butt dial a burger from your GrubHub app. Problem solved!

But one person's paradise is another's purgatory, and all the super-convenient food delivery apps and restaurant reservation sites and proliferating juice and smoothie bars—where food is reduced to the most quickly consumed form possible—have only served to speed the race of calories into our bodies. I envy Great-Grandma and the muscles she built grinding that chuck steak and chopping those vegetables. Today, we just drink our lunch—and then go to the gym to work up some calorie burn because life is so damn convenient.

Consider this: When I wrote the *Eat This Not That! Restaurant Survival Guide*, in 2010, I reported on how Americans were getting 33 percent of their calories from outside the home—up from less than 20 percent in the 1980s. And it's not just because we're spending more time in restaurants.

The Great Recession changed the way we eat. When everyone was too worried about the future to book that trip to the Bahamas, we instead looked to little indulgences to feed our passions. And one of the places we indulged ourselves was food. Look at how our food is behaving differently.

It's Driving to Us!

THE FOOD TRUCK industry has grown by 12 percent each year since 2009—again, perhaps in part as a response to the recession. Eating indulgent food, eating more local, and eating on the go—especially when lunch hours are squeezed and bosses are angsty—are three trends that coalesce around the idling food truck. America's 3,900 food trucks take in $804 million in revenue, but some analysts see this as a $2.7 billion industry within the decade.

It's Getting Baked Beforehand

DOES IT COUNT as "food shopping" if you go to a supermarket and buy a takeout dinner there, instead of at a takeout joint? More and more, supermarkets aren't selling us fixin's, they're selling us food that's already been fixed. Every year, Americans swing by the grocery store and pick up 450 million rotisserie chickens; in one year alone, Costco sold 68 million of them.

That's a trend that's only going to grow. According to one survey, 78 percent of millennials brought home prepared foods from the supermarket in the last month. Only 57 percent of seniors did the same. As our cooking skills erode, so too does our ability to control exactly what it is we're eating.

It's Coming at Us Through Our Phones!

SIXTY-NINE PERCENT of Americans have used a mobile device to order delivery food. The growth of GrubHub and other delivery apps has made ordering takeout so simple that there's no reason to go through the hassle and inconvenience of trekking to the grocery store and buying food—even if someone's already cooked it for you.

And Then Going Back Out Through Our Phones!

SHARING AND COLLECTING images of our meals has become a national pastime—one in four Americans say they photograph their meals. In a one-month survey of social media users, 29 million Americans posted a photo of their meal at a restaurant. Pinterest reports that food-related content is its top category, with 57 percent of users posting food shots. One food industry report showed that over a two-week period, Instagram users posted 48,000 photos

from just 30 of the nation's top restaurants. And once our friends start sharing their awesome restaurant meals, it makes us wonder why we should bother slaving over a hot stove.

It's Showing Us to Our Tables Faster

GONE ARE THE DAYS when you had to call five different restaurants to find an open reservation, and then slip the maître d' 20 bucks to get a decent table. Today, one in five restaurant reservations are made online, up from just 12 percent a few years ago. Fifteen million people use OpenTable.com every month. By taking the stress, guesswork, and fear of rejection out of dining out, sites like OpenTable are also removing one more reason to stay at home and cook.

Numbers Munching

Eight hundred sixty-seven people just like you responded to the most recent *Eat This, Not That!* poll and shared what was going on in their heads—and in their bellies. The surprising facts? Almost half of us are on a diet, yet more than half of us have no idea how many calories were in our last meal …

When was the last time you ate a meal at a restaurant?

LAST 24 HOURS	**33%**
LAST WEEK	**46%**
LAST MONTH	**14%**
MORE THAN A MONTH AGO	**7%**

Do you know how many calories were in your meal there?

 YES **28%**
 NO **71%**

Are you concerned with counting calories?

 YES **73%**
 NO **26%**

Are you currently on a diet?

 YES **46%**
 NO **53%**

In a recent study in the *Journal of the American Medical Association,* researchers looked at the nutrition facts of a typical breakfast, lunch, and dinner from 19 chain restaurants. Their findings were pretty stunning. While only 45 percent of respondents in our poll say they're okay with a restaurant meal that tops 1,000 to 1,200 calories, the average restaurant meal (and remember, this includes breakfasts!) contains:

↘ **1,128** CALORIES

or about 56 percent of a person's daily calorie intake

↘ **2,269 MG** SODIUM

or 95 percent of a person's daily intake

↘ **58 G** FAT

or 89 percent of a person's daily intake

A 2013 survey of foods at popular restaurants found dishes at:

PERKINS,
ON THE BORDER,
CHEESECAKE FACTORY,
FRIENDLY'S,
APPLEBEE'S,
BERTUCCI'S
UNO PIZZERIA & GRILL

that *exceeded* 1,800 calories per serving—the total number of calories an adult woman should eat in an entire day.

How many calories are too many for a restaurant meal?

500–800	**10%**
800–1,000	**45%**
1,000–1,200	**28%**
1,200–1,500	**10%**
MORE THAN 1,500	**7%**

FOODS PREPARED BY RESTAURANTS, CATERERS, AND OTHER SOURCES NOW ACCOUNT FOR 43 PERCENT OF OUR CALORIES, UP FROM 33 PERCENT JUST FIVE YEARS AGO. ON ANY GIVEN DAY, A THIRD OF AMERICANS HAVE EATEN AT A RESTAURANT. IN THE 1980S, ONLY 20 PERCENT OF OUR CALORIES CAME FROM OUTSIDE THE HOME.

What aspect of food are you most concerned about?

CHEMICAL ADDITIVES **28%**

CALORIES **25%**

SUGAR **12%**

CARBS **11%**

SODIUM **6%**

SATURATED FAT **5%**

OTHER **8%**

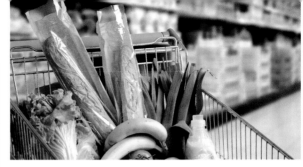

When you food shop, what's more important?

HEALTHY INGREDIENTS → 76%   PRICE → 23%

You've just learned that your favorite restaurant meal contains more calories than you should eat in an entire day. Your reaction is:

That's okay, it's a splurge
42%

I'm never eating that again
56%

Don't care
1%

Do you trust that foods labeled "organic" or "non-GMO" are what they say they are?

YES **40%**

NO **59%**

WHAT PROMISES ON FOOD PACKAGING ARE MOST LIKELY TO GET YOU TO PICK UP A PRODUCT?

Whole Grain	Organic	Fresh	Natural	A good source of fiber	Multigrain	A good source of omega-3	Low-Fat	Low-Carb	Light or Lite	Fat-free
41%	**40%**	**33%**	**28%**	**28%**	**20%**	**20%**	**17%**	**17%**	**15%**	**12%**

Look for "100% whole grain" on the label; even a "healthy" bread like Pepperidge Farm Light Style Soft Wheat is made with a mix of whole-wheat and white flour. Same holds true at restaurants: Panera's Whole Grain Loaf and Whole Grain Baguette are primarily enriched white flour.

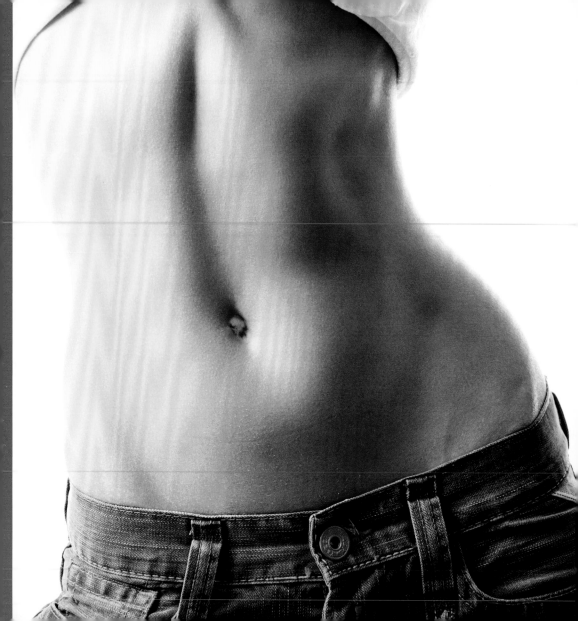

How to
LOSE WEIGHT
with This Book

THE BASIC BELIEF has always been that, for adults, calculating your potential weight gain is simple. It takes about 3,500 calories' worth of food to build a pound of body fat, and 3,500 calories' worth of activity to burn that pound off: Calories in minus calories out divided by 3,500 equals the number of pounds that a given meal or daily diet will help you to gain or lose.

In recent years, however, more and more researchers have looked at the increasingly robust American landscape and thought, "There's got to be more to it than this." And in fact there is. New research shows that too many calories, when combined with too little nutrition, can do more than just tip the scales of that weight-gain equation. When we overeat without giving our bodies the nutrients it needs—especially early in life—we trigger our fat genes to turn "on." Now our genetic propensity to gain weight is accelerated, and our bodies become much more efficient at converting incoming calories to fat. That's why some people seem to diet constantly but never lose weight—their fat genes are revving on high, and just reducing calories by cutting out certain food groups like all meat, or all carbs, or all foods that begin with the letter T, simply won't work.

Here's why that's good news: When we start swapping out egregiously bad foods and swapping in healthier versions, we can actually impact the behavior of our genes. While you can never fully turn them back "off," you can dim their powers. The better you eat, the more your fat genes deactivate. The more they deactivate, the more weight you lose—and it becomes a virtuous cycle. Weight loss leads to even greater weight loss.

But to start the process, you have to reduce calories in—without skipping meals or cutting out your favorite foods—while maintaining calories out. And that's what *Eat This, Not That!* is all about.

Understanding the Numbers

On the "calories out" side, we have your daily activities: cleaning house, standing in line at the post office, hauling groceries, and so on. Often, when people discover extra flab hanging around their midsections, they assume there's something wrong with this side of the equation. Maybe so, but more likely it's the front end of the equation— the "calories in" side—that's tipping the scale. That side keeps track of all the cookies, fried chicken, and piles of pasta you eat every day.

In order to maintain a healthy body weight, a moderately active female between the ages of 20 and 50 needs only about 1,800 calories per day, according to the Centers for Disease Control and Prevention. The average man fitting the same profile needs about 2,200 calories per day. Those numbers will fluctuate depending on whether you're taller or shorter than average, whether you run marathons or resist exercise like the plague. (For a more accurate assessment, use the calorie calculator at mayoclinic.com.)

The problem is, many of the foods that we consider "normal" servings are, in fact, so packed with calories that we can easily blow through that 1,800 to 2,200 figure in just one sitting. But if you'd come armed with *Eat This, Not That!*, you might have made different choices. If you'd ordered the Shrimp on the Barbie (no need to share, eat the whole thing), an Asian Sesame Salad with Seared Ahi and Sesame Vinaigrette, and then shared a Classic Cheesecake, you'd have each cut your calorie total to 969—a respectable dinner that's less than a third of what you might have eaten. Even if you only have date night once a week, that's enough for each of you to lose 31 pounds a year!

Here's the Math

Do This ↙

That's the magic of *Eat This, Not That!* Within these pages are literally hundreds of simple food swaps that will save you from 10 to 1,000 calories apiece. The more often you choose the "Eat This" foods over the "Not That" options, the quicker you'll notice layers of fat melting away from your body. Check this out:

THE MATH

3,050	calories in the big meal
—969	calories in meal swap
2,081	calories saved with swap
2,081	calories saved in swap
x 52	once a week for a year
108,212	calories saved per year
108,212	calories saved per year
÷3,500	calories per pound of fat
30.91	pounds saved per year!

3,050 minus 969 equals 2,081 calories you just saved. Once a week means 2,081 times 52, which equals 108,212 calories in a year. And since it takes 3,500 calories to produce a pound of body weight, simple division leads you to 30.91 pounds.

EXAMPLES

A cup of Apple Cinnamon Cheerios contains **160 calories.**

A cup of Cinnamon Burst Cheerios contains **110 calories.**

Alter your breakfast every morning and save 5 pounds this year!

Two tablespoons of Kraft Roka Blue Cheese dressing will cost you **120 calories.**

Bolthouse Farms Yogurt Dressing Chunky Blue Cheese is **just 35 calories.**

It's only 85 calories, what's the difference? But making one swap like this at home every day will *help you lose 9 pounds this year.*

WHAT'S HEALTHIER

The Premium Grilled Chicken Ranch BLT Sandwich at McDonald's, or their Premium Crispy Chicken Ranch BLT Salad?

Choose wrong and you've cost yourself **160 calories.** (Hint: It's the sandwich!) Make the right choice every day and drop nearly 17 pounds in a year!

A turkey sandwich from Panera Bread sounds like a reasonable lunch. But pass on the Sierra Turkey on Asiago Cheese Focaccia and opt instead for the Smoked Turkey Breast on Country.

Pretty much the same meal? Not when you're *saving 380 calories* by making the swap. A move like this at lunch five times a week *saves you more than 39 pounds* this year!

And the *Best* News Is . . .

THESE SWAPS AREN'T ISOLATED CALORIE SAVERS. IN THESE PAGES WE'LL SHOW YOU HOW TO SAVE CALORIES ON EVERYTHING FROM SOUPS TO SALADS, FROM RUBY TUESDAY TO T.G.I. FRIDAY'S, AND EVERY DAY IN BETWEEN.

8 SUPERFOODS

You Should Eat Every Day

WE ALL WANT to eat a "balanced" diet. But what does that mean in an era of 1,759-calorie burgers? (Your Pretzel Burger is not a good buy, Ruby Tuesday!) Or soups with three days' worth of sodium? (P.F. Chang's Hot & Sour—yep, we're pretty hot and sour!) Or coffee drinks with the equivalent of 42 sugar packets? (That's not cool, Dunkin' Vanilla Bean Coolatta!)

Eating a balanced diet in today's food landscape means that when you're surrounded by bad, you've got to maximize the good. We've chosen eight of the best foods to build your pantry around—a belly-filling, metabolism-revving, nutrient-maximizing mix of classic health-food favorites and twenty-first century superfoods.

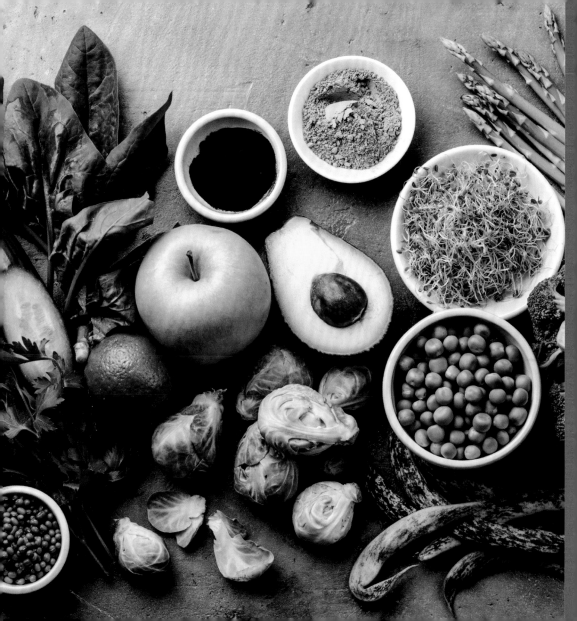

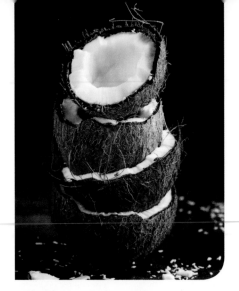

1/ Coconut Oil

One study from the *American Journal of Clinical Nutrition* found that subjects who ate coconut oil lost overall weight and belly fat faster than a group consuming the same amount of olive oil. The secret is in coconut's medium-chain triglycerides. Unlike the long-chain fatty acids in most oils, coconut oil is broken down immediately for use rather than stored, and has been found to speed up the metabolism. That's right—your body has trouble storing the calories in coconut oil and revs up its metabolism to burn them instead. Coconut oil's high smoke point makes it great for just about every dish from eggs to stir-fries, and a delicious substitute for butter when baking.

2/ Flax & Chia Seeds

One of the hallmarks of a balanced diet is to have a good ratio of omega-6 fatty acids to omega-3s. A 4:1 ratio would be ideal, but the modern American diet is more like 20:1. That leads to inflammation, which can trigger weight gain. But while eating a serving of salmon every day isn't exactly convenient, sprinkling these two seeds—among the most highly concentrated sources of omega-3s in the food world—into smoothies, salads, cereals, pancakes, or even desserts is as easy a diet upgrade as you can get. Animal studies suggest a

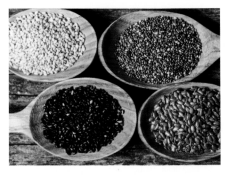

chia-rich diet can lower harmful LDL cholesterol and protect the heart, and a recent study in the journal *Hypertension* found that daily consumption of flax-seed-fortified bakery products reduced blood pressure in patients with peripheral artery disease. Best absorbed when ground, flax adds delicious nuttiness to oats, cereal, smoothies, and baked goods.

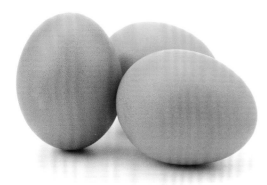

3/ **Eggs**

Eggs are the single best dietary source of the B vitamin choline, an essential nutrient used in the construction of all the body's cell membranes. Two eggs will give you half your day's worth; only beef liver has more. (And believe us, starting your day with a slab of beef liver does not make for a great morning.) Choline deficiency is linked directly to the genes that cause the accumulation of belly fat. Eggs can solve the problem: Research has shown dieters who eat eggs for breakfast instead of high-carb bagels have an easier time losing weight due to eggs' satiety value. At about 70 calories, a hard-boiled egg also makes an easy afternoon snack . . . just don't tell your coworkers; according to a personality analysis by the British Egg Industry Council, boiled-egg consumers tend to be disorganized! (Other findings: Fried egg fans have a high sex drive, and omelet eaters are self-disciplined.)

4/ **Apples** (skin on)

A medium-size apple, at about 100 calories and 4.5 grams of fiber per fruit, is one of the best snack options for anyone looking to slim down—but especially apple-shaped folks. A recent study at Wake Forest Baptist Medical Center found that for every 10-gram increase in soluble fiber eaten per day, visceral fat (that's dangerous belly fat) was reduced by 3.7 percent over five years. Participants who paired their apple-a-day habit with 30 minutes of exercise two to four times per week saw a 7.4 percent decrease in the rate of visceral fat accumulation over the same time period. But don't peel your apple if you want to peel off the pounds: A study conducted at the University of Western Australia found that the blushing varieties (such as Pink Ladies) had the highest level of antioxidant phenols, most of which are found in the skin. Applesauce isn't a worthy substitute.

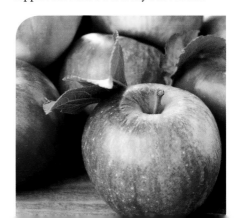

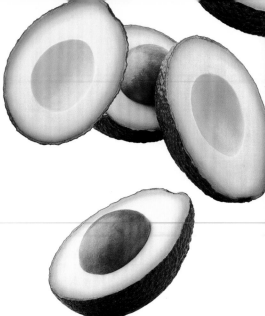

5/ **Cinnamon**

It may be the easiest nutrition upgrade of all: Put cinnamon on your toast. According to researchers, cinnamon contains powerful antioxidants called polyphenols proven to improve insulin sensitivity and, in turn, our body's ability to store fat and manage hunger cues. A series of studies printed in the *American Journal of Clinical Nutrition* found that adding a heaping teaspoon of cinnamon to a starchy meal may help stabilize blood sugar and ward off insulin spikes.

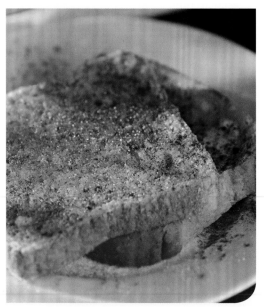

6/ **Avocado**

A scoop of guacamole is one of the most effective hunger-squashers known to man. In a study published in *Nutrition Journal*, participants who ate half a fresh avocado with lunch reported a 40 percent decreased desire to eat for hours afterward. At only 60 calories, a 2-tablespoon serving of guacamole (on top of eggs, salads, grilled meats, etc.) can provide the same satiety benefit with even more of a flavor punch. Just be sure when buying store-bought guac that avocados actually made it into the box (many are made without the real fruit)! We love Wholly Guacamole as a store brand.

7/Lettuce

Move over, King Kale. In a new William Paterson University study that compared the 47 top superfoods by nutrient volume, the trendy green came in a respectable—but unremarkable—15th on the list. Ranking higher: watercress, spinach, leafy green lettuce, and endive. Make yourself a bowl of simple leafy greens and splash on some olive oil. According to a Purdue University study, as little as 3 grams of monounsaturated fat can help the body absorb vegetables' carotenoids (those magic molecules that protect you from chronic diseases like cancer and heart disease). Pairing your lettuce with a scant tablespoon of olive oil–based vinaigrette is your best bet.

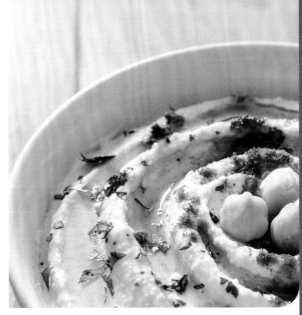

8/Hummus

A recent study published in the journal *Obesity* found people who ate a single serving a day of garbanzo beans or chickpeas (which form the basis of hummus) reported feeling 31 percent fuller than their beanless counterparts. Packed with fiber and protein, garbanzo beans have a low glycemic index, meaning that they break down slowly and keep you feeling full. The secret is to avoid hummus varieties made with tahini; sourced from sesame seeds, tahini has a high omega-6-to-omega-3 fatty acid ratio. Look for hummus that's olive oil–based.

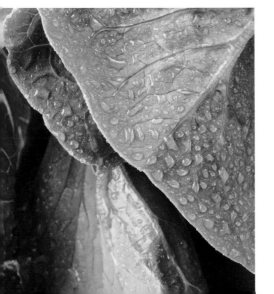

CHAPTER 1

EAT THIS, NOT THAT AT YOUR
FAVORITE
RESTAURANTS

SIMPLE WAYS TO EAT ALL YOUR FAVORITE FOODS— AND DODGE THE CALORIE BOMBS

HERE'S A NUMBER you should keep in mind: 43. That's the percentage of calories you're going to eat this year that will come from restaurants, catering companies, and other folks who, unlike you and your mom, don't really care very much about your health. So you'd better plan to be extra vigilant yourself.

And that's hard to do at a restaurant. Researchers call it the "special occasion mentality," and it sets in whenever we eat out at the local Applebee's or Arby's. Restaurants are where we celebrate our victories and drown our defeats—so it's worth it to splurge, right?

In this chapter, you'll discover exactly how not-so-special some of your restaurant favorites really are and some smart ways to ensure that the terrific spread at the buffet doesn't turn into a terrific spread at your waistline.

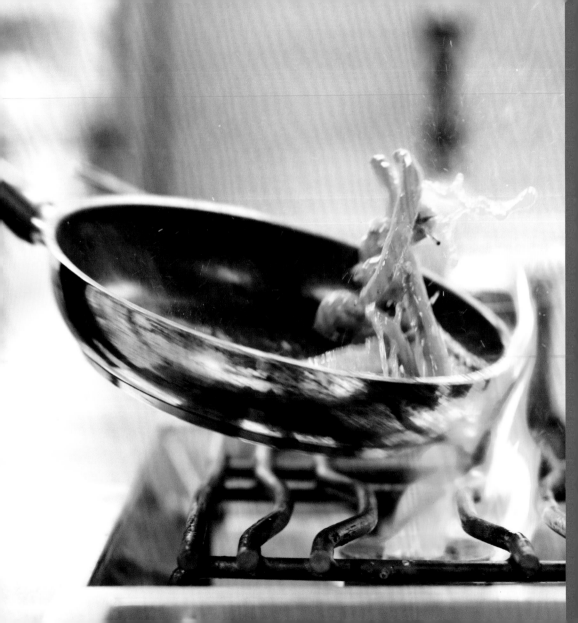

APPLEBEE'S

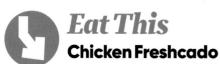

Eat This
Chicken Freshcado

CALORIES **440**

FAT **10 G** (2 G saturated)

SODIUM **1,250 MG**

Often healthy-sounding chicken dishes come coated in fatty breading, but the Freshcado is a welcome exception. Less than 25 percent of its calories come from fat, compared with nearly 50 percent for the pasta on the right.

OTHER PICKS

Roma Pepper Steak

510 CALORIES

27 G FAT (12 G saturated)

1,860 MG SODIUM

Classic Turkey Breast Sandwich
with side of fruit

650 CALORIES

29 G FAT (4.5 G saturated)

910 MG SODIUM

Garlic Mashed Potatoes

250 CALORIES

14 G FAT (2.5 G saturated)

600 MG SODIUM

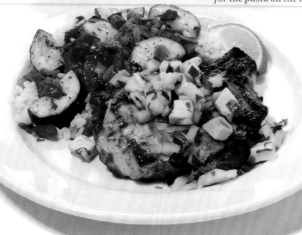

GRADE

D+

It's easy to see why it took Applebee's so many years to release its nutritional information. The 1,330-calorie Riblets Basket, the 1,390-calorie Oriental Chicken Salad, and the 2,370-calorie Appetizer Sampler are just a few of the little nightmares lurking on the menu. The bright spots on the menu include the steaks and the ever-expanding "Have It All" menu (despite some serious sodium issues).

SURVIVAL STRATEGY

Skip the meal-wrecking appetizers, pastas, and fajitas, and be very careful with salads, too; more than half of them top 1,000 calories. Concentrate on the excellent line of lean steak entrées, or anything from the fantastic 550-calorie-or-less "Have It All" menu.

OTHER PASSES

Steak Sizzling Skillet Fajitas

1,330 CALORIES

48 G FAT
(22 G saturated, 1 G trans)

5,240 MG SODIUM

Boneless Wings
with Honey BBQ Sauce

1,250 CALORIES

55 G FAT
(11 G saturated, 0.5 G trans)

SODIUM **3,060 MG**

Loaded Mashed Potatoes

460 CALORIES

31 G FAT (12 G saturated)

970 MG SODIUM

★

Oh, Applebee's: you had us fooled with "Chicken Broccoli." How could such a dish be bad? But the chain has noodled around and given us nearly two days' worth of saturated fat and more sodium than a human should consume in a whole day. Alfredo? More like "Saltfredo."

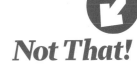

Not That!

Chicken Broccoli Pasta Alfredo

CALORIES **1,120**

FAT **55 G** (30 G saturated)

SODIUM **2,620 MG**

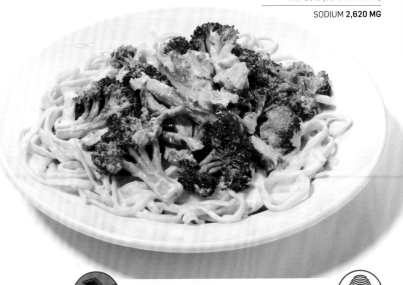

GUILTY PLEASURE

Garlic Mashed Potatoes

250 CALORIES

14 G FAT
(2.5 G saturated)

600 MG SODIUM

Mashed potatoes at sit-down chains are usually loaded with cream and butter, but Applebee's managed to make its version with fewer calories and fat grams than a baked potato or small Caesar salad.

HEALTH-FOOD FRAUD

Oriental Chicken Salad

1,390 CALORIES

98 G FAT
(15 G saturated, 1.5 G trans)

1,610 MG SODIUM

How can chicken on a bed of greens do this much damage? At first we assumed it was the fried chicken, but ordering it grilled only saves you 100 calories. The collision of crispy noodles and oily dressing in this Oriental salad leaves us totally disoriented!

19

ARBY'S

Eat This

Beef 'n Cheddar Classic

450 CALORIES

20 G FAT (6 G saturated)

1,310 MG SODIUM

★

What Arby's does best is roast beef, and maybe it should just stick to that plan. The totally decadent-sounding Beef 'n Cheddar Classic is a healthy serving of lean protein that won't blow your saturated-fat budget.

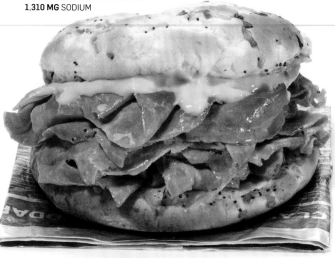

OTHER PICKS

Grand Turkey Club

480 CALORIES

24 G FAT (8 G saturated)

1,610 MG SODIUM

Roast Turkey Chopped Farmhouse Salad
with Balsamic Vinaigrette

360 CALORIES

25 G FAT (9 G saturated)

1,250 MG SODIUM

Potato Cakes
(small)

230 CALORIES

14 G FAT (2 G saturated)

460 MG SODIUM

GRADE

C+

Just a few years ago, you could pull up to the Arby's window, order a grilled chicken sandwich, and be pretty sure you were keeping lunch under 500 calories. But the chain took a step backward by eliminating its roast chicken line. Credit Arby's for nixing the trans fat from its frying oil years ago, but the restaurant doesn't offer a single side that hasn't had a long soak in a bath of hot oil.

SURVIVAL STRATEGY

You're not doing yourself any favors by ordering off the Market Fresh menu; that head-fake leads to dead ends like an 800-calorie Roast Turkey Ranch & Bacon Sandwich. A regular roast beef or Melt Sandwich will save you an average of nearly 300 calories over a Market Fresh sandwich.

OTHER PASSES

Angus Three Cheese & Bacon Sandwich

630 CALORIES

30 G FAT
(11 G saturated, 0.5 G trans)

2,220 MG SODIUM

Crispy Chopped Farmhouse Salad
with Honey Mustard Dressing

600 CALORIES

39 G FAT (10 G saturated)

1,250 MG SODIUM

Steakhouse Onion Rings

410 CALORIES

20 G FAT (3 G saturated)

1,690 MG SODIUM

★

With an average of 688 calories, Arby's healthy-sounding Market Fresh sandwiches are the worst items on the menu. This turkey option has roughly the same fillings as the club, but it packs nearly double the calories and fat. The honey-wheat bread alone contains a staggering 380 calories and the same amount of sugar as a Hostess Ho Ho.

Not That!

Market Fresh Roast Turkey, Ranch & Bacon Sandwich

800 CALORIES

35 G FAT
(9 G saturated, 0.5 G trans)

2,250 MG SODIUM

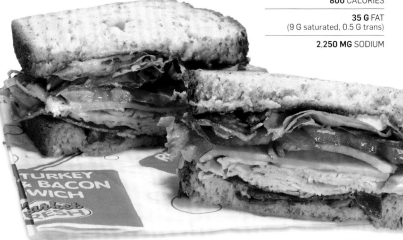

BEEF SANDWICH STACK-UP

Jr Roast Beef
210 CALORIES
8 G FAT

Bacon Beef 'n Cheddar
510 CALORIES
23 G FAT

French Dip and Swiss
540 CALORIES
23 G FAT

Beef 'n Cheddar Mid
560 CALORIES
27 G FAT

Roast Beef Classic
360 CALORIES
14 G FAT

Ham & Swiss Melt

300 CALORIES

9 G FAT
(3.5 G saturated)

1,030 MG SODIUM

EAT THIS APPROVED NOT THAT!

The best bang for your nutritional buck at Arby's. It not only is low in calories and fat, but also delivers 18 grams of protein to help keep hunger pangs at bay.

AU BON PAIN

Eat This

Grilled Chicken Sandwich

480 CALORIES

15 G FAT (2 G saturated)

1,230 MG SODIUM

★

Our kind of sandwich: substantial, flavorful, packed with 32 grams of protein and just 480 calories.

OTHER PICKS

Classic Chicken Salad Sandwich

450 CALORIES

12 G FAT (2 G saturated)

990 MG SODIUM

Chicken Gumbo Soup
(medium)

190 CALORIES

9 G FAT (1 G saturated)

930 MG SODIUM

Chocolate Dipped Cranberry Almond Macaroon

290 CALORIES

16 G FAT (13 G saturated)

25 G SUGARS

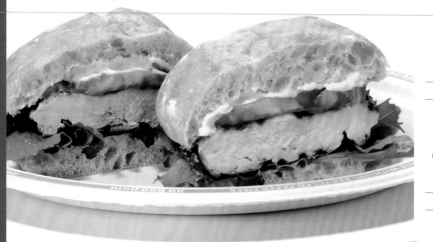

GRADE

B+

There are plenty of ways you could go wrong here, but Au Bon Pain couples an extensive inventory of healthy items with an unrivaled standard of nutritional transparency. Use the on-site nutritional kiosks to seek out one of dozens of paths to a sensible meal. Or simply opt for one of the excellent soups or salads, or pair two smaller items from the All Portions menu.

SURVIVAL STRATEGY

Banish bagels and baked goods from your breakfast routine and opt for eggs instead. As for lunch, soups are a great option and there are plenty of low-calorie options on the All Portions menu, but steer clear of the Mediterranean Power Pack.

OTHER PASSES

Black Angus Steak and Cheese Sandwich

840 CALORIES

46 G FAT (19 G saturated)

1,560 MG SODIUM

Chicken and Vegetable Stew
(medium)

340 CALORIES

19 G FAT (5 G saturated)

1,040 MG SODIUM

Double Chocolate Chunk Muffin

580 CALORIES

24 G FAT (7 G saturated)

49 G SUGARS

★

You think white meat is healthier than red meat? Think again. When it comes to deli slices, turkey, ham, and roast beef all pack about the same number of calories, fats, and protein per serving, which means when you're looking for the healthiest option, it all comes down to bread and condiments.

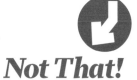

Not That!

Newport Turkey Sandwich

770 CALORIES

34 G FAT (14 G saturated)

1,790 MG SODIUM

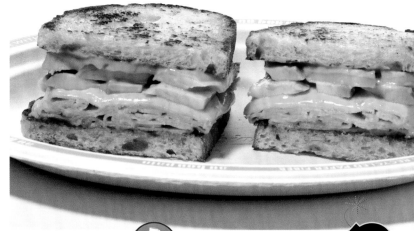

SIDE STACK-UP

Chicken Noodle Soup
110 CALORIES
2 G FAT

Beef Chili
300 CALORIES
13 G FAT

Turkey Chili
380 CALORIES
14 G FAT

Lobster Bisque
410 CALORIES
30 G FAT

Macaroni & Cheese
560 CALORIES
35 G FAT

Pecan Roll
43 G FAT (18 G saturated)
48 G SUGARS

740 CALORIE BOMB

You could eat two Double Chocolate Cupcakes and still not reach the calorie load of this pecan-encrusted disaster. Unless you want to cultivate rolls of your own, avoid this pastry at all costs.

BASKIN-ROBBINS

Eat This

Oreo Cookies'n Cream Ice Cream in a Cake Cone

(two 2.5-oz scoops)

345 CALORIES

18 G FAT (10 G saturated)

24 G SUGARS

★

Keep it simple at the scoop shop. Most BR flavors weigh in at fewer than 200 calories per scoop, so when you pile two of 'em on a 25-calorie cake cone, you get a classic American treat with a reasonable calorie load.

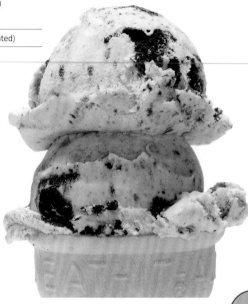

OTHER PICKS

Cappuccino Blast
Made with Soft Serve
(small)

190 CALORIES

6 G FAT (4.5 G saturated)

26 G SUGARS

Chocolate Chip Cookie Dough Ice Cream
(two 2.5-oz scoops in a cake cone)

385 CALORIES

18 G FAT (12 G saturated)

30 G SUGARS

Soft Serve Cookie Sandwich

180 CALORIES

5 G FAT (3 G saturated)

17 G SUGARS

GRADE

C−

Baskin-Robbins has a long tradition of carrying some of the worst frozen fare in the country. Sure, it shed its atrocious line of Premium Shakes, but it's going to take a lot more downsizing to earn a higher grade from us. The Premium Sundae line averages 1,055 calories, and even the average small Fruit Blast Smoothie contains 71 grams of sugars. If not for the frozen yogurt and sherbet, this grade would be even worse.

SURVIVAL STRATEGY

With choices like frozen yogurt, sherbet, and no-sugar-added ice cream, Baskin's lighter menu is the one bright spot in this otherwise dark world. Beyond that, look to the freezer for a Grab-N-Go treat. Stacked next to even a smoothie, these are great bets.

OTHER PASSES

Turtle Cappuccino Blast
(small)

510 CALORIES

---

14 G FAT (8 G saturated)

70 G SUGARS

Chocolate Chip Cookie Dough Shake
(medium)

980 CALORIES

---

42 G FAT (27 G saturated)

114 G SUGARS

Peanut Butter 'n Chocolate Ice Cream
(two 2.5-oz scoops in a cake cone)

425 CALORIES

---

26 G FAT (12 G saturated)

32 G SUGARS

Not That!
Oreo Layered Sundae

1,330 CALORIES

---

61 G FAT (31 G saturated, **1 G** trans)

146 G SUGARS

★

BR's Premium sundaes come with a premium price of about 1,055 calories a pop. We get why people are seduced by the decadence of a gluttonous sundae, but truth be told, you're essentially getting the same flavor as an ice cream cone at a much higher cost to your health.

CONE STACK-UP

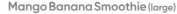

Cake Cone
25 CALORIES

---

0 G SUGARS

Sugar Cone
45 CALORIES

---

3 G SUGARS

Waffle Cone
130 CALORIES

---

11 G SUGARS

HEALTH-FOOD FRAUD

Mango Banana Smoothie (large)

880 CALORIES

---

3 G FAT

192 G SUGARS

Smoothies have a sterling reputation in nutritional circles, but unless they're made without added sugars and served in small doses, they're really just dessert in disguise. Case in point: This mango monstrosity has more sugar than half a dozen Snickers bars.

BEN & JERRY'S

Eat This

Banana Peanut Butter Greek Frozen Yogurt

(½ cup)

220 CALORIES

10 G FAT (3 G saturated)

22 G SUGARS

★

We were glad to see Ben & Jerry's introduce its new line of Greek frozen yogurt flavors this year. Greek fro yo offers the same creamy goodness of regular ice cream, minus most of the saturated fat.

OTHER PICKS

Vanilla Toffee Bar Crunch Ice Cream
(½ cup)

170 CALORIES

4 G FAT (2.5 G saturated)

20 G SUGARS

Super Pomegranate Smoothie
(large)

190 CALORIES

0 G FAT

36 G SUGARS

Cherry Garcia Ice Cream
(½ cup)

240 CALORIES

13 G FAT (9 G saturated)

23 G SUGARS

GRADE

C

What sets Ben & Jerry's apart from the competition amounts to more than just an affinity for jam bands and Hacky Sacks. The company remains committed to the quality of its ingredients. All dairy is hormone free and the chocolate, vanilla, and coffee ingredients are all Fair Trade Certified. From a strictly nutritional standpoint, though, it's still just an ice cream shop, and Ben & Jerry's average scoop is packed with more fat and sugar than most of its competitors.

SURVIVAL STRATEGY

With half of the calories of the ice cream, sorbet makes the healthiest choice on the menu. If you demand dairy, the frozen yogurt can still save you up to 100 calories per scoop.

Coconut Seven Layer Bar Ice Cream
(½ cup)

270 CALORIES

17 G FAT (10 G saturated)

21 G SUGARS

Blueberry Cream Smoothie
(large)

360 CALORIES

8 G FAT (2.5 G saturated)

55 G SUGARS

Chubby Hubby Ice Cream
(½ cup)

340 CALORIES

21 G FAT (11 G saturated)

25 G SUGARS

Not That!

Peanut Butter Cup Ice Cream
(½ cup)

360 CALORIES

24 G FAT (13 G saturated)

25 G SUGARS

★

Ben and/or Jerry managed to cram more than half a day's saturated fat into this peanut butter–chocolate bomb, making it the worst scoop on the menu, and one of the worst in America. The frozen yogurt on the opposite page is a much safer way to get your PB fix at B&J's.

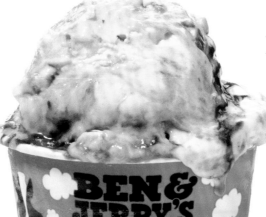

CELEBRITY ICE CREAM SHOWDOWN

Liz Lemon Greek Frozen Yogurt

180 CALORIES

4.5 G FAT (2.5 G saturated)

21 G SUGARS

Stephen Colbert's Americone Dream

280 CALORIES

16 G FAT (10 G saturated)

28 G SUGARS

Phish Food

290 CALORIES

14 G FAT (9 G saturated)

32 G SUGARS

ALL THIS OR THAT!

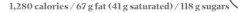

1,280 calories / 67 g fat (41 g saturated) / 118 g sugars

1 small Sorbet Splash

1 small Berry Vanilla shake

1 scoop of Chunky Monkey ice cream

and an Ice Cream Float

or Banana Split

BOB EVANS

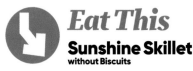

Eat This

Sunshine Skillet
without Biscuits

436 CALORIES

24 G FAT (10 G saturated)

1,410 MG SODIUM

★

An omelet with fewer than 500 calories is a rarity at American breakfast chains, but this open-faced version at Bob Evans requires fewer eggs, so the sausage, potato, and cheese fillings don't take it over the caloric edge.

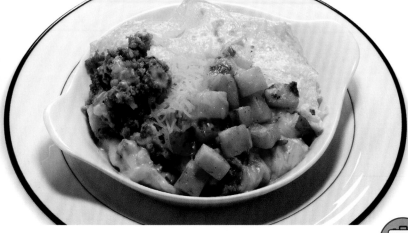

OTHER PICKS

Meat Loaf
with Mashed Potatoes and Green Beans

575 CALORIES

32 G FAT (15 G saturated)

2,225 MG SODIUM

The Farm Favorite Fried Chicken Sandwich

658 CALORIES

26 G FAT (8 G saturated)

1,578 MG SODIUM

Fruit & Yogurt Plate and Cup of Oatmeal

439 CALORIES

4 G FAT (0 G saturated)

78 MG SODIUM

GRADE

C−

No menu in America is more perplexing than Bob's. On one hand, the Ohio-based chain offers up an array of great entrées and side options, making it easy to cobble together a well-balanced meal. On the other, the menu is littered with land mines like 1,200-calorie multigrain pancakes and 1,000-calorie chicken salads. Until Mr. Evans shows us some consistency, we'll be showing him a lousy report card.

SURVIVAL STRATEGY

Breakfast should consist of staples like oatmeal, eggs, fruit, and yogurt (with maybe a slice or two of bacon); for lunch and dinner, stick with grilled chicken or fish paired with one of the non-fried vegetable sides. Or opt for one of Bob's perfectly portioned Savory Size entrées.

28

★

Ordering à la carte is usually your best strategy at big breakfast chains, but a couple of misguided choices can take your custom creation into dangerous territory. Switch the sausage to bacon and the hash browns to home fries, and you'll bring this meal down to a much more reasonable 418 calories.

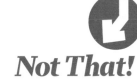

Not That!

2 Scrambled Eggs
with 3 Sausage Links and Hash Browns

884 CALORIES

56 G FAT (14 G saturated)

2,124 MG SODIUM

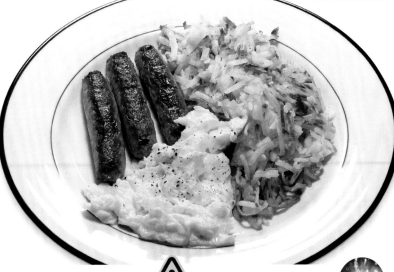

Many of the breakfast items come with a side of two biscuits, which may feel like a bonus to hungry eaters, but the damage is often worse than the breakfast itself. Remember, it's these items—the bread basket, the chips and salsa, the "free" biscuits—that do the most damage to your waistline.

MENU MAGIC

Opting for mashed potatoes over french fries at Bob Evans will save you more than 300 calories and 12 grams of fat. But be warned: This strategy won't work its magic everywhere. Many chains jack their mashed taters with copious amounts of cream and butter.

BURGER KING

Eat This

Bacon Cheeseburger Deluxe

290 CALORIES

14 G FAT (6 G saturated, 0.5 G trans)

720 MG SODIUM

You like bacon? You like cheese? You like burgers? At BK, your problem is solved. Even its Bacon Double Cheeseburger clocks in at fewer than 400 calories. Just stay away from the entire Whopper family and anything too gimmicky, like the Extra Long BBQ Burger.

OTHER PICKS

Tendergrill Chicken Sandwich

410 CALORIES

16 G FAT (2.5 G saturated)

830 MG SODIUM

Chicken Strips
(3 pieces)

340 CALORIES

17 G FAT (2.5 G saturated)

1,130 MG SODIUM

BK Breakfast Muffin Sandwich
(Sausage, Egg, and Cheese)

430 CALORIES

26 G FAT (8 G saturated)

1,140 MG SODIUM

GRADE

C-

BK invites you to "Take a Break from Boredom." You will definitely not be bored when you look down in panicked horror at the bathroom scale. The rule of thumb at Burger King is to be suspicious of anything that was invented after Taylor Swift was born: Newfangled options like 400-calorie wraps, sugar-loaded smoothies, and coffee drinks with nearly as many calories as a Whopper only make eating well more difficult. Thankfully, standbys like the Whopper Jr., basic hamburgers, and apple slices give you a way out.

SURVIVAL STRATEGY

Start your day with a Muffin Sandwich. For lunch, match the regular hamburger, the Whopper Jr., or the Tendergrill Sandwich with apple slices and water, and you'll escape for about 700 calories.

OTHER PASSES

Chicken Apple & Cranberry Garden Fresh Salad
with Tendercrisp Chicken and Dressing

680 CALORIES

42 G FAT (9 G saturated)

1,010 MG SODIUM

Tendercrisp Chicken Sandwich

640 CALORIES

36 G FAT (6 G saturated)

1,270 MG SODIUM

Double Croissan'wich
(Sausage, Egg, and Cheese)

790 CALORIES

57 G FAT
(21 G saturated, 1 G trans)

1,630 CALORIES

★

BK recently joined its Golden Arches rival in offering specialty burgers designed to imitate the more substantial burgers offered by sit-down chains. The problem? These pseudo-gourmet burgers translate into nothing more than bigger portions (a.k.a. bigger calorie loads). BK is not the place to go gourmet.

Not That!

A.1. Ultimate Bacon Cheeseburger

850 CALORIES

51 G FAT (22 G saturated, **3 G** trans)

1,480 MG SODIUM

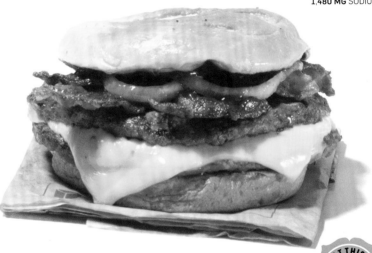

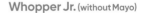
ALL THIS OR THAT!

1,160 calories

1 Hamburger
Chicken Strips (3 pieces)
Onion Rings (small)
and
a Strawberry Sundae

or

1,080 calories

Triple Whopper with Cheese

Whopper Jr. (without Mayo)

240 CALORIES

10 G FAT
(3.5 G saturated)

410 MG SODIUM

Sans mayo, the Whopper Jr. is a star beyond just the realm of Burger King. Order it solo for a solid snack or pair it with Chicken Tenders or a side garden salad for a satisfying meal.

EAT THIS APPROVED NOT THAT!

Eat This

Original BBQ Chicken Pizza

(3 slices)

535 CALORIES

13.5 G FAT (7.5 G saturated)

1,445 MG SODIUM

★

With no shortage of pastas and salads that break the 1,000-calorie mark, eating a few slices of pizza is your safest move at CPK. Chicken makes a great low-calorie, high-protein topper, and this is among the lightest pies on the menu.

GRADE

D+

CPK's sneakiest trick is to make its "healthy" thin-crust pizzas somehow more caloric than its regular pies. A Five Cheese + Fresh Tomato Hand-Tossed will actually cost you nearly 200 calories per pie less than the Margherita Crispy Thin Crust. Oh, and if you order whole-wheat crust? Add another 140 calories. Salads range from 530 calories up to 1,500 for the Moroccan-Spiced Chicken—nearly what an adult woman should eat in a whole day.

SURVIVAL STRATEGY

Pair something from the nutrition-packed Lite Adventures menu with a cup of soup (Shrimp Scampi Zucchini Fettuccine with a cup of Dakota Smashed Pea + Barley brings you in at 640 calories), or split a Hawaiian pizza with your date.

HEN

OTHER PASSES

The Meat Cravers Pizza
(3 slices)

795 CALORIES

38 G FAT (16 G saturated)

2,310 MG SODIUM

Avocado Club Egg Rolls

1,190 CALORIES

82 G FAT (20 G saturated)

2,280 MG SODIUM

Tuscan Hummus
with Wheat Whole Grain Pita

970 CALORIES

33 G FAT (0.5 G saturated)

1,520 MG SODIUM

★

That's right, you could eat an entire BBQ Chicken Pizza and still not come close to the calorie count of this salad. Time and again CPK manages to take some of the world's healthiest ingredients—like avocados and black beans—and serve them up in dishes that sport eye-popping calorie counts.

Not That!

The Original BBQ Chicken Chopped Salad with Avocado
(full)

1,250 CALORIES

81 G FAT (19 G saturated)

1,800 MG SODIUM

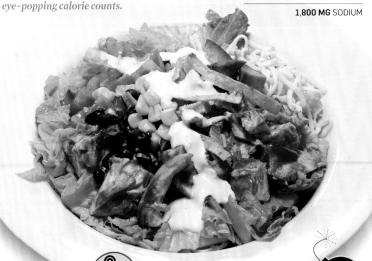

1,630 CALORIE BOMB

CRUST SELECTOR				
Crispy Thin	**Hand-Tossed Original**	**Hand-Tossed Wheat Whole Grain**	**Chicken Piccata**	In the upside-down world of CPK, the healthier a dish sounds, the more caloric it probably is. That's the case with Chicken Piccata, which packs a full day's worth of sodium along with its 1,630 calories.
570 CALORIES	**580** CALORIES	**720** CALORIES		
3 G FAT (0 G saturated)	**2.5 G** FAT (0 G saturated)	**12 G** FAT (0 G saturated)	**78 G** FAT (24 G saturated)	
1,250 MG SODIUM	**1,250 MG** SODIUM	**1,110 MG** SODIUM	**2,140 MG** SODIUM	

CARL'S JR.

Eat This
Single Teriyaki Burger

630 CALORIES

29 G FAT (11 G saturated)

1,060 MG SODIUM

★

Certainly not the healthiest drive-thru burger around, but other than the ultra-basic Big Hamburger, it's the only beef burger on the menu that falls below 670 calories. Plus, the grilled pineapple topper adds a gourmet twist you won't find at most fast-food joints.

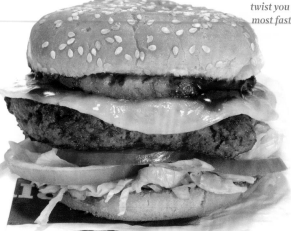

GRADE

C+

Carl's Jr. may have the raciest ads in fast-food land, but some of its offerings are downright respectable, starting with its line of 500-calorie-or-less turkey burgers and Chicken Stars, the chain's version of nuggets that clock in at just over 40 calories apiece. Still, many of the burgers deliver twice the calories of a Big Mac, and almost everything on the breakfast menu makes for a bad morning.

SURVIVAL STRATEGY

Opt for any of the salads, but make sure you choose the low-fat balsamic dressing (35 calories) and not the blue cheese (320 calories). The Charbroiled BBQ Chicken Sandwich or any of the turkey burgers make healthy options. Breakfast? Eat at home.

OTHER PASSES

Charbroiled Santa Fe Chicken Sandwich

560 CALORIES

27 G FAT (7 G saturated)

1,290 MG SODIUM

Big Country Breakfast Burrito

720 CALORIES

43 G FAT (18 G saturated)

1,380 MG SODIUM

Sweet Potato Fries
(small)

360 CALORIES

17 G FAT (3 G saturated)

590 MG SODIUM

★

From jumbo patties to superfluous toppings, excess is the standard at Carl's Jr. Case in point: The double whammy of Special Sauce and mayo makes this basic double cheeseburger one of the worst you'll find.

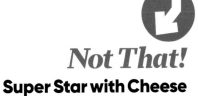

Not That!
Super Star with Cheese

930 CALORIES

56 G FAT (23 G saturated)

1,540 MG SODIUM

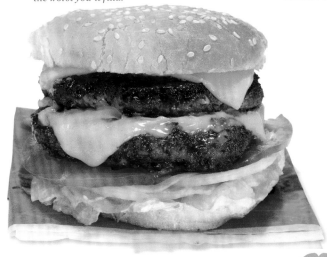

TEST TUBE FOODS

Breakfast Burger

800 CALORIES

43 G FAT
(18 G saturated, 1 G trans)

1,380 MG SODIUM

Smash a plate of eggs, bacon, and hash browns between two buns and you get a breakfast sandwich that's nearly three times the calories of an Egg McMuffin.

Charbroiled Turkey Burgers
(4 varieties)

480 TO **500** CALORIES

14 TO **22 G** FAT
(**4.5** TO 6 G saturated)

960 TO **1,150 MG** SODIUM

In 2011, we worked with Carl's to design a line of lean, juicy turkey burgers with toppings like teriyaki and guacamole.

THE CHEESECAKE FAC**T**

Eat This
Factory Burger

740 CALORIES

N/A **G** FAT (16 G saturated)

1,020 MG SODIUM

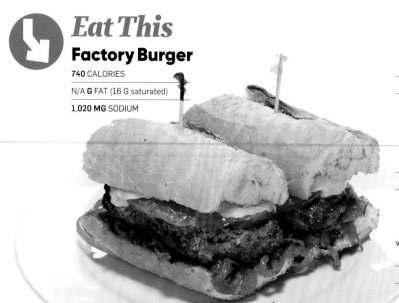

OTHER PICKS

Grilled Mahi

470 CALORIES

N/A **G** FAT (5 G saturated)

390 MG SODIUM

Vietnamese Shrimp Summer Rolls

660 CALORIES

N/A **G** FAT (2 G saturated)

1,680 MG SODIUM

Giant Belgian Waffle
with Strawberries, Pecans, Cream

740 CALORIES

N/A **G** FAT (7 G saturated)

930 MG SODIUM

★

You'll seldom find a burger at any sit-down chain with fewer than 800 calories, so to find one at the most calorie-infested restaurant in the country is quite a feat. But be warned: With an average of 1,290 calories, the other burgers on the menu are more in line with the Cheesecake Factory's standard fare.

GRADE

F

The Cheesecake Factory stands nearly alone in its brazen refusal to reveal what's really in its food. And for good reason: In a recent survey of the most caloric restaurant foods in America, Cheesecake Factory scored 5 of the top 10! It made some progress when it introduced its SkinnyLicious menu, but most entrées still come with quadruple-digit calorie counts. Once again, the Cheesecake Factory retains the title of Worst Restaurant in America.

SURVIVAL STRATEGY

Your best survival strategy is to turn your car around and head home. Failing that, skip pasta, specialties, combos, and sandwiches at all costs. Split a pizza or a salad, or look to the SkinnyLicious menu.

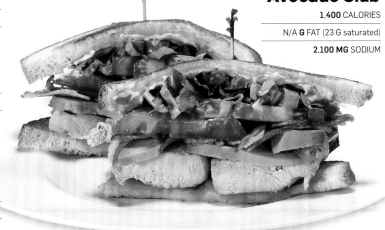

...ORY

OTHER PASSES

Miso Salmon
1,670 CALORIES

N/A **G** FAT (39 G saturated)

2,420 **MG** SODIUM

Thai Lettuce Wraps
1,030 CALORIES

N/A **G** FAT (6 G saturated)

2,350 **MG** SODIUM

French Toast with Grilled Ham
1,570 CALORIES

N/A **G** FAT (51 G saturated)

3,100 **MG** SODIUM

Not That!

Grilled Chicken and Avocado Club
1,400 CALORIES

N/A **G** FAT (23 G saturated)

2,100 **MG** SODIUM

★

Only in the bizarro world of the Cheesecake Factory could a grilled chicken sandwich house nearly double the calories of a burger. We're consistently baffled by the chain's ability to cram staggering amounts of calories, fat, and salt into ordinary-sounding dishes. Add fries and you're looking at nearly 2,000 calories on a single plate.

2,290 CALORIE BOMB

Bistro Shrimp Pasta

N/A G FAT (73 G saturated)

820 **MG** SODIUM

This is an unhealthy head-fake if ever we've seen one. With more than an entire day's worth of calories and more than three days' worth of saturated fat, the normally low-fat, low-cal shrimp is primed to turn you into a jumbo.

PASTA STACK-UP

Shrimp with Angel Hair
850 CALORIES

2 **G** saturated FAT

Pasta Marinara
1,210 CALORIES

3 **G** saturated FAT

Garlic Noodles
1,500 CALORIES

22 **G** saturated FAT

Pasta Carbonara
2,130 CALORIES

81 **G** saturated FAT

CHICK-FIL-A

Eat This

Chick-fil-A Chicken Sandwich

440 CALORIES

16 G FAT (3.5 G saturated)

1,400 MG SODIUM

★

You'll rarely find anything deep-fried on this side of the page, but Chick-fil-A's classic sandwich is a surprisingly modest indulgence. You can go even lighter by ordering it grilled, but if you hanker for fried chicken, there are much worse ways you could get your fix.

OTHER PICKS

Grilled Chicken Sandwich

320 CALORIES

5 G FAT (1.5 G saturated)

800 MG SODIUM

Bacon, Egg, and Cheese Biscuit

450 CALORIES

23 G FAT (11 G saturated)

1,040 MG SODIUM

Hearty Breast of Chicken Soup

130 CALORIES

3 G FAT (1 G saturated)

790 MG SODIUM

GRADE

A-

Chick-fil-A ranks among the best of the country's major fast-food establishments, thanks to a line of low-calorie chicken sandwiches and an impressive roster of healthy sides like yogurt parfaits and various salads. But the menu does seem to be inching ever upward in the calorie and sodium departments. Any more movement and this A- becomes a B.

SURVIVAL STRATEGY

Instead of nuggets or strips, look to the grilled chicken sandwiches or the classic fried chicken sandwich. And sub in a healthy side—a salad or soup—for the standard fried fare. Just don't supplement your meal with a shake—none has fewer than 500 calories.

OTHER PASSES

Chicken Salad Sandwich

500 CALORIES

20 G FAT (4 G saturated)

1,120 MG SODIUM

Sausage, Egg, and Cheese Biscuit

670 CALORIES

45 G FAT (19 G saturated)

1,340 MG SODIUM

Chicken Cool Wrap
with Avocado Lime Ranch Dressing

650 CALORIES

45 G FAT (10 G saturated)

1,420 MG SODIUM

★

A prime example of how fast-food chains turn salads into junk food. High-fat toppings like fried chicken and shredded cheese make this salad one of the most caloric entrées on the menu.

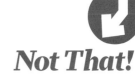

Not That!

Cobb Salad
with Avocado Lime Ranch Dressing

740 CALORIES

54 G FAT (12 G saturated)

1,890 MG SODIUM

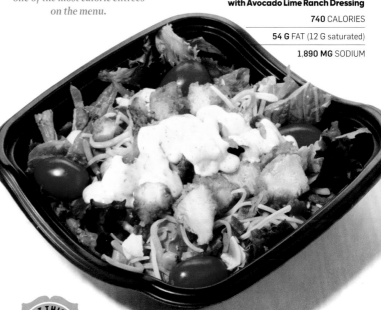

EAT THIS APPROVED NOT THAT!

Grilled Market Salad

200 CALORIES

5 G FAT (2 G saturated)

570 MG SODIUM

A seriously healthy salad with berries, apples, red cabbage, and carrots, all on top of a bed of mixed greens. The grilled chicken and a sprinkling of blue cheese loads you up with 23 grams of protein for a mere 5 grams of fat. We couldn't have designed a better muscle-up, slim-down food ourselves.

COOKIE STACK-UP

Chocolate Chunk Cookie

330 CALORIES

27 G SUGARS

Cookie Sundae

400 CALORIES

52 G SUGARS

Cookies & Cream Milkshake
(small)

520 CALORIES

69 G SUGARS

CHILI'S

Eat This

Classic Sirloin
with Sweet Corn on the Cob, Butter, and Steamed Broccoli

(6 oz)

520 CALORIES

19 G FAT (5.5 G saturated)

2,280 MG SODIUM

★

At Chili's—where the average burger plate packs more than 1,700 calories— creating your own steak combo is the safest way to meet your meat craving. Just be sure to stay away from 400-calorie accompaniments like the fries and Loaded Mashed Potatoes.

OTHER PICKS

Sweet Potato Fries

800 CALORIES

48 G FAT (8 G saturated)

1,080 MG SODIUM

Margarita Grilled Chicken

610 CALORIES

16 G FAT (4 G saturated)

2,450 MG SODIUM

Caribbean Salad
with Grilled Chicken

680 CALORIES

27 G FAT (4.5 G saturated)

1,150 MG SODIUM

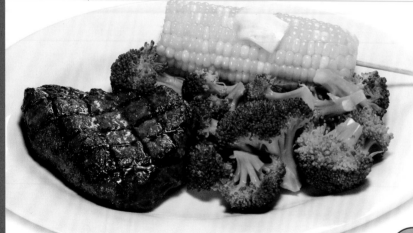

GRADE

D+

Chili's serves up some of the country's saltiest, fattiest, most calorie-laden fare, from tacos and salads to baby back ribs. Worst among the offenders are the burgers, fajitas, and appetizers, including the 1,760-calorie Texas Cheese Fries. The Lighter Choices menu is Chili's attempt at healthier meals, but with only a handful of options and a sky-high average sodium count, nothing at Chili's will make you look particularly hot.

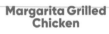

SURVIVAL STRATEGY

There's not too much to choose from after you eliminate the ribs, burgers, fajitas, and starters. Try a salad or the Make It a Combo section. Pair a Spicy Garlic and Lime Grilled Shrimp skewer with Margarita Chicken or sirloin and a side of black beans.

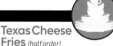

OTHER PASSES

Classic Nachos
(large)

1,190 CALORIES

81 G FAT (43 G saturated)

2,990 MG SODIUM

Monterey Chicken

940 CALORIES

51 G FAT (19 G saturated)

3,560 MG SODIUM

Boneless Buffalo Chicken Salad

1,030 CALORIES

68 G FAT (14 G saturated)

3,730 MG SODIUM

★

Veggies and some healthy guac can't save this burger from the Chili's treatment: huge portions, fatty sauces, and a heaping pile of greasy fries. Two days' worth of sodium will have you thirsting for another round of drinks. Hmm, coincidence?

Not That!

Guacamole Burger
with Homestyle Fries

1,680 CALORIES

87 G FAT (26 G saturated)

4,590 MG SODIUM

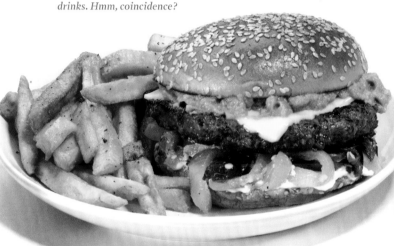

SALT LICK

Southern Smokehouse Burger with Fries

5,500 MG SODIUM

1,960 CALORIES

A typical Chili's burger plate packs a shameful 4,500 milligrams of sodium, and this disaster is the worst of the lot. Putting even more pressure on your arteries is a calorie load greater than what an adult woman should eat in an entire day.

APPETIZER STACK-UP

Classic Nachos
(regular)

820 CALORIES

56 G FAT

Loaded Potato Skins

1,110 CALORIES

78 G FAT

Texas Cheese Fries *(half order)*

1,270 CALORIES

89 G FAT

Skillet Queso with Chips

1,590 CALORIES

97 G FAT

41

Eat This

Soft Corn Tortilla Tacos
with Steak, Cheese, Lettuce, and Fresh Tomato Salsa

525 CALORIES

14 G FAT (7 G saturated)

1,040 MG SODIUM

Unlike most chains, Chipotle offers soft corn tortillas; three taco-size corn wraps have no fat, 6 grams fiber, and just 210 calories. That means twice the fiber and none of the fat found in the flour variety.

OTHER PICKS

Burrito Bowl
with Barbacoa Beef, Black Beans, Cheese, Lettuce, and Fresh Tomato Salsa

410 CALORIES

15.5 G FAT (7.5 G saturated)

1,480 MG SODIUM

Salad
with Chicken, Black Beans, Cheese, and Fresh Tomato Salsa

430 CALORIES

15.5 G FAT (8 G saturated)

1,265 MG SODIUM

Guacamole and Crispy Corn Taco Shell
(side order, 3 shells)

410 CALORIES

26.5 G FAT (6 G saturated)

360 MG SODIUM

GRADE

C

We've always commended Chipotle for the integrity of its ingredients and the flexibility of its menu. And the recent addition of a vegan protein option, Sofritas, in some of its outlets is a big nutritional step forward. But this burrito bar could still do a lot better. After years of telling people to avoid the meal-wrecking chips (570 calories), flour burrito tortillas (300 calories), and vinaigrette (270 calories), we have a challenge for Chipotle: Offer a smaller version of your belly-busting burrito.

SURVIVAL STRATEGY

Chipotle is all about customization. With fresh salsa, beans, lettuce, and grilled vegetables, you can get a nutritionally solid meal. Choose a bowl over a burrito, skip the white rice and sour cream, and you'll do just fine.

ILL

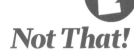

Not That!

Burrito with Steak, Black Beans, Cilantro-Lime Rice, Cheese, Sour Cream, and Roasted Chili-Corn Salsa

1,090 CALORIES

40 G FAT (15 G saturated)

2,195 MG SODIUM

★

Chipotle prides itself on serving "food with integrity." We appreciate the chain's commitment to high-quality ingredients, but all the integrity in the world won't make sour cream less fattening or giant flour tortillas less caloric.

OTHER PASSES

Soft Flour Tacos
with Barbacoa Beef, Black Beans, Cheese, Lettuce, and Fresh Tomato Salsa

685 CALORIES

23 G FAT (10.5 G saturated)

1,050 MG SODIUM

Salad
with Chicken, Black Beans, Cheese, and Vinaigrette

680 CALORIES

40.5 G FAT (12.5 G saturated)

1,615 MG SODIUM

Chips
with Fresh Tomato Salsa

590 CALORIES

27 G FAT (3.5 G saturated)

920 MG SODIUM

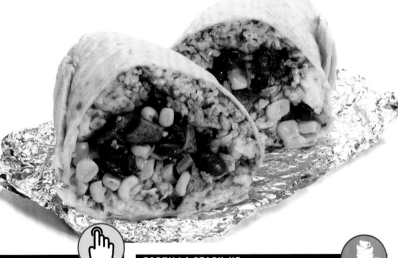

SALSA SELECTOR

Green Tomatillo *(2 oz)*
20 CALORIES
250 MG SODIUM

Fresh Tomato *(3.5 oz)*
20 CALORIES
500 MG SODIUM

Red Tomatillo *(2 oz)*
25 CALORIES
500 MG SODIUM

Roasted Chili-Corn *(3.5 oz)*
80 CALORIES
330 MG SODIUM

TORTILLA STACK-UP

Soft Corn Tortilla *(3)*
210 CALORIES
0 G FAT

Crispy Corn Taco Tortilla *(3)*
210 CALORIES
7.5 G FAT

Flour Taco Tortilla *(3)*
255 CALORIES
7.5 G FAT

Flour Burrito Tortilla
300 CALORIES
10 G FAT

DAIRY QUEEN

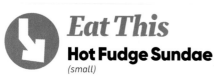

Eat This
Hot Fudge Sundae
(small)

300 CALORIES

10 G FAT (8 G saturated)

36 G SUGARS

★

A hot fudge sundae was once the epitome of decadence, but thanks to the invention of candy-infused soft-serve disasters like the Blizzard to your right, traditional sundaes are often the most prudent treats at big ice cream chains.

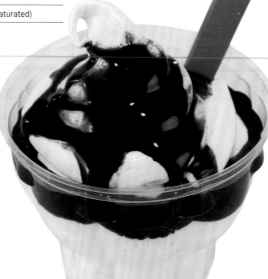

OTHER PICKS

Original Cheeseburger

380 CALORIES

19 G FAT (8 G saturated)

930 MG SODIUM

Grilled Chicken Sandwich

360 CALORIES

16 G FAT (2.5 G saturated)

1,040 MG SODIUM

DQ Sandwich

190 CALORIES

5 G FAT (3 G saturated)

18 G SUGARS

GRADE

C–

By offering a few decent sandwiches, a Mini Blizzard, and reasonable-size 300-calorie sundaes, DQ has inched their way into C territory. Still, a wide array of bad burgers, bulging chicken baskets, and blindingly sweet concoctions leave plenty of room for error. Here's a look at one hypothetical meal: a Mushroom Swiss Burger with regular onion rings and a small Snickers Blizzard—a hefty 1,530 calories.

SURVIVAL STRATEGY

Your best offense is a solid defense: Skip elaborate burgers, fried sides, and specialty ice cream concoctions. Order a Grilled Chicken Sandwich or an Original Cheeseburger, and if you must have a treat, stick to a soft-serve cone or a small sundae.

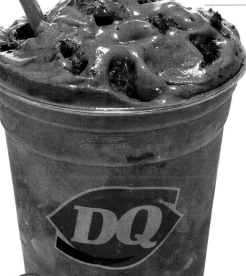

OTHER PASSES

¼ Pound GrillBurger
with Cheese

520 CALORIES

28 G FAT
(11 G saturated, 1 G trans)

1,100 MG SODIUM

Iron Grilled Turkey Sandwich

550 CALORIES

23 G FAT (7 G saturated)

1,510 MG SODIUM

Buster Bar

460 CALORIES

28 G FAT (16 G saturated)

36 G SUGARS

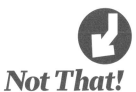

Not That!

Georgia Mud Fudge Blizzard
(small)

660 CALORIES

34 G FAT (13 G saturated, 0.5 G trans)

61 G SUGARS

★

Same fudgy flavor with more than triple the fat and roughly double the sugar and calories. Blizzard, McFlurry, 31° Below— whatever you call it, it's not worth the caloric investment.

1,250 CALORIE BOMB

Corn Dog with Fries
(regular)

620 CALORIES

30 G FAT
(5.5 G saturated)

1,180 MG SODIUM

A battered and deep-fried hot dog doesn't exactly scream "healthy," but compared with DQ's 1,200-calorie basket meals, this corn-dog-and-fry combo is surprisingly sensible.

Chicken Strip Basket with Country Gravy

(6 strips)

65 G FAT
(10 G saturated, 0.5 G trans)

3,210 MG SODIUM

This bird basket houses more calories than a Bacon Cheese Grill Burger with a large order of fries.
Here's some quick math:
Fried chicken + a pile of greasy fries + a cup of creamy gravy + 2 slices of butter-drenched toast = one of the worst chicken meals in America.

DENNY'S

Eat This

Grand Slam with 2 Eggs, 2 Strips of Turkey, Bacon, an English Muffin, and Seasonal Fruit

510 CALORIES

26 G FAT (6 G saturated)

822 MG SODIUM

★

Eggs, bacon, and fruit is a sensible way to start the morning anywhere you eat. It's when you buy into some sort of fancy barbarian breakfast behemoth that things go awry— as you can see on the opposite page. Rule: If it has a clever name, it's not a clever choice.

OTHER PICKS

Fit Fare Sirloin Steak

590 CALORIES

12 G FAT (5 G saturated, **0.5** trans)

1,370 MG SODIUM

Pancake Puppies
(6 pieces)

490 CALORIES

8 G FAT (2 G saturated)

1,020 MG SODIUM

Veggie Skillet

340 CALORIES

11 G FAT (2 G saturated)

1,360 MG SODIUM

GRADE

C−

At least Denny's deserves kudos for giving its calorically overleveraged breakfasts descriptive names that alert us to their dangers. The Lumberjack Slam will hit you with the force of 1,000 calories, and while the Peanut Butter Cup Pancake Breakfast may boast 1,500 calories, at least no one can claim they didn't see that one coming. Fortunately, Denny's offers a small Fit Fare menu with calorie counts under 600.

SURVIVAL STRATEGY

There are two ways to hack the Denny's calorie system. One is to build your own, and choose lean proteins, fruits, and vegetables, like the Grand Slam above. The other is to fake your ID and order off the 55+ Menu, as Senior versions tend to have about 15 percent fewer calories.

OTHER PASSES

Prime Rib Philly Melt
(without sides)

670 CALORIES

34 G FAT (13 G saturated)

2,010 MG SODIUM

Zesty Nachos

1,320 CALORIES

65 G FAT (34 G saturated)

2,260 MG SODIUM

Ultimate Skillet

740 CALORIES

56 G FAT (17 G saturated)

1,470 MG SODIUM

★

A healthy diet means no more than 65 grams fat and 2,400 grams sodium in a day. But starting off your morning with a Slamwich puts you out over your nutritional skis before you even finish your morning coffee. It may well be the worst breakfast sandwich in the country, and the single worst way to start your day.

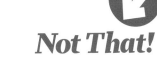

Not That!

The Grand Slamwich
with Hash Browns

1,340 CALORIES

89 G FAT
(28 G saturated, **1 G** trans)

3,390 MG SODIUM

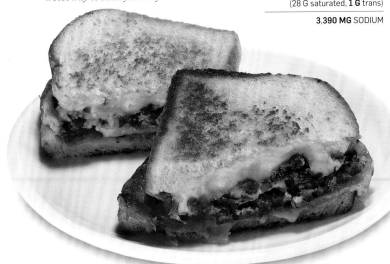

| TEST TUBE FOODS | |

Brooklyn Spaghetti & Meatballs

1,220 CALORIES

61 G FAT
(21 G saturated, 0.5 G trans)

2,460 MG SODIUM

Just spaghetti & meatballs, like Mom made, but with a day's worth of salt and fat into the pot.

| STARCH STACK-UP |

Hash Browns
210 CALORIES

2 G FIBER

Grits
with Margarine
220 CALORIES

3 G FIBER

Oatmeal
with milk and brown sugar
240 CALORIES

3 G FIBER

Toast
with Margarine *(2 slices)*
270 CALORIES

1 G FIBER

Buttermilk Pancakes *(2)*
340 CALORIES

2 G FIBER

47

DOMINO'S

Eat This

Brooklyn Style Crust Grilled Chicken and Jalapeño Pepper Pizza
(2 slices, large pie)

540 CALORIES

22 G FAT (10 G saturated)

1,700 MG SODIUM

★

Designing your own pie is the best approach at Domino's— or any pizza chain, for that matter— and this is one of the healthiest custom creations you can order. The Brooklyn crust is among the chain's lightest, and grilled chicken is one of the leanest meat toppings on the menu.

OTHER PICKS

Hand Tossed Crust Chorizo and Bacon Pizza
(2 slices, large pie)

620 CALORIES

24 G FAT (10 G saturated)

1,530 MG SODIUM

Crunchy Thin Crust Sliced Sausage, Onions, and Green Peppers Pizza
(2 slices, large pie)

480 CALORIES

26 G FAT (9 G saturated)

890 MG SODIUM

Fire Chicken Wings
(4)

200 CALORIES

13 G FAT (3.5 G saturated)

1,350 MG SODIUM

GRADE

B

Domino's has been busy these past few years, first successfully rolling out bolder sauce and better-seasoned dough, then adding the new Artisan line of pizzas, which, along with the Crunchy Thin Crust pizzas, provide some of the lightest slices in America. But there is still plenty of trouble afoot at the pizza juggernaut—namely, a line of high-calorie specialty pies and breadsticks and Domino's appalling line of pasta bread bowls and oven-baked sandwiches.

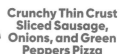

SURVIVAL STRATEGY

The more loaded a pie is at Domino's, the fewer calories it tends to pack. That's because more vegetables and lean meats mean less space for cheese. It doesn't hold true for greasy meats, so choose wisely.

OTHER PASSES

Hand Tossed Crust MeatZZa Feast Pizza
(2 slices, large pie)

760 CALORIES

---

38 G FAT (16 G saturated)

2,060 MG SODIUM

Italian Sausage Marinara Breadbowl Pasta

1,470 CALORIES

---

53 G FAT (20 G saturated)

2,770 MG SODIUM

Stuffed Cheesy Bread
(4)

555 CALORIES

---

22 G FAT
(12 G saturated, 1 G trans)

---

960 MG SODIUM

★

This is why specialty pizzas fail our nutrition test. You have essentially the same flavor as the pizza on the left, but superfluous additions like multiple cheeses and a whey-infused crust translate to nearly 160 additional calories and 12 extra grams of fat. The novelty's just not worth it.

Not That!

Hand Tossed Crust Buffalo Chicken American Legends Pizza
(2 slices, large pie)

700 CALORIES

---

34 G FAT (17 G saturated)

1,760 MG SODIUM

TEST TUBE FOODS

Chicken Carbonara Breadbowl Pasta

1,480 CALORIES

---

57 G FAT
(24 G saturated)

2,220 MG SODIUM

Domino's already doubled down on carbs with this bready pasta vessel, but by brushing it with an oil blend, the chain adds 44 supernatural ingredients like "disodium inosinate" and "lipolyzed butter oil" to the mix. Consider this a science experiment gone horribly wrong.

ALL THIS OR THAT!

860 calories

9 pieces Boneless Chicken
1 slice medium Crunchy Thin Crust Ham Pineapple Pizza
and
1 Garden Fresh Salad with Light Italian dressing

 or

Italian Sausage and Peppers Sandwich

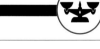

49

DUNKIN'

Eat This

Sugar Raised Donut and Iced Latte with Skim Milk
small

300 CALORIES

14 G FAT (6 G saturated)

14 G SUGARS

★

Dunkin' serves similar-sounding foods with wildly different health implications. Choose a Crumb doughnut and a medium Coolatta and this same approach could yield a 1,000-calorie breakfast. But this sugar-dusted doughnut and Iced Latte make a low-cal, albeit low-nutrition, start to your day.

OTHER PICKS

Apple 'n Spice Donut

270 CALORIES

14 G FAT (6 G saturated)

8 G SUGARS

Caramel Mocha Iced Coffee
with Cream
(medium)

260 CALORIES

9 G FAT (6 G saturated)

36 G SUGARS

Oatmeal Raisin Cookie

160 CALORIES

5 G FAT (2.5 G saturated)

19 G SUGARS

GRADE

B

The doughnut king cast out the trans fats in 2007, and it's been pushing the menu toward healthier options ever since— including the DDSmart Menu, which emphasizes the menu's nutritional champions. With a line of low-fat and protein-packed flatbread sandwiches, there's no excuse to settle for bagels, muffins, doughnuts, and oversweetened coffee drinks, which are as bad as ever.

SURVIVAL STRATEGY

Use the DDSmart Menu as a starting point, or stick to the sandwiches served on flatbread or English muffins. Beware: Beverages like Coolattas and souped-up coffee drinks can do even more damage than the food here, so keep your joe as plain as possible.

OTHER PASSES

Apple Crumb Donut

490 CALORIES

18 G FAT (9 G saturated)

49 G SUGARS

Coffee Coolatta
with Cream
(medium)

600 CALORIES

35 G FAT
(22 G saturated, 1 G trans)

65 G SUGARS

Chocolate Chip Muffin

550 CALORIES

21 G FAT (6 G saturated)

50 G SUGARS

★

Another reminder of why bagels are shaped like zeroes: They offer no real nutritional value whatsoever. Even if you went for reduced-fat cream cheese, you'd still be consuming 150 calories more than the doughnut-latte combo to the left.

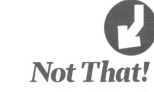

Not That!

Sesame Seed Bagel
with Plain Cream Cheese

500 CALORIES

19.5 G FAT
(10 G saturated, 0.5 G trans)

880 MG SODIUM

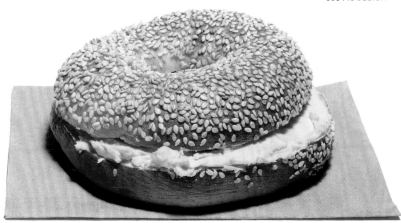

ICED COFFEE DECODER			**MUNCHKIN MOSHPIT**			
Regular Iced Coffees	**Flavored Iced Coffees**		**Cinnamon Cake**		**Glazed Cake**	
10 TO 250 CALORIES	110 TO 350 CALORIES		60 CALORIES		70 CALORIES	
UP TO 35 GRAMS OF SUGARS	UP TO 48 GRAMS OF SUGARS		3 G SUGARS		4 G SUGARS	
Regular Iced Latte	**Flavored Iced Lattes**		**Glazed Chocolate Cake**		**Jelly Filled**	
70 TO 240 CALORIES	170 TO 450 CALORIES		70 CALORIES		80 CALORIES	
UP TO 20 GRAMS OF SUGARS	UP TO 68 GRAMS OF SUGARS		4 G SUGARS		2 G SUGARS	

FIVE GUYS

Eat This

Little Bacon Burger
with Lettuce, Ketchup, and Onions

594 CALORIES

33 G FAT
(14.5 G saturated)

805 MG SODIUM

★

What's in a name? At Five Guys, apparently not much. The chain's regular burgers are doubles and its "Little" burgers are singles. The menu is high in calories and low in choices, so if you want to escape without consuming more than 600 calories, stick with a Little Burger topped with either cheese or bacon (but not both!).

GRADE

C

Without much more than burgers, hot dogs, and french fries on the menu, it's difficult to find anything nutritionally redeeming about Five Guys. The only option geared toward health-conscious consumers is the Veggie Sandwich. The burgers range from 480 to 920 calories, so how you order can make a big difference to your waistline. Keep your burgers small, choose your topping wisely, and skip the fries.

SURVIVAL STRATEGY

The regular hamburger is actually a double, so order a Little Hamburger and load up on the vegetation. Or skip the patty entirely and play around with the huge variety of toppings—it's not hard to create a solid sandwich.

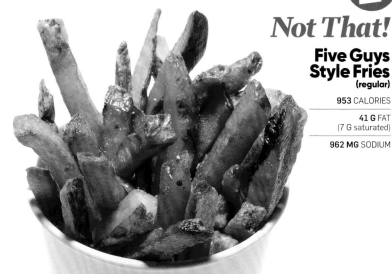

OTHER PASSES

Hamburger
700 CALORIES

43 G FAT (19.5 G saturated)

430 MG SODIUM

Cheese Dog
615 CALORIES

41 G FAT (19 G saturated)

1,440 MG SODIUM

Grilled Cheese
470 CALORIES

26 G FAT (9 G saturated)

715 MG SODIUM

Not That!

Five Guys Style Fries
(regular)

953 CALORIES

41 G FAT
(7 G saturated)

962 MG SODIUM

★

Why this comparison? Because it shows that often a meal's biggest mistakes are nestled on the side. Even if you upgrade to the bigger burger— which has 780 calories—and skip the fries, you'll save yourself 400 calories.

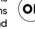

ALL THIS OR THAT!

100 calories

Cheese
Onions
Grilled Mushrooms
and
A.1. Steak Sauce

or

Mayonnaise

{250K}

Number of possible burger combinations you could order at Five Guys

MEET YOUR MATCH

1,474 calories

Five Guys
Style Fries
(large)

=

29
Wendy's
Chicken
Nuggets

HARDEE'S

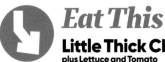

Eat This

Little Thick Cheeseburger
plus Lettuce and Tomato

440 CALORIES

23 G FAT (9 G saturated)

1,150 MG SODIUM

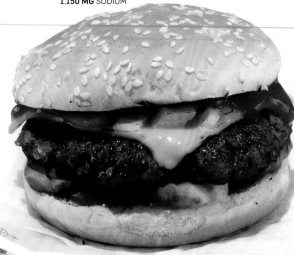

★
Don't be limited by the confines of the drive-thru menu. Fast-food restaurants usually let you alter your burger at no extra cost, and the single best way to exercise your right to customize is to pile on the produce. The simple addition of lettuce and tomato makes a basic burger much more substantial.

OTHER PICKS

Charbroiled BBQ Chicken Sandwich

330 CALORIES

6 G FAT (0 G saturated)

1,160 MG SODIUM

Hand Breaded Chicken Tenders
(3 pieces)

260 CALORIES

13 G FAT (2.5 G saturated)

770 MG SODIUM

Ham, Egg & Cheese Biscuit

450 CALORIES

24 G FAT (8 G saturated)

1,440 MG SODIUM

GRADE

C

Hardee's earns its reputation as one of the most perilous fast-food chains by continuing to sire one crazily caloric burger after the next (and by failing to offer many impressive breakfast options). A recent line of lean turkey burgers has, sadly, been rolled back to just one, leaving diners with fewer options to squash their hunger without breaking the caloric bank.

SURVIVAL STRATEGY

The Sunrise Croissant and the Frisco Breakfast Sandwich are two of your best options in the early hours. For lunch, look to the roast beef, the Big Hot Ham 'N' Cheese, or the Charbroiled BBQ Chicken Sandwich.

OTHER PASSES

Charbroiled Chicken Club Sandwich

540 CALORIES

31 G FAT (8 G saturated)

1,510 MG SODIUM

Natural-Cut French Fries
(medium)

490 CALORIES

24 G FAT (4.5 G saturated)

970 MG SODIUM

Loaded Breakfast Burrito

580 CALORIES

30 G FAT (12 G saturated)

1,320 MG SODIUM

★

And here's what you get when you leave your nutritional fate up to the fast-food gods. This is essentially the exact same burger as the one on the left—same size patty, same bun, similar toppings— but a generous blob of mayo costs you in both calories and cents.

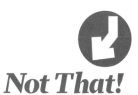

Not That!

¼ lb. Little Thickburger

580 CALORIES

39 G FAT (12 G saturated)

1,190 MG SODIUM

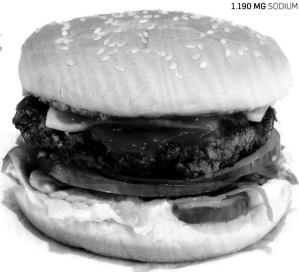

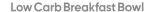

GUILTY PLEASURE

Jumbo Chili Dog

370 CALORIES

25 G FAT (8 G saturated)

1,210 MG SODIUM

Ironically, the Jumbo Chili Dog is one of the smallest threats at Hardee's. With 15 grams of protein and fewer calories than all but the smallest burger, you could do a lot worse than this spicy dog.

HEALTH-FOOD FRAUD

Low Carb Breakfast Bowl

660 CALORIES

52 G FAT (20 G saturated)

1,550 MG SODIUM

Sure, it's low-carb, but it's nearly a day's worth of fat. This meal is like putting the entire barnyard—chickens, cows, and pigs—onto one heart-stopping combination of eggs, ham, two types of sausage, bacon, and a triple dose of cheese.

IHOP

Eat This
Two × Two × Two with Bacon

680 CALORIES

39 G FAT (13 G saturated, 0.5 G trans)

1,790 MG SODIUM

★

There are two ways to leave IHOP with your belt still buckled: Choose one of the Simple & Fit items or stick to the basics. This no-frills dish isn't winning any health-food awards, but it's a pretty conservative breakfast compared with IHOP's typical 1,000-calorie fare. Just remember to go easy on the syrup.

OTHER PICKS

Honey-Lime Chicken Salad

410 CALORIES

21 G FAT (4 G saturated)

1,160 MG SODIUM

Simple & Fit Blueberry Harvest Grain 'N Nut Combo

500 CALORIES

24 G FAT (4 G saturated)

1,250 MG SODIUM

Double BLT

690 CALORIES

48 G FAT (12 G saturated)

2,139 MG SODIUM

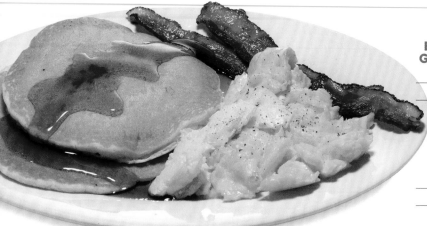

GRADE

D

IHOP was one of the last chains to release its nutritional numbers, and given the national-debt-level calorie counts on much of its menu, we see why. Factor in the new line of bacon burgers and the absolute worst breakfast menu in America and it's hard to find much to like about IHOP. The best thing we can say is that lunch and dinner aren't nearly as calamitous as breakfast.

SURVIVAL STRATEGY

IHOP's full name includes the word "cake," and it seems to take that seriously, piling on the carbs at every turn. You'll have a hard time finding a breakfast with fewer than 700 calories. Stick to the Simple & Fit menu, where you'll find a small selection of healthier items.

OTHER PASSES

Crispy Chicken Cobb Salad with Grilled Chicken

1,130 CALORIES

89 G FAT
(27 G saturated, 1.5 G trans)

2,880 MG SODIUM

Whole Wheat Pancake with Bananas and Sausage

990 CALORIES

60 G FAT
(17 G saturated, 0.5 G trans)

1,780 MG SODIUM

Ham and Egg Melt

1,190 CALORIES

75 G FAT
(37 G saturated, 1.5 G trans)

2,800 MG SODIUM

★

Sounds innocuous enough, yet it packs nearly a third more calories and fat of the Two × Two × Two. The principal difference between this plate and the breakfast on the opposite page is the double dose of starch. It's never a good idea to double up on empty carbs, especially when one of them comes in the form of oil-drenched potatoes.

Not That!

Quick Two-Egg Breakfast with Bacon

910 CALORIES

58 G FAT (19 G saturated, 0.5 G trans)

1,420 MG SODIUM

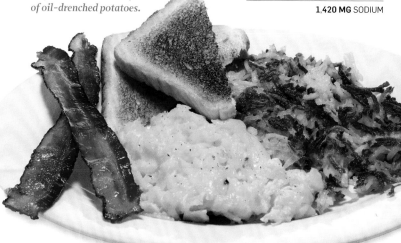

4 FLAPJACKS STACK-UP

Original Buttermilk
624 CALORIES
17 G SUGARS

Double Blueberry
690 CALORIES
37 G SUGARS

Chocolate Chip
730 CALORIE
32 G SUGARS

Strawberry Banana
760 CALORIES
41 G SUGARS

Harvest Grain 'N Nut
740 CALORIES
34 G SUGARS

CINN-A-STACK
900 CALORIES
61 G SUGARS

New York Cheesecake
1,100 CALORIES
53 G SUGARS

53

The number of breakfast entrées with more than 1,000 calories

JAMBA JUICE

Eat This

Banana Berry Smoothie
(Make It Light, 22 oz)

240 CALORIES

0.5 G FAT (0 G saturated)

44 G SUGARS

★
Make It Light smoothies, like this berry option, have up to half the sugar of the chain's Classic creations. Consider them the smartest options at the healthiest smoothie shop in the country.

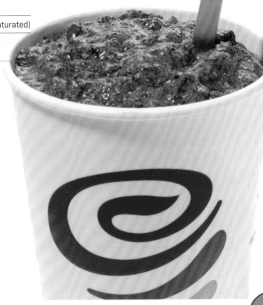

OTHER PICKS

Mega Mango Smoothie
(16 oz)

230 CALORIES

0 G FAT (0 G saturated)

52 G SUGARS

Blueberry & Blackberry Oatmeal

290 CALORIES

3.5 G FAT (1 G saturated)

25 G SUGARS

Spinach 'N Cheese Breakfast Wrap

240 CALORIES

8 G FAT (6 G saturated)

1 G SUGARS

GRADE

A−

Jamba Juice makes more than a few faux-fruit blends—beverages unnecessarily weighed down with sherbet, sorbet, and other added sugars—but its menu has a ton of real-deal smoothies, as well. Jamba's incredible line of Fruit & Veggie smoothies and its low-calorie food menu are unrivaled by other American chains. But order what's on the opposite page and you could be drinking down the equivalent of more than 24 packets of sugar.

SURVIVAL STRATEGY

For a perfectly guilt-free treat, opt for a Jamba Light or an All Fruit Smoothie in a 16-ounce cup. And unless you're looking to put on weight for your latest movie role, don't touch the Peanut Butter Moo'd or any of the other Creamy Treats.

Mango-a-Go-Go Smoothie
(16 oz)

300 CALORIES

1.5 G FAT (0 G saturated)

66 G SUGARS

Coconut Water Pina Colada
(medium)

380 CALORIES

8 G FAT (7 G saturated)

68 G SUGARS

Sweet Belgian Waffle

310 CALORIES

15 G FAT (8 G saturated)

21 G SUGARS

Not That!

Strawberry Surf Rider
(regular, 22 oz)

450 CALORIES

1.5 G FAT (0.5 G saturated)

98 G SUGARS

★

Smoothies have a reputation as a health food, but sugary add-ins turn many frozen-fruit blends into glorified desserts. The fruit in this cup is mixed with sherbet— no wonder it has more sugar than two McDonald's Hot Fudge Sundaes.

STEALTH HEALTH

Berry UpBEET
(Original size, 22 fl oz)

340 CALORIES

56 G SUGARS

13 G FIBER

True to their name, Jamba's Fruit & Veggie smoothies contain nothing but fruit, fruit juice, and vegetable juice. This berry option packs the most belly-filling fiber, but all four of the flavors are decent—not to mention tasty—ways to meet your veggie quota.

TWISTED DOUGH TORNADO

Cheddar Tomato Twist
240 CALORIES

3 G SUGARS

Cheesy Pretzel
310 CALORIES

6 G SUGARS

Sourdough Parmesan Pretzel
410 CALORIES

4 G SUGARS

Apple Cinnamon Pretzel
380 CALORIES

14 G SUGARS

Pesto Twist
290 CALORIES

3 G SUGARS

KFC

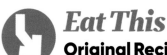

Fried chicken isn't anyone's idea of a healthy meal, but the Colonel's classic recipe has surprisingly conservative nutrition stats. We defy you to find a fast-food burger meal with two starchy sides for fewer than 600 calories and 6 grams of saturated fat.

Eat This

Original Recipe Chicken Breast
with Mashed Potatoes and Gravy and Sweet Kernel Corn

540 CALORIES

18.5 G FAT (4 G saturated)

1,660 MG SODIUM

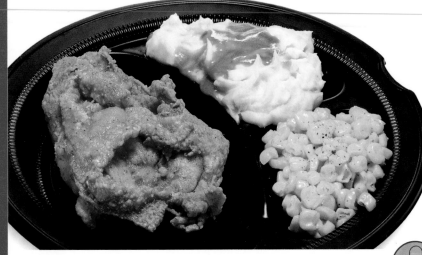

OTHER PICKS

Doublicious
with Original Recipe Fillet

530 CALORIES

27 G FAT (7 G saturated)

1,390 MG SODIUM

Hot Wings Value Box

490 CALORIES

27 G FAT (4.5 G saturated)

1,290 MG SODIUM

Sweet Life Chocolate Chip Cookie

160 CALORIES

8 G FAT (3.5 G saturated)

22 G SUGARS

GRADE

B+

Hold on a second! KFC gets a B+? Surprisingly enough, KFC has more than a few things going for it. The menu's crispy bird bits are offset by skinless chicken pieces, low-calorie sandwich options, and a host of sides that come from beyond the fryer. Plus, the fact that KFC has stuck with its grilled chicken line shows that it's determined to cast aside the Kentucky fried nutritional demons of their past.

SURVIVAL STRATEGY

Avoid the bowls and potpies, and choose your chicken wisely: The difference between an Original Recipe breast and an Extra Crispy is 170 calories; order Kentucky Grilled and you'll save another 100 calories. Then adorn your plate with one of the Colonel's healthy sides.

OTHER PASSES

Crispy Twister

620 CALORIES

32 G FAT (6 G saturated)

1,260 MG SODIUM

EC Thigh Value Box

660 CALORIES

41 G FAT (7 G saturated)

1,560 MG SODIUM

Cafe Valley Bakery Mini Chocolate Chip Cake

300 CALORIES

12 G FAT (2.5 G saturated)

35 G SUGARS

This is the single worst option on KFC's menu. Chunky Chicken Pot Pie is stuffed with veggies and never touches the deep fryer, but it remains one of the worst chicken dishes of all time. The main calorie culprit is its buttery shell, but the creamy sauce that binds the filling together certainly doesn't help matters.

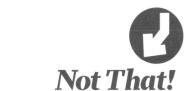

Not That!
Chunky Chicken Pot Pie

790 CALORIES

45 G FAT (37 G saturated)

1,970 MG SODIUM

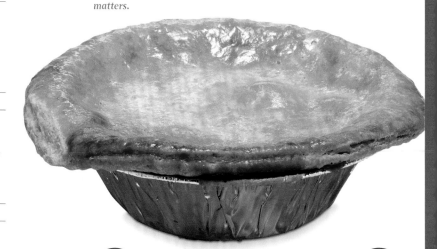

HEALTHY SIDES SMACKDOWN

Green Beans
25 CALORIES
0 G FAT (0 G saturated)

Corn on the Cob
(3")
70 CALORIES
0.5 G FAT (0 G saturated)

Sweet Kernel Corn
100 CALORIES
5 G FAT (0.5 G saturated)

Cole Slaw
170 CALORIES
10 G FAT (1.5 G saturated)

CHICKEN STACK-UP

Kentucky Grilled Chicken
80 TO 220 CALORIES
4 TO **10 G** FAT

Original Recipe
120 TO 320 CALORIES
2 TO **21 G** FAT

Extra Crispy
160 TO 490 CALORIES
10 TO **29 G** FAT

Spicy Crispy
150 TO 520 CALORIES
10 TO **34 G** FAT

KRISPY KREME

Eat This
Original Glazed Doughnut

190 CALORIES

11 G FAT (5 G saturated)

10 G SUGARS

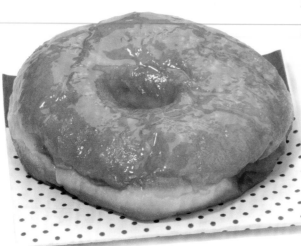

★

If you're coming to Krispy Kreme for health food, you're missing the point. But if you want a quick sugar fix without too much caloric damage, the simplest doughnuts are the best solution.

OTHER PICKS

Cinnamon Bun Doughnut

222 CALORIES

12 G FAT (5 G saturated)

13 G SUGARS

Deep Chocolate Cone

310 CALORIES

9 G FAT (6 G saturated)

33 G SUGARS

Iced Latte
with 2% Milk
(20 fl oz)

180 CALORIES

7 G FAT (4.5 G saturated)

18 G SUGARS

GRADE

In some parts of the United States, Krispy Kreme has expanded its food menu beyond doughnuts. The bad news is that most of the new additions are primarily sugar calories—mostly bagels—the same type of nutrient-devoid, carb-heavy fare the bakery has always specialized in. The rule of thumb at Krispy Kreme is to avoid anything that's filled with custard, cream, or whatever the berry flavoring is made from. A simple round doughnut is the closest you'll get to a square meal.

SURVIVAL STRATEGY

To stay under 500 calories, keep your doughnuts simple and your coffee drinks even more so. The Kreme's specialty drinks are sweeter than a YouTube puppy video.

OTHER PASSES

Classic Cinnamon Roll

670 CALORIES

38 G FAT
(18 G saturated, 1 G trans)

41 G SUGARS

Chocolate Kool Kreme Shake

750 CALORIES

24 G FAT
(16 G saturated, 0.5 G trans)

90 G SUGARS

Vanilla Iced Coffee
(20 fl oz)

540 CALORIES

2.5 G FAT (1.5 G saturated)

125 G SUGARS

★

You came for a doughnut. Have a doughnut. Don't fritter your time away on this meteorite-shaped lump of sugar and fat.

Not That!

Apple Fritter

400 CALORIES

20 G FAT (9 G saturated)

28 G SUGARS

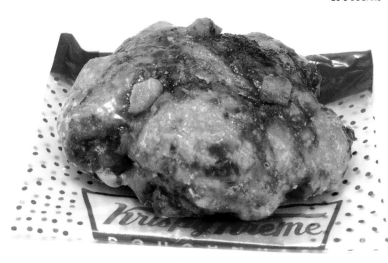

DOUGHNUT DECODER

Doughnut Holes
(4 holes)

190 TO **210** CALORIES

AS MUCH AS **11 G** FAT

Original or Sugar

200 CALORIES

12 G FAT

Cinnamon

210 TO **290** CALORIES

AS MUCH AS **16 G** FAT

Cake

230 TO **290** CALORIES

AS MUCH AS **14 G** FAT

Iced
(but not filled)

240 TO **280** CALORIES

AS MUCH AS **14 G** FAT

Filled

290 TO **350** CALORIES

AS MUCH AS **20 G** FAT

MEET YOUR MATCH

126 g sugars

Hazelnut Iced Coffee
(20 fl oz)

=

14 Sugar Doughnuts

McDONALD'S

Eat This

Premium Grilled Chicken Ranch BLT Sandwich

450 CALORIES

15 G FAT (4.5 G saturated)

1,230 MG SODIUM

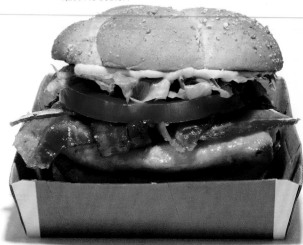

The beauty of a grilled chicken breast: Its super-low calorie count leaves room for splurge-worthy toppings like bacon and ranch dressing. Just be sure to stay away from the Crispy version of this sandwich. The price you pay for going fried over grilled at Mickey D's is an extra 160 calories and 13 grams of fat.

OTHER PICKS

McDouble

380 CALORIES

17 G FAT
(8 G saturated, 1 G trans)

840 MG SODIUM

Chicken McNuggets
with Tangy Barbecue Sauce
(6)

330 CALORIES

18 G FAT (3 G saturated)

800 MG SODIUM

Bacon, Egg & Cheese McGriddles

460 CALORIES

21 G FAT (9 G saturated)

1,250 MG SODIUM

GRADE

B+

The world-famous burger baron has come a long way since the publication of *Fast Food Nation*—at least nutritionally speaking. The trans fats are gone from its oils, the number of calorie bombs has been reduced, and there are more healthy options, such as salads and yogurt parfaits, than ever. Still, too many of the breakfast and lunch items top the 500-calorie mark, and the dessert menu is a total mess.

SURVIVAL STRATEGY

At breakfast, look no further than the Egg McMuffin—it remains one of the best ways to start your day in the fast-food world. Grilled chicken and Snack Wraps make for a sound lunch. Splurge on a Big Mac or Quarter Pounder, but only if you skip the fries and soda.

OTHER PASSES

Cheeseburger
(2)

580 CALORIES

---

22 G FAT
(10 G saturated, 1 G trans)

1,360 MG SODIUM

Southwest Crispy McWrap

670 CALORIES

---

33 G FAT
(8 G saturated, 0.5 G trans)

1,480 MG SODIUM

Bacon, Egg & Cheese Bagel

620 CALORIES

---

31 G FAT
(11 G saturated, 0.5 G trans)

1,480 MG SODIUM

★

Fried chicken and ranch dressing have caused the downfalls of countless fast-food meals. Here, these high-risk toppings result in a chicken dish with more calories and fat than a Quarter Pounder with Cheese.

Not That!

Premium Crispy Chicken Ranch BLT Sandwich

610 CALORIES

---

28 G FAT (6 G saturated)

1,400 MG SODIUM

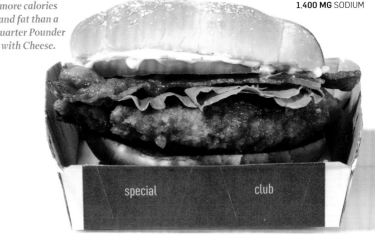

special   club

HEALTH-FOOD FRAUD

Mango Pineapple Smoothie
(small)

210 CALORIES

0.5 G FAT

---

40 MG SODIUM

---

46 G SUGAR

Even a small version of Ronald's smoothie has more sugar than a Hot Caramel Sundae. Smoothies tend to be health-food imposters at most major chains, and at Mickey D's it's no different.

Egg McMuffin

300 CALORIES

---

13 G FAT
(5 G saturated)

---

750 MG SODIUM

Few on-the-go breakfasts offer a better balance of protein, carbs, and fat than McDonald's legendary breakfast sandwich.

OLIVE GARDEN

Eat This

Lasagna Primavera with Grilled Chicken

560 CALORIES

29 G FAT (7 G saturated)

1,700 MG SODIUM

★

Most of Olive Garden's chicken pastas are high in carbs and doused in heavy sauces, but this dish gets its flavor and substance from lean meat and ricotta cheese. The result is one of the few pasta dishes in America with fewer than 700 calories.

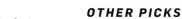

OTHER PICKS

Caprese Flatbread

600 CALORIES

34 G FAT (10 G saturated)

1,430 MG SODIUM

Baked Tilapia
with Shrimp

360 CALORIES

12 G FAT (6 G saturated)

980 MG SODIUM

Chicken Meatballs

260 CALORIES

9 G FAT (3 G saturated)

910 MG SODIUM

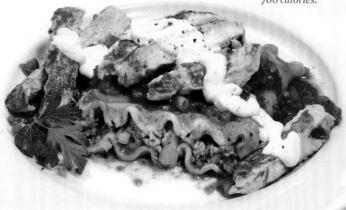

GRADE

D+

Olive Garden is in desperate need of a menu makeover. The chicken and beef entrées are saddled with huge calorie and fat counts, the seafood is swimming in sodium, and the average dinner-size plate of pasta packs a staggering 976 calories. All of this is before you tack on the breadsticks and salad. Olive Garden cooks need to learn to lay off the oil and the salt; then maybe we'll bump them up to a C.

SURVIVAL STRATEGY

Most pasta dishes are burdened with at least a day's worth of sodium and more than 1,000 calories, but the Lighter Italian Fare menu goes easier on your waistline. As for chicken and seafood, stick with the Herb-Grilled Salmon. And lay off the breadsticks!

OTHER PASSES

Grilled Chicken Flatbread

760 CALORIES

44 G FAT (15 G saturated)

1,500 MG SODIUM

Seafood Alfredo

1,210 CALORIES

71 G FAT
(42 G saturated, 1.5 G trans)

3,200 MG SODIUM

Artichoke Fritti

650 CALORIES

31 G FAT (15 G saturated)

1,430 MG SODIUM

★

Other than the choice of noodles, what's the difference between this plate and the lasagna? The simple addition of garlic cream sauce gives it almost double the calories and nearly three times the saturated fat.

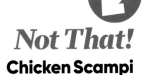

Not That!

Chicken Scampi

1,310 CALORIES

76 G FAT (20 G saturated)

1,850 MG SODIUM

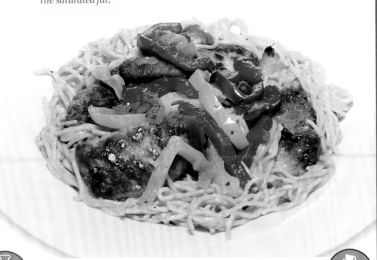

TEST TUBE FOODS

Lasagna Fritta

1,070 CALORIES

71 G FAT
(29 G saturated,
1.5 G trans)

1,650 MG SODIUM

Olive Garden's battered, deep-fried lasagna invention will set you back a day's worth of saturated fat. Just because you can deep-fry something doesn't mean you should.

SOUP STACK-UP

Minestrone

110 CALORIES

1.5 G FAT
(0 G saturated)

840 MG SODIUM

Pasta e Fagioli

180 CALORIES

6 G FAT
(0 G saturated)

840 MG SODIUM

Zuppa Toscana

220 CALORIES

15 G FAT
(0 G saturated)

840 MG SODIUM

Chicken & Gnocchi

250 CALORIES

14 G FAT
(5 G saturated)

1,400 MG SODIUM

OUTBACK STEAKHOUSE

Eat This

Victoria's Filet with Baked Potato
with Sour Cream and Grilled Asparagus
(8 oz without Crumb Topping)

620 CALORIES

20 G FAT (8 G saturated)

1,200 MG SODIUM

★

You're at Outback Steakhouse, so order steak. A lean slab of beef paired with some veggies and a baked potato is one of the safest—not to mention most satisfying—meals on the menu. Just be sure to forgo the crumb topping, or you'll add more than 200 calories to your steak.

OTHER PICKS

Sweet Glazed Pork Tenderloin
with Baked Potato with Sour Cream and Fresh Steamed French Green Beans

625 CALORIES

15 G FAT (7 G saturated)

1,672 MG SODIUM

Simply Grilled Mahi
with Rice Garnish and Steamed Veggies
(8 oz)

475 CALORIES

7 G FAT (3 G saturated)

1,178 MG SODIUM

Asian Sesame Salad
with Seared Ahi and Sesame Vinaigrette

490 CALORIES

37.8 G FAT (4.3 G saturated)

1,243 MG SODIUM

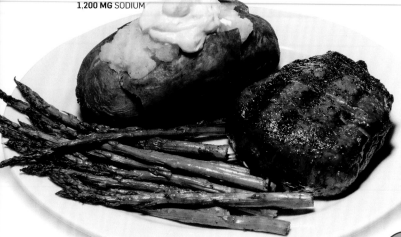

GRADE

C+

Outback has made some respectable strides in recent years, lightening up existing fare (the Alice Springs Chicken Quesadilla shrank from 2,140 calories down to 1,554) and offering a range of items under 500 calories. Many of the steaks now fall below 800 calories, and more than half of the side dishes come in under 350 calories.

SURVIVAL STRATEGY

Start with a small Seared Ahi Tuna (331 calories), then have the decadent-sounding Sirloin and Grilled Shrimp (494 calories). If you skip the bread and house salad (590 calories) and choose steamed veggies as your side, you can escape for fewer than 1,000 calories.

OTHER PASSES

Baby Back Ribs
with Garlic Mashed Potatoes
(½ order)

986 CALORIES

60 G FAT (24 G saturated)

1,953 MG SODIUM

Hearts of Gold Mahi
with Fresh Seasonal Mixed Veggies

694 CALORIES

29 G FAT (17 G saturated)

1,624 MG SODIUM

Aussie Chicken Cobb Salad
with Crispy Chicken and Thousand Island Dressing

1,296 CALORIES

100 G FAT (31 G saturated)

2,023 MG SODIUM

★

Burgers can be a sensible, protein-packed meal, but sit-down chains squash their nutritional potential by serving them up in jumbo portions alongside heaping piles of fried potatoes. All of the burger-and-fry combos at Outback pack more than 1,000 calories.

Not That!

The Outback Burger and Sweet Potato Fries
with American Cheese

1,235 CALORIES

72 G FAT (33 G saturated)

2,007 MG SODIUM

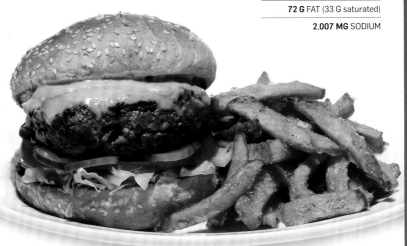

EAT THIS
APPROVED
NOT THAT!

Grilled Shrimp on the Barbie

312 CALORIES

19.7 G FAT
(4.6 G saturated)

587 MG SODIUM

On too many chain menus, the word "appetizer" is nothing but a formality—1,000-calorie nachos and plates of french fries smothered in cheese and bacon are hardly a way to warm up the appetite. A true appetizer should be light on fat and low in calories so you're not stuffed when your entrée arrives. This shrimp plate delivers.

MEET YOUR MATCH

1,919 calories

Wings with Mild Sauce

=

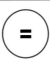

16 KFC Original Recipe Chicken Drumsticks

PANDA EXPRESS

Eat This

Kung Pao Chicken Entrée
with Steamed Rice and Mixed Veggies

690 CALORIES

18.5 G FAT (3 G saturated)

1,450 MG SODIUM

★

All of the nonbreaded chicken entrées at Panda are fair game. Pairing them with a rice-and-vegetable combo makes for a respectable meal, but if you ditch the rice altogether and go straight to veggies, you'll save an extra 155 calories.

OTHER PICKS

Golden Treasure Shrimp

230 CALORIES

10 G FAT (1.5 G saturated)

250 MG SODIUM

Chicken Pot Stickers
(3)

220 CALORIES

6 G FAT (1.5 G saturated)

250 MG SODIUM

Fortune Cookies
(3)

96 CALORIES

0 G FAT

9 G SUGARS

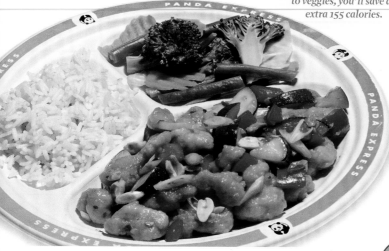

GRADE

C+

Oddly enough, it's not the wok-fried meat or the viscous sauces that do the most harm on this menu—it's the more than 400 calories of rice and noodles that form the foundation of each meal. Scrape these starches from the plate, and Panda Express starts to look a lot healthier. Only one entrée item has more than 500 calories, and there's hardly a trans fat on the menu. Problems arise when multiple entrées and sides start piling up on one plate, though, so bring some self-restraint to the table.

SURVIVAL STRATEGY

Avoid these entrées: Orange Chicken, Sweet & Sour Chicken, Beijing Beef, and anything with pork. Then swap in Mixed Veggies for the scoop of rice.

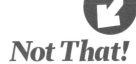

OTHER PASSES

Honey Walnut Shrimp

370 CALORIES

23 G FAT (4 G saturated)

470 MG SODIUM

Chicken Egg Rolls
(2)

400 CALORIES

24 G FAT (8 G saturated)

780 MG SODIUM

Chocolate Chunk Cookie

160 CALORIES

7 G FAT (3 G saturated)

14 G SUGARS

★

Never go all starch for your side. The Chow Mein contributes more than half of this plate's calories, and the Orange Chicken's crispy breading and sugary sauce finish it off.

Not That!
Orange Chicken Entrée
with Chow Mein

910 CALORIES

40 G FAT (7.5 G saturated)

1,600 MG SODIUM

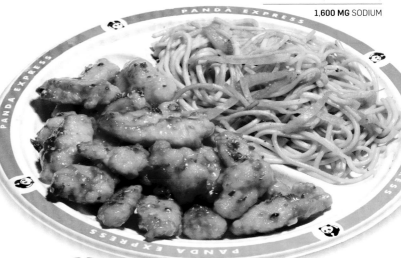

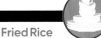

Broccoli Beef

120 CALORIES

9 G FAT
(1.5 G saturated)

660 MG SODIUM

The lowest-calorie entrée on Panda's menu, Broccoli Beef is a standout. Pair an order with an appetizer and you'll have a satisfying meal for a scant amount of calories. P.F. Chang's version, by comparison, packs 870 calories and more than 4,500 milligrams of sodium.

SIDE STACK-UP

Mixed Veggies

70 CALORIES

0.5 G FAT

Steamed Rice

380 CALORIES

0 G FAT

Fried Rice

470 CALORIES

19 G FAT

Chow Mein

490 CALORIES

22 G FAT

PANERA BREAD

Eat This

Half Asiago Roast Beef and Half Classic Salad
with Asian Sesame Vinaigrette

475 CALORIES

23 G FAT (8.5 G saturated)

990 MG SODIUM

★
At 700 calories, the full version of this sandwich is one of the most caloric on the menu, but when you cut it in half and pair it with a light side salad, you have a balanced lunch on your hands. What's better, this trick works with almost every sandwich at Panera.

OTHER PICKS

Smoked Turkey Breast on Country

430 CALORIES

3.5 G FAT (1 G saturated)

1,790 MG SODIUM

Full Strawberry Poppyseed & Chicken Signature Salad

350 CALORIES

13 G FAT (1.5 G saturated)

290 MG SODIUM

Breakfast Power Sandwich

340 CALORIES

15 G FAT (7 G saturated)

710 MG SODIUM

GRADE

B−

Panera's menu still features a roster of mostly great salads and soups, and between the 340-calorie Power Sandwich and the steel-cut oatmeal, a first-rate breakfast is there for the taking. But only 6 out of 18 sandwiches have 600 or fewer calories, and the bakery puts out little not tainted by refined carbs. Even its "whole-wheat" bread is more than 50 percent white flour. Until we see real progress, this B- is as good as Panera can hope for.

SURVIVAL STRATEGY

For breakfast, choose between the Egg & Cheese breakfast sandwich and the 310-calorie granola parfait. Skip the stand-alone sandwich lunch. Instead, pair soup and a salad, or order the soup and half-sandwich combo.

72

OTHER PASSES

Sierra Turkey
on Asiago Cheese Focaccia

810 CALORIES

37 G FAT (9 G saturated)

1,950 MG SODIUM

Full Roasted Turkey Fuji Apple Signature Salad

550 CALORIES

34 G FAT (7 G saturated)

620 MG SODIUM

Asiago Cheese Bagel with Bacon

610 CALORIES

28 G FAT
(13 G saturated, 0.5 G trans)

1,350 MG SODIUM

★

The trouble here isn't the eggs or bacon, it's the high-fat festival of ranch dressing and Gorgonzola cheese crumbles. You still get plenty of greens and protein with the meal on the opposite page, and you'll take in half the fat.

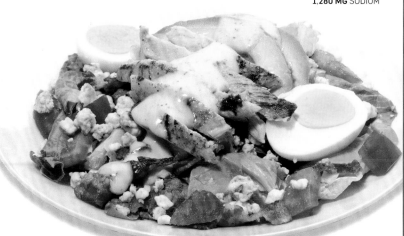

Not That!

Chicken Cobb
with Avocado and Buttermilk Ranch

710 CALORIES

53 G FAT (16 G saturated)

1,280 MG SODIUM

GUILTY PLEASURE

Pumpkin Muffie

290 CALORIES

11 G FAT
(2 G saturated)

26 G SUGARS

Lop off the bottom of a muffin and you get a pretty good treat. A regular pumpkin muffin, for example, has double the calories and sugars as this mini muffin. Plus, the top is the tastiest part.

TEST TUBE FOODS

Sourdough Bread Bowl

590 CALORIES

2.5 G FAT
(0 G saturated)

1,210 MG SODIUM

Sure, you could eat your lunch out of a bowl made entirely of bread. You could also eat your breakfast off of a pancake plate, but why would you? Bread bowls are just another wacky invention designed to get your novelty neurons firing, and they offer nothing but empty carbs.

PAPA JOHN'S

Eat This

The Works Original Crust Pizza and Chickenstrips with Cheese Dipping Sauce

(1 slice, large pie, and 3 strips)

400 CALORIES

26 G FAT (8.5 G saturated)

1,060 MG SODIUM

The best defense is a good offense, so start the meal off with a few pieces of belly-filling protein in the form of wings or chicken strips. Consider it insurance against scarfing too many slices later on in the meal.

OTHER PICKS

Spinach Alfredo Original Crust Pizza
(2 slices, medium pie)

400 CALORIES

16 G FAT (7 G saturated)

1,000 MG SODIUM

Sausage Original Crust Pizza
(2 slices, medium pie)

480 CALORIES

22 G FAT (9 G saturated)

1,200 MG SODIUM

Honey Chipotle Wings
(2)

190 CALORIES

12 G FAT (3 G saturated)

730 MG SODIUM

GRADE

We're glad that Papa John's struck its disastrous pan crust pizza from the menu. But with it also went its whole-wheat crust option. Now, very little separates Papa from the rest of the pizza competition. It still has some high-quality toppings, but they're nothing you can't get elsewhere. What hasn't changed? The breadsticks still deliver far too many calories, and the Special Garlic sauce can wreck even the healthiest slice.

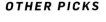

SURVIVAL STRATEGY

As with any other pizza place, it's best to start with a thin base, ask for light cheese, and cover it with anything other than sausage, pepperoni, or bacon. The Spinach Alfredo remains the pie to pick at Papa John's.

OTHER PASSES

Tuscan Six Cheese Thin Crust Pizza
(2 slices, large pie)

640 CALORIES

26 G FAT (12 G saturated)

1,600 MG SODIUM

The Meats Thin Crust Pizza
(2 slices, large pie)

620 CALORIES

38 G FAT (14 G saturated)

1,420 MG SODIUM

Parmesan Breadsticks
(2)

340 CALORIES

10 G FAT (1.5 G saturated)

720 MG SODIUM

★

Chicken fingers are no health food, but at least they have protein on their side. Cheesesticks, on the other hand, are nothing but empty carbs smothered in saturated fat. And the garlic dip? That little cup supplies 40 percent of this meal's fat count.

Not That!

Spicy Italian Original Crust Pizza and Cheesesticks with Special Garlic Dipping Sauce
(1 slice, large pie, and 2 sticks)

715 CALORIES

43 G FAT (13.5 G saturated)

1,720 MG SODIUM

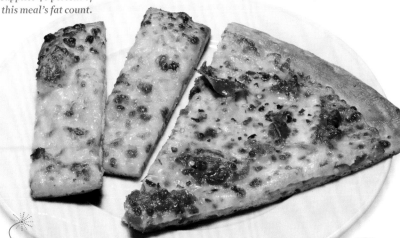

560 CALORIE BOMB

Cinnapie
(4 sticks)

19 G FAT (6 G saturated)

39 G SUGARS

After a dinner of refined carbs, do you really need more of the same? Just four of these cinnamon sticks pretty much guarantee that your delivered dinner will cross the 1,000-calorie mark.

1 CUP DIPPING SAUCE STACK-UP

Buffalo Sauce	Cheese Sauce	Special Garlic
15 CALORIES	**40** CALORIES	**150** CALORIES
0.5 G FAT	**3.5 G** FAT	**17 G** FAT

Pizza Sauce	Honey Mustard	Blue Cheese
20 CALORIES	**150** CALORIES	**160** CALORIES
1 G FAT	**15 G** FAT	**16 G** FAT

75

PERKINS

Eat This

Steak Medallions and Portabella Mushrooms Dinner
with Broccoli and Garlic Butter

520 CALORIES

29 G FAT (8 G saturated)

1,050 MG SODIUM

★

The fat's a bit high, but this 7-ounce steak dinner is about as good as it gets at problem-riddled Perkins. Scrap the dinner roll, or you'll add on another 120 calories.

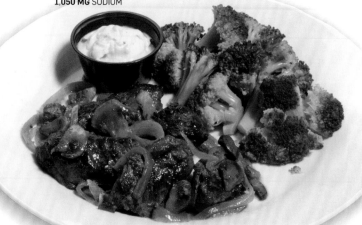

OTHER PICKS

French Dip Sandwich

610 CALORIES

31 G FAT (9 G saturated)

2,150 MG SODIUM

Classic Eggs and Bacon
with Breakfast Potatoes and Seasonal Fresh Fruit

610 CALORIES

37 G FAT (11.5 G saturated)

1,220 MG SODIUM

White Chocolate Macadamia Nut Cookie

340 CALORIES

19 G FAT (8 G saturated)

14 G SUGARS

GRADE

D

Of the more than 90 dishes at Perkins, only five qualify for the Calorie Counter menu. Outside of that you'll find entrées with more than 4,000 milligrams of sodium, pasta plates with more than 100 grams of fat, and an all-day omelet menu that averages more than 1,500 calories per order. Currently the chain has stores in 34 states. Hopefully it cleans up its nutritional act before it hits the other 16.

SURVIVAL STRATEGY

Stick with the steak pictured here or choose something off the Calorie Counter menu. Elsewhere on the menu, unexpected calories lurk at every turn. Even the Grilled Salmon with Broccoli, a dish that seems impossible to screw up, packs 750 calories.

OTHER PASSES

Triple Decker Club Sandwich

890 CALORIES

55 G FAT (11 G saturated)

2,070 MG SODIUM

Smoked Bacon & Ham Omelette
with Hash Browns and Seasonal Fresh Fruit

1,410 CALORIES

73 G FAT (23.5 G saturated)

3,380 MG SODIUM

Banana Nut Mammoth Muffin
with Whipped Butter Blend

700 CALORIES

40 G FAT (9 G saturated)

42 G SUGARS

★

White-meat turkey is one of the lightest meats you can have on your plate. Unfortunately, smothering it in gravy and heavy dressing and pairing it with too many starchy extras cancels out any benefit you get from the lean protein. Keep it simple at Perkins.

Not That!

Butterball Turkey & Dressing
with Mashed Potatoes with Gravy and Broccoli and Cranberry Sauce

810 CALORIES

37 G FAT (12 G saturated)

2,440 MG SODIUM

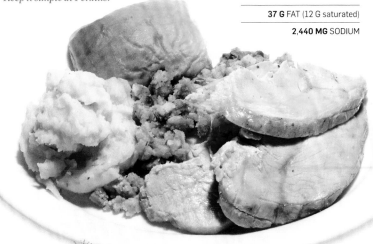

1,390 CALORIE BOMB

Country Sausage Biscuit Platter

90 G FAT
(46 G saturated)

3,680 MG SODIUM

Two sausage and cheese biscuits, two eggs, a pile of fried potatoes, a stack of bacon, and a smothering of cream gravy combine to give you a plate with nearly two days' worth of saturated fat and sodium. The scariest part? This isn't the worst breakfast plate on the menu! (That honor goes to their 1,860-calorie Southern Fried Chicken Biscuit Platter.)

SIDE STACK-UP

Sautéed Spinach
70 CALORIES
3.5 G FAT

Mashed Potatoes
150 CALORIES
7 G FAT

Buttered Corn
150 CALORIES
8 G FAT

Baked Potato
Lite Sour Cream
210 CALORIES
2.5 G FAT

P.F. CHANG'S

Eat This

Shrimp
with Lobster Sauce

360 CALORIES

18 G FAT (3.5 G saturated)

2,700 MG SODIUM

★

The Chang's seafood menu ranges from the cream-soaked Shrimp with Candied Walnuts (1,380 calories) all the way down to sensible plates like the 240-calorie Shanghai Shrimp with Garlic Sauce and the lean crustacean creation pictured here. Heavy sauces and crispy breading are the downfall of the higher-cal picks, so beware.

OTHER PICKS

Ginger Chicken
with Broccoli

460 CALORIES

10 G FAT (2 G saturated)

2,320 MG SODIUM

Ahi Tuna
with Avocado

320 CALORIES

14 G FAT (2 G saturated)

530 MG SODIUM

Sweet and Sour Pork

710 CALORIES

25 G FAT (6 G saturated)

1,460 MG SODIUM

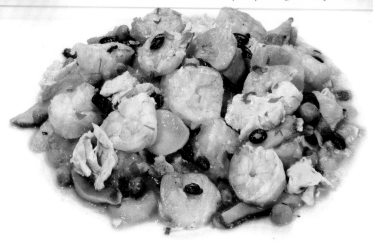

GRADE

C–

It's now considerably easier to put together a nutritionally respectable meal at P.F. Chang's than it was a few years ago, thanks in part to a solid line of low-calorie salads. But noodle dishes and nearly anything from the grill still come with dangerously high fat and calorie counts, while the entire menu is saltier than a Chris Rock monologue.

SURVIVAL STRATEGY

Order a lean appetizer like dumplings or the Seared Ahi Tuna for the table, and resolve to avoid anything that's prepared breaded. Servings are generous enough that you can even split one of the more reasonable entrées between two people.

OTHER PASSES

Kung Pao Chicken
1,070 CALORIES

64 G FAT (10 G saturated)

2,410 MG SODIUM

Spicy Eggplant Side
1,010 CALORIES

88 G FAT (13 G saturated)

3,790 MG SODIUM

Chang's Pork Fried Rice
1,370 CALORIES

41 G FAT (8 G saturated)

2,130 MG SODIUM

★

Compared with most fish, the tilapia used in this dish contains very little heart-healthy omega-3 fats. Rolled in deep-fried breading, this not-great protein becomes the star of When Bad Fats Happen to Good People.

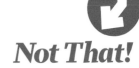

Not That!

Hunan-Style Hot Fish
1,000 CALORIES

43 G FAT (7 G saturated)

3,460 MG SODIUM

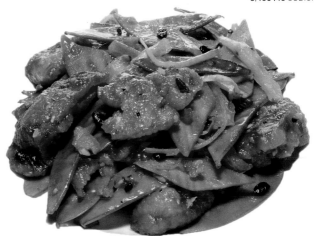

MENU MAGIC

A simple way to shave calories off your Chang's plate: Scratch the rice and get a small order of nutrient-packed vegetables instead. Almost any vegetable side will save you more than 100 calories over a side of brown rice. One exception: Don't touch the Spicy Eggplant Side!

SALT LICK

Hot & Sour Soup
(bowl)

7,980 MG SODIUM

380 CALORIES

11 G FAT (3 G saturated)

Would you like some soup with your salt? There's more than five days' worth of sodium in this simple bowl of broth, making it the single saltiest restaurant food we've ever come across—and it's only a side dish!

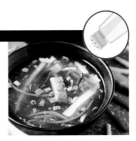

PIZZA HUT

Eat This
All American Traditional Hot Wings
(8)

320 CALORIES

20 G FAT (6 G saturated)

1,160 MG SODIUM

★
We know, it's called Pizza Hut. But we have a point here: You could eat an entire plateful of wings and still not reach the calorie count of a single slice of most of the Hut's specialty pies. We'd rather have the wings.

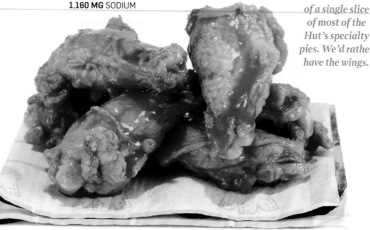

OTHER PICKS

Pepperoni Thin 'N Crispy Pizza
(2 slices, medium pie)

420 CALORIES

20 G FAT (9 G saturated)

1,400 MG SODIUM

Chicken Supreme Personal Pan Pizza

590 CALORIES

21 G FAT (8 G saturated)

1,370 MG SODIUM

Lemon Pepper Traditional Wings
(2)

150 CALORIES

10 G FAT (2 G saturated)

430 MG SODIUM

GRADE

C

In an attempt to push the menu beyond slices, Pizza Hut expanded into pastas, salads, and something called a P'Zone. Sound like an improvement? Think again. Calzone-like P'Zones all pack more than 1,000 calories each. The salads aren't much better, and the pastas are actually worse. The thin crust and Fit 'N Delicious pizzas offer sub-200-calorie slices, and the bone-in wings are a solid start to any meal. Combine those elements and you'll do just fine.

SURVIVAL STRATEGY

This is not the place for pasta. A pan of Chicken Alfredo packs more than 1,000 calories. The key to the Hut lies in the crust: Pan Pizzas cost you 80 more calories per slice over Thin 'N Crispy, and 40 more per slice than the Stuffed Crust.

OTHER PASSES

Pepperoni
P'Zone Pizza
with Marinara Dipping Sauce

980 CALORIES

32 G FAT (14 G saturated)

2,340 MG SODIUM

Ultimate
Cheese Lover's
Stuffed Crust Pizza
(2 slices, 14" large pie)

680 CALORIES

30 G FAT (16 G saturated)

2,070 MG SODIUM

Garlic Parmesan
Bone-Out Wings
(2)

260 CALORIES

19 G FAT (3.5 G saturated)

710 MG SODIUM

★
*You can love
meat without
taking in half a
day's saturated
fat with one
slice of pizza.
Specialty pizzas
are an excuse
to go crazy with
a ton of high-fat
toppings that do
virtually nothing
for flavor and
increase your
calorie load
considerably.
At Pizza Hut,
don't be a Lover,
be a fighter.*

Not That!
Meat Lover's Pizza
(1 slice, 14" large pan pizza)

470 CALORIES

28 G FAT (10 G saturated)

1,150 MG SODIUM

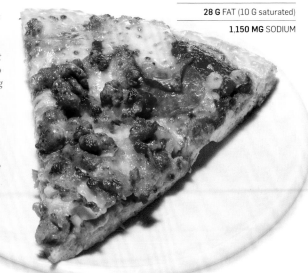

TEST TUBE FOODS

Garlic Parmesan Bone-Out Wings
(6)

780 CALORIES

57 G FAT
(10.5 G saturated)

2,130 MG SODIUM

Ever seen a chicken without bones? Of course not. Mother Nature put them there for a reason, and it wasn't so multinational food corporations could go removing them for their own twisted purposes. These freakish "bone-out" wings have twice as many calories as Pizza Hut's traditional wings.

BREAD STACK-UP

Breadstick	Cheese Breadstick	Stuffed Pizza Roller
140 CALORIES	**170** CALORIES	**230** CALORIES
5 G FAT (1 G saturated)	**6 G** FAT (2.5 G saturated)	**10 G** FAT (4.5 G saturated)
260 MG SODIUM	**390 MG** SODIUM	**630 MG** SODIUM

RED LOBSTER

Eat This

Wood-Grilled Shrimp

Two shrimp skewers served over rice, with choice of side

320 CALORIES

9 G FAT (2 G saturated)

1,850 MG SODIUM

★

The Red Lobster menu has a substantial selection of lean protein options, and the Lighthouse menu allows you to mix and match them with healthful sides. We'd love to see the cooks take it easy with the salt shaker, but for 320 calories, you still end up with a pretty impressive meal.

OTHER PICKS

Walt's Favorite Shrimp
with broccoli

590 CALORIES

24 G FAT (2 G saturated)

3,200 MG SODIUM

Southwest-Style Tacos with Grilled Shrimp

630 CALORIES

25 G FAT (3.5 G saturated)

2,230 MG SODIUM

Garden Salad
with Red Wine Vinaigrette
(side order)

150 CALORIES

6.5 G FAT (0 G saturated)

580 MG SODIUM

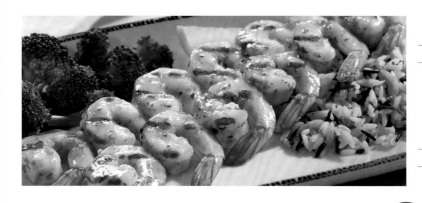

GRADE

A-

Compared with the other major sit-down chains, Red Lobster looks like a paradigm of sound nutrition. The new Lighthouse menu features grilled options like the meal pictured here, and the menu is long on low-calorie, high-protein entrées and reasonable vegetable-based sides. That's why Red Lobster is one of America's healthiest chain restaurants. The only flaw you'll find is an overreliance on the deep fryer and the salt shaker.

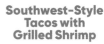

SURVIVAL STRATEGY

Avoid calorie-heavy Cajun sauces, combo dishes, and anything labeled "crispy." And tell the waiter to keep those biscuits for himself. You'll never go wrong with simple broiled or grilled fish and a vegetable side.

OTHER PASSES

Parrot Isle Jumbo Coconut Shrimp

880 CALORIES

60 G FAT (15 G saturated)

1,860 MG SODIUM

Crispy Calamari and Vegetables

1,650 CALORIES

109 G FAT (12 G saturated)

4,170 MG SODIUM

Caesar Salad
with Caesar Dressing
(side order)

570 CALORIES

57 G FAT (10.5 G saturated)

1,140 MG SODIUM

★

We don't know who Alfredo is, but he must love butter. And salt. With nearly two days' worth of sodium and almost as many calories as an adult woman should eat in a day, this crab dish isn't worth shelling out for.

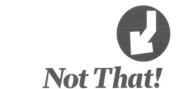

Not That!

Crab Linguine Alfredo
(full)

1,600 CALORIES

90 G FAT (37 G saturated)

3,840 MG SODIUM

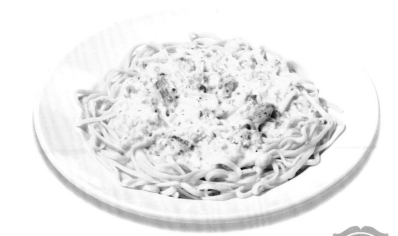

ALL THIS OR THAT!

1,530 calories

New England Clam Chowder
(bowl)
**Wood-Grilled Tilapia
Garlic-Grilled Shrimp
and Caramel Cheesecake**

 or

Bar Harbor Lobster Bake

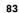

Fresh Fish Menu

Red Lobster may have built its name on crustaceans, but it's the daily rotating selection of fresh fish that represents why this is still the best sit-down chain in America. Try any of the fish (minus the cobia) blackened or grilled with a side of pineapple salsa for an amazing low-cal meal.

ROMANO'S MACARONI

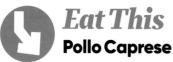

Eat This
Pollo Caprese

560 CALORIES

N/A G FAT (11 G saturated)

1,250 MG SODIUM

★

Crispy breading and creamy sauces cause the undoing of many of this country's chicken-and-pasta combos, but this refreshing entrée contains neither. It's the only way to have pasta and protein on your plate at Romano's for fewer than 700 calories.

OTHER PICKS

Lobster Ravioli

600 CALORIES

N/A G FAT (21 G saturated)

1,490 MG SODIUM

~~Goat Cheese Peppadew Peppers~~

350 CALORIES

N/A G FAT (6 G saturated)

710 MG SODIUM

Tiramisu

600 CALORIES

N/A G FAT (24 G saturated)

65 MG SODIUM

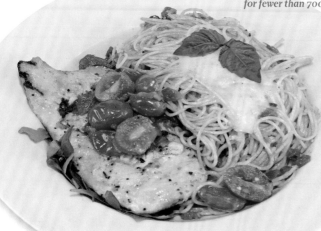

GRADE

C−

In 2010, we commended Macaroni Grill's efforts to revamp a pretty miserable menu by cutting calories and adding menu items such as rosemary spiedinis. Shortly thereafter— because no good deed goes unpunished—new ownership swept in to undo most of the progress from before. Lean proteins and prudent pastas have been traded in for the same cheesy, fatty fare it put out so many years ago. It was great while it lasted.

⊞ SURVIVAL STRATEGY

The Flatbreads, Pasta, and Classics menus are all serious trouble. Instead, opt for a soup-and-salad combo or a Create Your Own pasta with spaghetti, red sauce, and as many vegetables as you can fit in the bowl. Split a bowl of gelato and call it a day.

GRILL

Shrimp Portofino
1,120 CALORIES

N/A G FAT (36 G saturated)

1,700 MG SODIUM

Crispy Fresh Mozzarella
820 CALORIES

N/A G FAT (16 G saturated)

210 MG SODIUM

Homemade Chocolate Cake
940 CALORIES

N/A G FAT (29 G saturated)

570 MG SODIUM

★

Romano's doesn't make its ingredients public, so we're not sure how roasted chicken and potatoes can bear such a shameful nutritional profile, but knowing it contains more than half a day's calories and nearly a day's worth of sodium is reason enough not to order it.

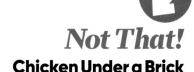

Not That!
Chicken Under a Brick

1,590 CALORIES

N/A G FAT (31 G saturated)

2,040 MG SODIUM

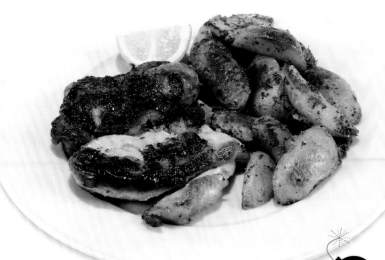

2,040 CALORIE BOMB

SIDESWIPED

Flatbreads!

1,210–1,420 CALORIES

Having embraced its mission of making America's beaches just plain uglier, Romano's recently launched Fatbreads, "the anti-flatbread. Fat on crust. Fat on toppings." Fat on your body. The most industriously caloric of the four is the Farmhouse, which comes with pepperoni, bacon, and prosciutto, plus three types of cheese and dipping sauce.

Mama's Trio

N/A G FAT (53 G saturated)

4,160 MG SODIUM

Mama's Trio has the saturated fat content of the Three Tenors. A combination of chicken Parmesan, lasagna Bolognese, and cannelloni Bolognese, it's cheese on meat and meat on cheese, wrapped in a noodle coffin.

RUBY TUESDAY

Eat This

Asiago Peppercorn Sirloin
with Garlic Cheese Biscuit and Fresh Steamed Broccoli

535 CALORIES

23 G FAT

1,810 MG SODIUM

★

With a cut as lean as sirloin, even a cheesy and indulgent topping keeps you well within the limits of a sensible dinner.

OTHER PICKS

Hickory Bourbon Chicken

250 CALORIES

5 G FAT

720 MG SODIUM

Top Sirloin and Lobster Tail

461 CALORIES

25 G FAT

1,337 MG SODIUM

Fried Mozzarella
(per serving)

135 CALORIES

8 G FAT

420 MG SODIUM

GRADE

C-

The chain built its reputation on a hearty selection of hamburgers. The problem is, the burgers average 75 grams of fat—100 percent of your recommended daily limit. And now that Ruby Tuesday has finally released full sodium counts, it's apparent it's been harboring one of the saltiest menus in America. But with the addition of the Fit & Trim and Petite menus in recent years, Ruby's earns a slight bump up on its report card.

SURVIVAL STRATEGY

Solace lies in the three S's: sirloin, salmon, and shrimp all make for relatively innocuous eating, especially when paired with one of Ruby Tuesday's half-dozen healthy sides, such as roasted spaghetti squash and fresh green beans.

OTHER PASSES

Avocado Turkey Burger

1,381 CALORIES	
77 G FAT	
2,763 MG SODIUM	

Ribs and Crispy Popcorn Shrimp

1,030 CALORIES	
55 G FAT	
2,335 MG SODIUM	

Queso & Chips
(per serving)

288 CALORIES	
18 G FAT	
489 MG SODIUM	

★

Mistakes were made. In this case, pairing the super fatty rib-eye cut with a baked potato that comes standard with fatty toppings.

Not That!

Rib Eye with Baked Potato
with Butter and Sour Cream

1,254 CALORIES	
85 G FAT	
1,096 MG SODIUM	

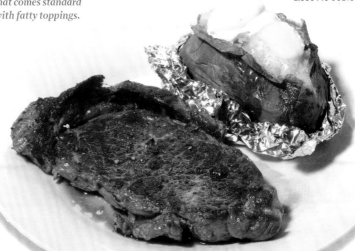

HEALTH-FOOD FRAUD

Avocado Grilled Chicken Sandwich

1,311 CALORIES	
64 G FAT	
2,833 MG SODIUM	

Ruby's makes a habit of corrupting healthy ingredients with fatty toppers and jumbo portions. A sandwich based on lean protein and avocado should be a nutritional no-brainer, but this plate has almost the same calorie count as a Triple Prime Burger.

SIDE STACK-UP

Mashed Potatoes
267 CALORIES

15 G FAT

Sweet Potato Fries
330 CALORIES

12 G FAT

French Fries
480 CALORIES

24 G FAT

Loaded Baked Potato
566 CALORIES

29 G FAT

STARBUCKS

Eat This
Reduced Fat Turkey Bacon Breakfast sandwich

230 CALORIES

6 G FAT (2.5 G saturated)

560 MG SODIUM

Lean protein from the bacon and egg meets its perfect accompaniment in the relatively low-carb English muffin. That's a powerful nutritional punch for a mere 230 calories.

OTHER PICKS

Iced Vanilla Latte
with 2% Milk
(Grande)

190 CALORIES

4 G FAT (2 G saturated)

28 G SUGARS

Chicken & Hummus Bistro Box

270 CALORIES

8 G FAT (1 G saturated)

520 MG SODIUM

Marshmallow Dream Bar

240 CALORIES

5 G FAT (3 G saturated)

23 G SUGARS

GRADE

B+

Once upon a time, Starbucks was a fine place for coffee, but a dangerous place for fancy drinks and food. But recent years have seen the introduction of a solid line of breakfast and lunch sandwiches, oatmeal, wraps, parfaits, and snack plates, making this coffee shop a reliable place to tame a growling stomach on the go. Just ignore the carb-fueled confections. As for the drinks? Unless you keep it simple, they can do some damage.

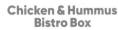

SURVIVAL STRATEGY

There's no beating a regular cup of joe or unsweetened tea, but if you need a specialty fix, stick with fat-free milk, sugar-free syrup, and no whipped cream. As for food, go with the Perfect Oatmeal or an Egg White, Spinach, and Feta Wrap.

OTHER PASSES

Iced White Chocolate Mocha
with 2% Milk
(Grande, No Whipped Cream)

340 CALORIES

9 G FAT (6 G saturated)

52 G SUGARS

Cheese & Fruit Bistro Box

480 CALORIES

28 G FAT
(10 G saturated, 0.5 G trans)

470 MG SODIUM

Old-Fashioned Glazed Doughnut

480 CALORIES

27 G FAT (13 G saturated)

30 G SUGARS

★

It's time you learned the truth: Muffins are icing-less cupcakes. It doesn't matter what healthy ingredients they boast—blueberries, zucchini, carrots, nuts, bran—they're just flour, eggs, butter, and sugar, and they'll leave you hungry shortly after you eat them. How do we know that? Because this muffin has 20 grams of sugar and not even a full gram of fiber.

Not That!

Carrot Cake Muffin with Pecans

370 CALORIES

20 G FAT (4 G saturated)

170 MG SODIUM

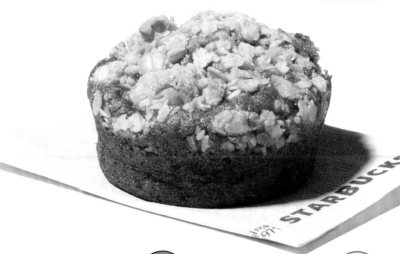

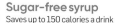

ESPRESSO DRINK STACK UP
(Grande, 16 oz)

Caffe Americano	Espresso	Caffe Mocha
15 CALORIES	**5** CALORIES	**260** CALORIES
0 G SUGARS	**0 G** SUGARS	**34 G** SUGARS
Cappuccino	**Caffe Latte**	
120 CALORIES	**190** CALORIES	
10 G SUGARS	**17 G** SUGARS	

CALORIE-CUTTING LINGO

Sugar-free syrup
Saves up to 150 calories a drink

Skinny
Uses sugar-free syrup and fat-free milk

Hold the whip
Cuts the cream and saves you up to 110 calories
Nonfat uses fat-free milk instead of whole or 2%

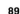

89

STEAK 'N SHAKE

Eat This

Double Steakburger
with Cheese

440 CALORIES

25 G FAT (11 G saturated)

590 MG SODIUM

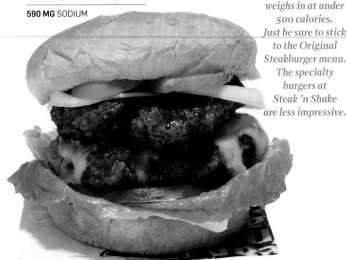

★

This is one of the only drive-thrus in the country where a substantial double-stacked cheeseburger weighs in at under 500 calories. Just be sure to stick to the Original Steakburger menu. The specialty burgers at Steak 'n Shake are less impressive.

OTHER PICKS

Guacamole Single Steakburger

380 CALORIES

21 G FAT
(7 G saturated, 0.5 G trans)

650 MG SODIUM

Grilled Chicken Salad
with Reduced Fat Berry Balsamic Vinaigrette

320 CALORIES

11.5 G FAT (3.5 G saturated)

1,020 MG SODIUM

Oreo Ice Cream Sandwich

240 CALORIES

10 G FAT (4 G saturated)

19 G SUGARS

GRADE

B-

For a chain named after two of the most precarious foods on the planet, Steak 'n Shake could be far more dangerous. A single Steakburger with Cheese delivers a modest 330 calories, and not a single salad exceeds 600. Too bad we can't make a similar claim about the shakes. Even the smalls commonly eclipse 600 calories, and at least one—the regular M&M shake—has more sugar than four Klondike Bars.

SURVIVAL STRATEGY

Go ahead and order a burger, but keep it simple. If you're feeling extra hungry, add a second steak patty for 110 calories. What you want to avoid are the tricked-out chili dishes. Anything entrée-size will saddle you with 830 to 1,220 calories.

OTHER PASSES

Wisconsin Buttery Steakburger

700 CALORIES

47 G FAT
(21 G saturated, 1.5 G trans)

760 MG SODIUM

Grilled Chicken Taco Salad
with Ranch Dressing

740 CALORIES

60 G FAT
(12.5 G saturated, 0.5 G trans)

2,020 MG SODIUM

Cookies 'n Cream Milk Shake
(small)

570 CALORIES

18 G FAT (11 G saturated)

74 G SUGARS

★

*"Melt" is code for extra cheese
and butter-drenched bread,
and when you're already dealing with
ground beef and cheese, that kind
of excess is just plain unnecessary.*

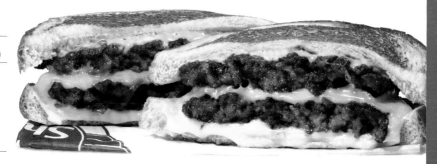

Not That!
Frisco Melt

750 CALORIES

53 G FAT (17 G saturated)

1,160 MG SODIUM

1,220 CALORIE BOMB

Chili Deluxe
(bowl)

74 G FAT
(39 G saturated,
1.5 G trans)

2,560 MG SODIUM

At its best, chili is a lean protein- and fiber-packed respite from the fatty offerings on most American menus. But chili is only as lean as the meat that goes into it. Steak 'n Shake must use some ridiculously high-fat beef to produce a cheese-topped chili bowl with the same number of calories and more saturated fat than two (!) Triple Steakburgers with Cheese.

MEET YOUR MATCH

105 g sugars

Chocolate Chip Pancakes **=** 29 Chips Ahoy! Original cookies

SUBWAY

Eat This

Steak and Cheese Toasted Sandwich and Veggie Delite Salad
with Honey Mustard Dressing
(6")

490 CALORIES

12 G FAT
(4.5 G saturated)

1,350 MG SODIUM

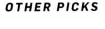

★
Nearly identical sandwiches with one critical difference: The Philly on the opposite page has 120 extra calories and triple the saturated fat. The choice is yours.

OTHER PICKS

Turkey Breast and Ham
with double meat
(6")

280 CALORIES

4 G FAT (1 G saturated)

730 MG SODIUM

Subway Club
with Avocado
(6")

370 CALORIES

10 G FAT (2 G saturated)

800 MG SODIUM

Black Forest Ham, Egg, and Cheese Flatbread
(2)

400 CALORIES

16 G FAT (5 G saturated)

1,180 MG SODIUM

GRADE

A

Subway is the first major fast-food chain to carry avocado (now available at breakfast, too), and all the heart-healthy fats found within, in every one of its 26,688 US stores. And in 2014, the chain removed the creepy plastic dough conditioner azodicarbonamide from its breads and upped its level of whole grains. If the chain weren't already America's healthiest chain, it certainly is now.

SURVIVAL STRATEGY

Trouble lurks in three areas at Subway: 1) hot subs, 2) foot-longs, 3) chips and soda. Stick to 6-inch cold subs made with ham, turkey, roast beef, or chicken. Load up on veggies, and be extra careful about your condiment choices.

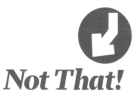
OTHER PASSES

Cold Cut Combo
(6")

360 CALORIES

12 G FAT (3.5 G saturated)

1,030 MG SODIUM

Chicken & Bacon Ranch Melt

570 CALORIES

28 G FAT
(10 G saturated, 0.5 G trans)

1,050 MG SODIUM

Sriracha Chicken Melt Salad
with Ranch Dressing

880 CALORIES

49 G FAT (10.5 G saturated)

1,470 MG SODIUM

The Big Philly Cheesesteak Toasted Sandwich and Veggie Delite Salad
with Ranch Dressing
(6")

770 CALORIES

41 G FAT
(12.5 G saturated)

1,760 MG SODIUM

★
Subway does a lot of things better than other sandwich shops, but ranch dressing ain't one of 'em. The salad dressing alone accounts for more than 30 percent of this meal's calories.

CONDIMENT CATASTROPHE

All Sandwiches

Subway's numbers are good, but the calorie counts don't include condiments. Mayo and ranch will each cost you 110 calories and up to 12 grams of fat. Stick to veggies, mustard, and light mayonnaise.

12
The number of 6-inch subs with fewer than 350 calories

STEALTH HEALTH

Ordering 9-Grain Wheat or Honey Oat bread instead of a white roll will increase your fiber load by four or five times, respectively. Fiber keeps you fuller longer; an *American Journal of Clinical Nutrition* study found that eating more fiber-packed whole grains resulted in less belly fat compared with a diet high in refined grains.

T.G.I. FRIDAY'S

Eat This

Balsamic-Glazed Chicken Caesar Salad

500 CALORIES

31 G FAT (7 G saturated)

1,340 MG SODIUM

★

"Caesar" is usually a nutritional red flag, but the dressing here is a Caesar vinaigrette, a less creamy take on the classic. Other than the Low-Fat Balsamic Vinaigrette, it's one of the only Friday's dressings with fewer than 210 calories, and the lightest of all Friday's entrée salads.

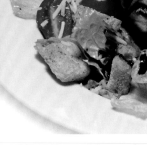

OTHER PICKS

Petite Sirloin with Crispy Shrimp

640 CALORIES

20 G FAT (9.5 G saturated)

2,110 MG SODIUM

Sizzling Chicken and Shrimp

530 CALORIES

14 G FAT (3 G saturated)

1,680 MG SODIUM

Thai Pork Tacos

280 CALORIES

14 G FAT (3.5 G saturated)

700 MG SODIUM

GRADE

D

After much analysis, we've finally figured out the real acronym here: Tremendous-Gut-Inducing Friday's. While Friday's has reintroduced our favorite part of the menu, the small portions option (the Taste & Share menu), it still turns too many healthy-sounding dishes into nutritional nuclear attacks. How does Pan-Seared Flounder break the 1,100-calorie mark? That's more than two Big Macs! But if you're a steak lover who can get along with a healthy side dish, you actually have plenty of options.

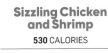

SURVIVAL STRATEGY

Danger is waiting in every crack and corner of Friday's menu. Your best bets? The grilled salmon, or perhaps a Black Angus steak (either the Petite Sirloin or the FlatIron).

OTHER PASSES

Jack Daniel's Black Angus Rib-Eye & Grilled Shrimp Scampi

1,150 CALORIES

42 G FAT (15 G saturated)

2,490 MG SODIUM

Friday's Shrimp

730 CALORIES

48 G FAT (15 G saturated)

2,870 MG SODIUM

Tuscan Spinach Dip

1,110 CALORIES

71 G FAT (15 G saturated)

1,650 MG SODIUM

★

What's the difference between one chicken salad and another? Primarily the dressing: The Avocado Vinaigrette delivers nearly 25 percent of the Yucatan's calories.

Not That!

Chipotle Yucatan Chicken Salad

840 CALORIES

60 G FAT (21 G saturated)

1,560 MG SODIUM

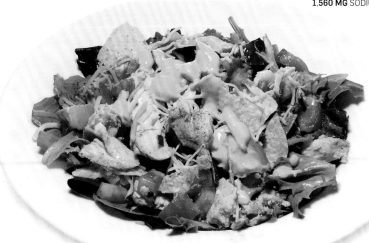

STEAK STACK-UP

Petite Sirloin	10 oz Sirloin	Rib-Eye
370 CALORIES	590 CALORIES	560 CALORIES
23 G FAT	44 G FAT	32 G FAT
Flat Iron	Jack Daniel's Rib-Eye	Jack Daniel's Sirloin
380 CALORIES	690 CALORIES	720 CALORIES
27 G FAT	22 G FAT	34 G FAT

ALL THIS OR THAT!

2,070 calories

Rib-Eye
Grilled Lobster Tail
Sweet Potato Fries
Triple Berry Smoothie
Tomato Mozzarella Salad
and Oreo Madness

or

Blue Cheese
Stacked Burger

UNO PIZZERIA & GRILL

Eat This

Margherita Flatbread Artisan Crust Pizza

(½ pie)

445 CALORIES

14.5 G FAT (7.5 G saturated)

750 MG SODIUM

★

The only way to get your pizza fix at Uno without ingesting 1,000 or more calories in one sitting is to eat half of a thin-crust pizza. The Margherita pie is the lightest option.

OTHER PICKS

Roasted Eggplant, Spinach & Feta
Traditional Flatbread
(½ pie)

440 CALORIES

16 G FAT (5.5 G saturated)

815 MG SODIUM

Baked Spinoccoli Chicken

360 CALORIES

14 G FAT (7 G saturated)

1,440 MG SODIUM

Red Bliss Mashed Potatoes

270 CALORIES

14 G FAT (3.5 G saturated)

650 MG SODIUM

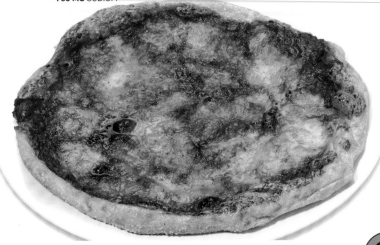

GRADE

D+

Uno strikes a curious (if not altogether healthy) balance between oversize sandwiches and burgers, lean grilled steaks and fish entrées, and one of the world's most calorie-dense foods, deep-dish pizza, which Uno's invented. It may pride itself on its nutrition transparency, but the only thing that's truly transparent is that there are far too many dishes here that pack 1,000 calories or more.

SURVIVAL STRATEGY

Stick with flatbread instead of deep-dish pizzas—this one move could save you close to 1,000 calories at a sitting. Beyond that, turn to the steak and seafood parts of the menu, or else Uno is going to give you an unhealthy dose.

OTHER PASSES

Wild Mushroom & White Cheddar
Traditional Flatbread
(½ pie)

640 CALORIES

39.5 G FAT (13.5 G saturated)

1,120 MG SODIUM

Chicken Milanese

850 CALORIES

56 G FAT (12 G saturated)

2,370 MG SODIUM

Mediterranean Farro Salad
with Honey Lime Dressing

520 CALORIES

39 G FAT (9 G saturated)

990 MG SODIUM

★

An average "individual" pizza at Uno houses an astonishing 1,800 calories. The thick, oily crust is obviously the culprit, but we're still baffled as to how the chain manages to fit that much fat into a small circle of dough. It's impressive— in the worst possible way.

Not That!

Prima Pepperoni Individual Deep Dish Pizza
with Traditional Crust

1,750 CALORIES

121 G FAT (33 G saturated)

3,010 MG SODIUM

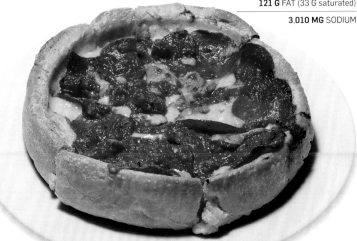

HEALTH-FOOD FRAUD

Farmer's Market Individual Pizza
with Nine Grain Crust

1,490 CALORIES

91 G FAT (25 G saturated)

1,950 MG SODIUM

This is the lightest individual pizza on Uno's menu, which is like being the least-wealthy Kardashian sister. The Nine Grain dough has nearly the same amounts of calories and fat as the Traditional deep dish crust. Stay away.

ATTACK OF THE APPETIZER

Pizza Skins

2,070 CALORIES

140 G FAT (48 G saturated, 1 G trans)

3,050 MG SODIUM

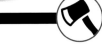

Uno's pizza crust is already the worst in the country, so we're not surprised that filling it with potatoes, bacon, cheese, and sour cream results in a catastrophe.

WENDY'S

Eat This

Chicken Nuggets
with Barbecue Sauce
(10)

450 CALORIES

30 G FAT
(7 G saturated)

870 MG SODIUM

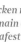

Chicken nuggets remain one of the safest options at the drive-thru. You get a higher protein-to-bread ratio compared with a sandwich, and you avoid the need for high-calorie toppings. This is the largest order of nuggets Wendy's offers, and it still has fewer calories than the majority of sandwiches on the menu.

QUALITY NATURAL-CUT FRIES WITH SEA SALT IS OUR RECIPE

OTHER PICKS

Double Stack

460 CALORIES

25 G FAT
(12 G saturated, 1.5 G trans)

1,280 MG SODIUM

Ultimate Chicken Grill

370 CALORIES

7 G FAT (1.5 G saturated)

880 MG SODIUM

Chocolate Frosty
(small)

340 CALORIES

9 G FAT (6 G saturated)

46 G SUGARS

GRADE

B

Scoring a decent meal at Wendy's is just about as easy as scoring a bad one, and that's a big compliment to pay a burger joint. Options such as chili and apple slices offer the side-order variety that's missing from less-evolved fast-food chains. Plus, Wendy's offers a handful of Jr. Burgers that stay below 400 calories. Where Wendy's errs is in the trans fats and the roster of double- and triple-patty burgers. The ongoing bacon obsession doesn't help either.

SURVIVAL STRATEGY

Choose a grilled chicken sandwich or a wrap—they don't exceed 320 calories. Or opt for a small burger and pair it with chili or a side salad.

OTHER PASSES

Dave's Hot 'N Juicy Quarter Pound Single

580 CALORIES

31 G FAT
(13 G saturated, 1.5 G trans)

1,220 MG SODIUM

Bacon and Cheese Baked Potato

540 CALORIES

23 G FAT
(11 G saturated, 0.5 G trans)

890 MG SODIUM

Chocolate Frosty Shake
(small)

540 CALORIES

13 G FAT
(8 G saturated, 1 G trans)

98 G SUGARS

★

Specialty sandwiches are usually tricked out with tons of unnecessary extras. In this case, bacon, cheese, ranch sauce, and a buttered bun combine to make a chicken sandwich with nearly as many calories as a Baconator. Order it with grilled chicken to bring it down to a much more reasonable 580 calories.

Not That!

Asiago Ranch Homestyle Chicken Club

670 CALORIES

32 G FAT
(9 G saturated)

1,610 MG SODIUM

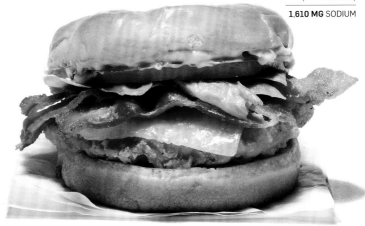

BACON BURGER DECODER

Junior Bacon Cheeseburger	Pretzel Bacon Cheeseburger	Baconator	Son of Baconator
370 CALORIES	**680** CALORIES	**940** CALORIES	**660** CALORIES
21 G FAT (8 G saturated, 0.5 G trans)	**36 G** FAT (15 G saturated, 1.5 G trans)	**57 G** FAT (23 G saturated, 2.5 G trans)	**36 G** FAT (14 G saturated, 1.5 G trans)

HIDDEN DANGER ⚠

Trans Fats

Most processed beef contains trace amounts of trans fats, but Wendy's beef is loaded with the stuff. Even a basic Quarter-Pound Cheeseburger has 1.5 grams, nearly as much as the American Heart Association recommends you eat in an entire day.

CHAPTER 2

AT THE
SUPERMARKET

UNPACK A LOAD OF GROCERIES THAT WILL
BOOST YOUR HEALTH—AND TRIM YOUR WAIST

EVERYBODY LOVES FOOD. Everybody loves shopping. And yet, oddly, nobody loves food shopping, despite the fact that we make an average of 1.6 trips a week to buy groceries.

Maybe that's why more and more of our grocery shopping is happening at places other than grocery stores. (Target, Walmart, Walgreens, CVS and Costco are the top non-supermarket stops for folks buying their foodstuffs.) And while a recent survey found that alternative grocery stores can be cheaper (up to 20 percent cheaper at a Walmart Supercenter or SuperTarget, compared to Giant or Safeway), the sprawl of groceries is making it harder than ever to find what we're looking for.

Regardless of whether you're ordering groceries online, slipping into the local bodega, or standing behind a line of people who are utterly confused by "self-checkout," a cheat sheet to guide you through the questionable claims and hyper bolic come-ons of modern food packaging is an invaluable resource. So dive into the following pages and prepare to be amazed. One seemingly insignificant swap—starting your day with Quaker Reduced-Sugar Oatmeal instead of Quaker Granola Oats & Honey—can save you 300 calories every morning. That's enough to save you more than 31 pounds this year alone!

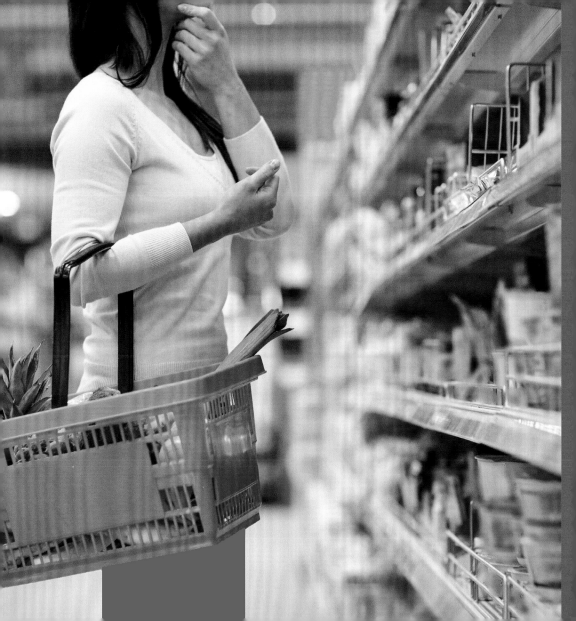

SWEET CEREALS

Eat This

Kellogg's Froot Loops
(1 cup)

110 CALORIES

1 G FAT
(0.5 G saturated)

135 MG SODIUM

3 G FIBER

12 G SUGARS

★

It's still not exactly a health food, but the denigrated Froot Loops has a similar fiber-to-sugar ratio to the health-conscious Kashi, and far fewer calories.

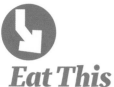

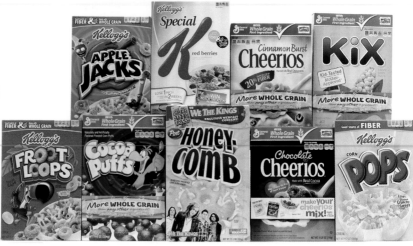

OTHER PICKS

KELLOGG'S
Apple Jacks
(1 cup)
110 CALORIES
1 G FAT (0.5 G saturated)
130 MG SODIUM
3 G FIBER / **12 G** SUGARS
The whole-grain corn flour adds just enough fiber to offset the sugar.

KELLOGG'S
Special K Red Berries
(1 cup)
110 CALORIES
0 G FAT
190 MG SODIUM
3 G FIBER / **9 G** SUGARS
This cereal employs wheat bran to up the fiber count and dried strawberries for sweetness.

GENERAL MILLS
Cinnamon Burst Cheerios
(1 cup)
120 CALORIES
2 G FAT (0 G saturated)
125 MG SODIUM
3 G FIBER / **9 G** SUGARS
All the cholesterol-busting power of oat bran with just a touch of sweetness.

GENERAL MILLS
Kix
(1 cup)
CALORIES **88**
1 G FAT (0 G saturated)
144 MG SODIUM
2.5 G FIBER / **2.5 G** SUGARS
Kix just might be the safest of all the sweetened kids' cereals. Try it with blueberries.

GENERAL MILLS
Cocoa Puffs
(1 cup)
133 CALORIES
2 G FAT (0 G saturated)
200 MG SODIUM
2.5 G FIBER / **13.5 G** SUGARS
General Mills has slowly added more whole grains to all of its Big G cereals.

POST
Honeycomb
(1 cup)
87 CALORIES
0.5 G FAT (0 G saturated)
120 MG SODIUM
0.5 G FIBER / **7 G** SUGARS
We'd love more fiber, but at least Post keeps the sugar and calories down.

GENERAL MILLS
Chocolate Cheerios
(1 cup)
133 CALORIES
2 G FAT (0 G saturated)
200 MG SODIUM
2.5 G FIBER / **12 G** SUGARS
Two of the first five ingredients are whole grains.

KELLOGG'S
Corn Pops
(1 cup)
120 CALORIES
0 G FAT
105 MG SODIUM
3 G FIBER / **9 G** SUGARS
Following General Mills' lead, Kellogg's began bulking up its fiber profile in 2009.

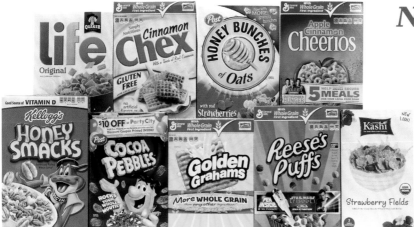

OTHER PASSES

Not That!

Kashi Strawberry Fields

(1 cup)

200 CALORIES

0 G FAT

190 MG SODIUM

3 G FIBER

11 G SUGARS

★

This is one of Kashi's biggest flops. Strawberry Fields features white rice instead of the 7 Whole Grain blend found in many of its cereals.

QUAKER
Life
(1 cup)
160 CALORIES
2 G FAT (0 G saturated)
213 MG SODIUM
2.5 G FIBER / **8 G** SUGARS
Life isn't the worst cereal on the shelf, but it does pack in more than three times as much sugar as fiber.

GENERAL MILLS
Cinnamon Chex
(1 cup)
160 CALORIES
3 G FAT (0 G saturated)
240 MG SODIUM
1 G FIBER / **11 G** SUGARS
This cereal delivers more than 130 calories of pure carbohydrates.

POST
Honey Bunches of Oats
with Real Strawberries
(1 cup)
160 CALORIES
2 G FAT (0 G saturated)
167 MG SODIUM
3 G FIBER / **11 G** SUGARS
Heavy on the carbs.

GENERAL MILLS
Apple Cinnamon Cheerios
(1 cup)
160 CALORIES
2 G FAT (0 G saturated)
153 MG SODIUM
2.5 G FIBER / **13 G** SUGARS
Worse than most junk cereal.

KELLOGG'S
Honey Smacks
(1 cup)
133 CALORIES
0.5 G FAT (0 G saturated)
53 MG SODIUM
1.5 G FIBER / **20 G** SUGARS
This is among the most sugar-loaded boxes in the cereal aisle.

POST
Cocoa Pebbles
(1 cup)
160 CALORIES
1 G FAT (1 G saturated)
227 MG SODIUM
0 G FIBER / **13 G** SUGARS
Not just devoid of fiber, but also soaked with hydrogenated oils.

GENERAL MILLS
Golden Grahams
(1 cup)
160 CALORIES
1 G FAT (0 G saturated)
320 MG SODIUM
2.5 G FIBER / **13.5 G** SUGARS
Loaded with sugar, lacking fiber, and saturated with sodium.

GENERAL MILLS
Reese's Puffs
(1 cup)
213 CALORIES
4 G FAT (0.5 G saturated)
213 MG SODIUM
1 G FIBER / **13.5 G** SUGARS
Oxford researchers rated this the unhealthiest cereal in the supermarket.

WHOLESOME CEREALS

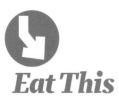

Eat This

Kellogg's Raisin Bran Cinnamon Almond

(1 cup)

CALORIES **160**	
1 G FAT (0 G saturated)	
176 MG SODIUM	
4 G FIBER	
14 G SUGARS	

★

Cinnamon is a worthwhile addition to any cereal. Studies show that it helps your body manage blood sugar. Most of the sugars here come from the coating on the raisins. Pick some out if you want to reduce your intake.

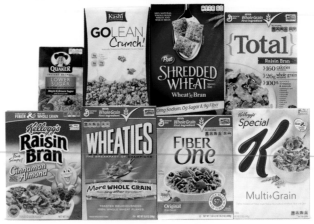

OTHER PICKS

QUAKER
Instant Oatmeal Lower Sugar Maple & Brown Sugar
(1 packet)
CALORIES **120**
2 G FAT (0 G saturated)
290 MG SODIUM
3 G FIBER / **4 G** SUGARS
It has a third of the sugar, but the same great taste. Promise.

KASHI
GoLean Crunch!
(1 cup)
CALORIES **250**
4 G FAT (0 G saturated)
133 MG SODIUM
10 G FIBER / **17 G** SUGARS
Ten grams of fiber goes a long way toward making up for the higher than ideal sugar content.

GENERAL MILLS
Wheaties
(1 cup)
CALORIES **133**
1 G FAT (0 G saturated)
253 MG SODIUM
4 G FIBER / **5 G** SUGARS
Being made with whole grains should be the minimum requirement for a cereal to land on your breakfast table. Anything less should be relegated to dessert.

POST
Shredded Wheat Spoon Size Wheat 'n Bran
(1 cup)
CALORIES **160**
1 G FAT (0 G saturated)
0 MG SODIUM
7 G FIBER / **0 G** SUGARS
Made with just whole-grain wheat and wheat bran— a pure base crying out for fresh blueberries or bananas.

GENERAL MILLS
Fiber One
(1 cup)
CALORIES **120**
2 G FAT (0 G saturated)
220 MG SODIUM
28 G FIBER / **0 G** SUGARS
Sprinkle over Greek yogurt instead of granola for a fiber- and protein-filled start to the day.

GENERAL MILLS
Total Raisin Bran
(1 cup)
CALORIES **160**
1 G FAT (0 G saturated)
180 MG SODIUM
5 G FIBER / **17 G** SUGARS
Among the many nutrients added to each serving in this box are an entire day's worth of calcium and vitamin E.

KELLOG'S
Special K Multi-Grain
(1 cup)
CALORIES **110**
0 G FAT (0 G saturated)
190 MG SODIUM
3 G FIBER / **6 G** SUGARS
The sugar count could be a little lower, but at least it has the fiber to back it up.

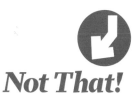

Not That!

Kellogg's Cracklin' Oat Bran
(1 cup)

267 CALORIES
9 G FAT (4 G saturated)
180 MG SODIUM
8 G FIBER
19 G SUGARS

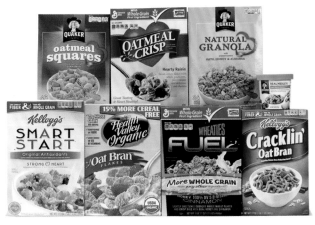

Nearly 20 grams of sugar alone make this cereal less than wholesome, but Cracklin' Oat Bran also comes with a massive glut of palm oil that loads this box with fat.

OTHER PASSES

QUAKER
Cinnamon Oatmeal Squares
(1 cup)
210 CALORIES
2.5 G FAT (0.5 G saturated)
190 MG SODIUM
5 G FIBER / 9 G SUGARS
Overloaded with sugar and cheap refined carbs like maltodextrin.

GENERAL MILLS
Oatmeal Crisp Hearty Raisin
(1 cup)
230 CALORIES
2.5 G FAT (0.5 G saturated)
120 MG SODIUM
5 G FIBER / 17 G SUGARS
Each bowl before adding milk has just 10 calories fewer than a McDonald's hamburger.

QUAKER
Natural Granola Oats & Honey
(1 cup)
420 CALORIES
10 G FAT (1 G saturated)
60 MG SODIUM
10 G FIBER / 26 G SUGARS
Rumors of granola's healthfulness have been vastly overstated. You'd be wise to keep it far away from your breakfast bowl.

QUAKER
Real Medleys Apple Walnut Oatmeal
(1 container)
290 CALORIES
8 G FAT (1 G saturated)
270 MG SODIUM
5 G FIBER / 22 G SUGARS
A full 30 percent of these calories come from sugar.

KELLOGG'S
Smart Start Strong Heart Original Antioxidants
(1 cup)
190 CALORIES
1 G FAT (0 G saturated)
210 MG SODIUM
3 G FIBER / 14 G SUGARS
What's so smart about a high-sugar, low-fiber cereal? We still don't know.

HEALTH VALLEY
Organic Oat Bran Flakes
(1 cup)
190 CALORIES
1.5 G FAT (0.5 G saturated)
190 MG SODIUM
4 G FIBER / 11 G SUGARS
Sugar outnumbers fiber nearly three to one.

GENERAL MILLS
Wheaties Fuel
(1 cup)
253 CALORIES
4 G FAT (0 G saturated)
187 MG SODIUM
10.5 G FIBER / 18.5 G SUGARS
Confusing this box with regular Wheaties will cost you nearly double the calories and nearly four times the sugar.

BREAKFAST BREADS

Eat This

Thomas' Light Multi-Grain English Muffins

(1 muffin, 57 g)

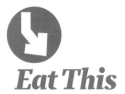

100 CALORIES

1 G FAT (0 G saturated)

180 MG SODIUM

26 G CARBOHYDRATES

8 G FIBER

★

Outside of green vegetables, you'll find very few foods that pack 8 grams of fiber into 100 calories. That makes this an unbeatable foundation for breakfast sandwiches.

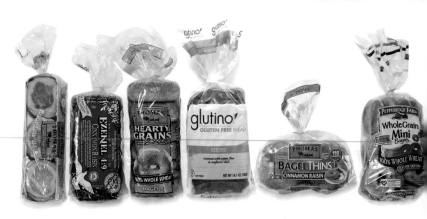

OTHER PICKS

FOOD FOR LIFE
Ezekiel 4:9 Sprouted 100% Whole Grain Cinnamon Raisin Bread
(1 slice, 34 g)
80 CALORIES
0 G FAT
65 MG SODIUM
18 G CARBOHYDRATES / **2 G** FIBER
Barley, millet, and spelt help boost fiber.

THOMAS'
Hearty Grains 100% Whole Wheat Bagels
(1 bagel, 95 g)
240 CALORIES
2 G FAT (0.5 G saturated)
400 MG SODIUM
49 G CARBOHYDRATES / **7 G** FIBER
One of the best bagels we've seen. Tons of fiber, plus 10 grams of protein in each serving.

GLUTINO
Seeded Bread
(1 slice, 29 g)
80 CALORIES
4.5 G FAT (0 G saturated)
120 MG SODIUM
10 G CARBOHYDRATES / **1 G** FIBER
Sunflower, flax, and poppy seeds give this bread a decent hit of healthy fats for hardly any calories.

THOMAS'
Bagel Thins Cinnamon Raisin
(1 bagel, 46 g)
110 CALORIES
1 G FAT (0 G saturated)
160 MG SODIUM
25 G CARBOHYDRATES / **5 G** FIBER
Switching to these is the best way to wean yourself off bagels. Try a swipe of peanut butter instead of cream cheese for a near-perfect snack.

PEPPERIDGE FARM
Whole Grain Mini Bagels 100% Whole Wheat
(1 bagel, 40 g)
100 CALORIES
0.5 G FAT (0 G saturated)
120 MG SODIUM
20 G CARBOHYDRATES / **3 G** FIBER
The perfect base for a ham and egg breakfast sandwich.

Not That!

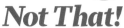

Sara Lee Original Made with Whole Grain English Muffins
(1 muffin, 66 g)

140 CALORIES

1 G FAT (0 G saturated)

210 MG SODIUM

27 G CARBOHYDRATES

2 G FIBER

★

The more fiber you work into your breakfast, the more likely you'll be to make it to lunch without experiencing hunger pangs. That means this muffin is a recipe for mid-morning cravings.

OTHER PASSES

THOMAS'
Plain Mini Bagels
(1 bagel, 43 g)
120 CALORIES
1 G FAT (0 G saturated)
210 MG SODIUM
24 G CARBOHYDRATES / **<1 G** FIBER
Once your palate is accustomed to whole grains, flavorless, nutritionless lumps of refined carbs like this will taste boring.

PEPPERIDGE FARM
Cinnamon Raisin Bagels
(1 bagel, 99 g)
270 CALORIES
1 G FAT (0 G saturated)
290 MG SODIUM
57 G CARBOHYDRATES / **3 G** FIBER
This bagel belongs on a dessert menu, not a breakfast table.

FOOD FOR LIFE
Gluten-Free Multi-Seed Rice Bread
(1 slice, 50 g)
120 CALORIES
1 G FAT (0 G saturated)
170 MG SODIUM
26 G CARBOHYDRATES / **1 G** FIBER
What this rice-and-tapioca concoction cuts in gluten it doesn't make up for in whole grains.

SARA LEE
Plain Deluxe Bagels
(1 bagel, 95 g)
260 CALORIES
1 G FAT (0 G saturated)
50 G CARBOHYDRATES / **2 G** FIBER
This is a wedge of refined carbohydrates, and as such, it will induce a blood sugar roller coaster that will wreak havoc on your energy reserves.

PEPPERIDGE FARM
Brown Sugar Cinnamon Swirl Bread
(1 slice, 38 g)
110 CALORIES
2 G FAT (0 G saturated)
140 MG SODIUM
21 G CARBOHYDRATES / **<1 G** FIBER
This bread contains five different forms of sugar.

HOT DOGS & SAUSAGE

 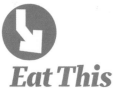

Eat This

Hebrew National 97% Fat Free Beef Franks

(1 frank, 45 g)

40 CALORIES

1 G FAT (0 G saturated)

520 MG SODIUM

6 G PROTEIN

★

There's no reason to fear hot dogs. A recent study from Kansas State University found that microwave-cooked hot dogs have fewer cancer-causing compounds than even rotisserie chicken. Stick with low-calorie brands and you're never far from a quick, healthy, and protein-packed meal.

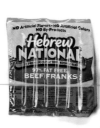 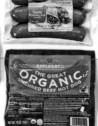 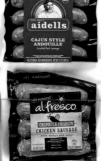 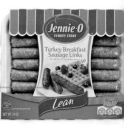

OTHER PICKS

JOHNSONVILLE
Chicken Sausage Chipotle Monterey Jack Cheese
(1 link, 85 g)
150 CALORIES
9 G FAT (2.5 G saturated)
650 MG SODIUM / **13 G** PROTEIN
We're glad to see the sausage behemoth get on board with the chicken variety.

AIDELLS
Cajun Style Andouille
(1 link, 85 g)
CALORIES **160**
11 G FAT (4 G saturated)
600 MG SODIUM / **15 G** PROTEIN
Remember Aidells. It's one of the most reliable purveyors in the deli fridge.

APPLEGATE FARMS
The Great Organic Uncured Beef Hot Dog
(1 frank, 56 g)
CALORIES **110**
8 G FAT (3 G saturated)
330 MG SODIUM / **7 G** PROTEIN
It looks and tastes like a classic ballpark frank, but without the dubious waste cuts or antibiotic-heavy meat.

AL FRESCO
Chipotle Chorizo Chicken Sausage
(1 link, 85 g)
CALORIES **140**
7 G FAT (2 G saturated)
420 MG SODIUM / **15 G** PROTEIN
Our love for Al Fresco runs deep. No company offers a wider variety of bold-flavored, low-calorie sausages.

JENNIE-O
Turkey Breakfast Sausage Links Lean
(2 links, 48 g)
65 CALORIES
4 G FAT (1 G saturated)
310 MG SODIUM / **8 G** PROTEIN
Cutting fat doesn't just drop the calorie count, it also makes more space for protein.

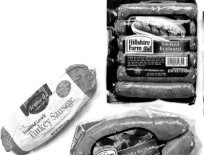
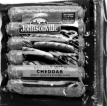

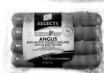

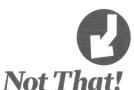

Not That!

Oscar Mayer Classic Light Beef Franks

(1 frank, 50 g)

---

60 CALORIES

3.5 G FAT (1.5 G saturated)

---

380 MG SODIUM

---

6 G PROTEIN

Hot dogs vary widely in terms of fat content, so it's important to flip the package and scan the ingredient statement. Case in point: You could eat three of the Hebrew National dogs on the opposite page and still not reach the fat load of these "light" franks.

OTHER PASSES

HILLSHIRE FARM
Smoked Bratwurst
(1 link, 66 g)
220 CALORIES
19 G FAT (7 G saturated)
520 MG SODIUM
7 G PROTEIN
More than 80 percent of
this brat's calories come from fat.

JOHNSONVILLE
Beddar with Cheddar
(1 link, 66 g)
210 CALORIES
18 G FAT (7 G saturated)
630 MG SODIUM
8 G PROTEIN
More calories, less protein,
and a hearty dose of MSG.

JENNIE-O
**Breakfast Lover's
Turkey Sausage**
(50 g)
90 CALORIES
5 G FAT (1.5 G saturated)
550 MG SODIUM
8 G PROTEIN
With "turkey" on the label
you should expect more from your
breakfast sausage.

HILLSHIRE FARM
Polska Kielbasa
(56 g)
180 CALORIES
16 G FAT (5 G saturated)
510 MG SODIUM
7 G PROTEIN
Both kielbasa and chorizo are spicy
ethnic sausages, but opt for Al Fresco
and you double up on protein while
cutting calories, fat, and sodium.

OSCAR MAYER
**Selects Angus Beef
Franks**
(1 frank, 50 g)
170 CALORIES
15 G FAT (6 G saturated)
370 MG SODIUM
6 G PROTEIN
Applegate provides a more protein-
packed dog for fewer calories and less
sodium and fat. This is an easy choice.

CONDIMENTS

Eat This

Kraft Mayo with Olive Oil

(1 Tbsp, 15 g)

35 CALORIES

3 G FAT (0 G saturated)

95 MG SODIUM

1 G SUGARS

★

A study published in the British Journal of Nutrition suggests that monounsaturated fatty acids might actually facilitate the breakdown of fat. The olive oil used in this jar has more than three times as many monounsaturates as the soybean oil used in regular mayo.

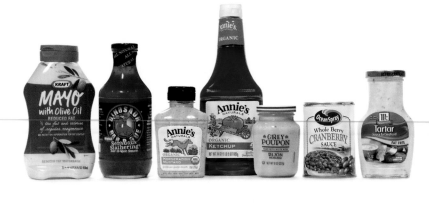

OTHER PICKS

DINOSAUR
Bar-B-Que Original Sensuous Slathering
(2 Tbsp, 31 g)

28 CALORIES
0 G FAT
177 MG SODIUM
6 G SUGARS

Two superfoods, tomatoes and yellow mustard, make up the base of this only slightly sweetened sauce. This is as good as barbecue gets.

ANNIE'S NATURALS
Organic Horseradish Mustard
(2 tsp, 10 g)

10 CALORIES
0 G FAT
120 MG SODIUM
0 G SUGARS

This bottle contains no ingredients that you wouldn't have in your kitchen.

ANNIE'S NATURALS
Organic Ketchup
(1 Tbsp, 17 g)

15 CALORIES
0 G FAT
130 MG SODIUM
4 G SUGARS

Go ahead and spring for organic. Research shows that organically raised tomatoes produce nearly twice as much cancer-fighting lycopene.

GREY POUPON
Classic Dijon
(1 tsp, 5 g)

0 CALORIES
0 G FAT
0 MG SODIUM
0 G SUGARS

Made mostly from mustard seeds, which are loaded with omega-3 fatty acids.

OCEAN SPRAY
Whole Berry Cranberry Sauce
(2 Tbsp, 35 g)

55 CALORIES
0 G FAT
5 MG SODIUM
11 G SUGARS

Not just for Thanksgiving anymore. Turn to cranberry sauce for a low-calorie, high-antioxidant sandwich companion.

MCCORMICK
Fat Free Tartar Sauce
(2 Tbsp, 32 g)

30 CALORIES
0 G FAT
250 MG SODIUM
5 G SUGARS

Although by no means a nutritious condiment, this light take on tartar does eliminate more than 100 calories per serving.

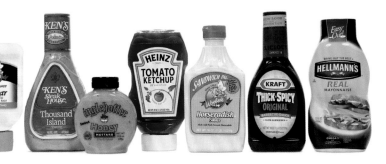

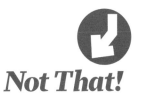

Not That!

Hellmann's Real Mayonnaise

(1 Tbsp, 13 g)

90 CALORIES

10 G FAT (1.5 G saturated)

90 MG SODIUM

0 G SUGARS

★

Aside from pure oil, mayonnaise is the most calorie-dense thing you can put on a sandwich. Every one of its 90 calories comes from low-quality fat. Choosing the olive oil version is one of the best swaps in the supermarket.

OTHER PASSES

WOEBER'S
Sweet & Tangy
Tartar Sauce
(2 Tbsp, 30 g)
140 CALORIES
14 G FAT (4 G saturated)
140 MG SODIUM
2 G SUGARS
Tartar sauce is little more than mayonnaise with relish stirred in. Go with a light version or switch to cocktail sauce.

KEN'S STEAK HOUSE
Thousand Island
Dressing
(2 Tbsp, 30 g)
140 CALORIES
13 G FAT (2 G saturated)
300 MG SODIUM
3 G SUGARS
Let there be no secrets about this sauce. Thousand Island is big on calories and low on nutrients.

INGLEHOFFER
Honey Mustard
(1 Tbsp, 15 g)
45 CALORIES
0 G FAT
105 MG SODIUM
6 G SUGARS
The first two ingredients are water and sugar, and corn syrup trails close behind.

HEINZ
Tomato Ketchup
(1 Tbsp, 17 g)
20 CALORIES
0 G FAT
160 MG SODIUM
4 G SUGARS
Switch to Annie's and you earn the benefits of organic tomatoes and eliminate the high-fructose corn syrup in Heinz's.

WOEBER'S
Sandwich Pal
Horseradish Sauce
(2 tsp, 10 g)
40 CALORIES
4 G FAT (1 G saturated)
60 MG SODIUM
0 G SUGARS
As used here, "sauce" means soybean oil and corn syrup.

KRAFT
Thick 'n Spicy Original
Barbecue Sauce
(2 Tbsp, 37 g)
70 CALORIES
0 G FAT
340 MG SODIUM
13 G SUGARS
High-fructose corn syrup is the primary ingredient, which is why this bottle delivers twice as much sugar as the Dinosaur sauce.

BREADS

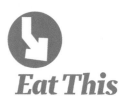

Eat This

Nature's Own Double Fiber Wheat Bread

(2 slices, 52 g)

200 CALORIES

3 G FAT (0 G saturated)

340 MG SODIUM

42 G CARBOHYDRATES

12 G FIBER

8 G PROTEIN

The high fiber content (40 percent of your daily intake from one sandwich) comes from the addition of inulin, a natural fiber made from chicory.

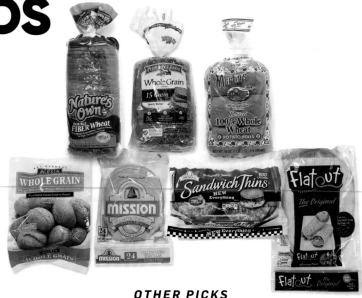

OTHER PICKS

PEPPERIDGE FARM
Whole Grain 15 Grain
(2 slices, 86 g)
200 CALORIES
4 G FAT (1 G saturated)
230 MG SODIUM
40 G CARBOHYDRATES / **8 G** FIBER
10 G PROTEIN
Five grams of protein and 4 grams of fiber per slice? Yes, please!

MARTIN'S
100% Whole Wheat Potato Rolls
(1 roll, 42.5 g)
100 CALORIES
1.5 G FAT (0 G saturated)
135 MG SODIUM
26 G CARBOHYDRATES
3 G FIBER / **7 G** PROTEIN
A perfect hot dog vessel. Whole wheat adds a potent fiber punch.

ALEXIA
Whole Grain Hearty Rolls
(1 roll, 43 g)
100 CALORIES
1 G FAT (0 G saturated)
200 MG SODIUM
18 G CARBOHYDRATES / **1 G** FIBER
4 G PROTEIN
Unless your roll has 100 calories or fewer, it has no place on the dinner table.

MISSION
Yellow Extra Thin Corn Tortillas
(2 tortillas, 37 g)
80 CALORIES
1 G FAT (0 G saturated)
7 MG SODIUM
16 G CARBOHYDRATES / **3 G** FIBER
2 G PROTEIN
Fiber-rich corn trumps flour every time in the tortilla battle.

ARNOLD
Sandwich Thins Flax & Fiber
(1 roll, 43 g)
100 CALORIES
1 G FAT (0 G saturated)
170 MG SODIUM
21 G CARBOHYDRATES / **5 G** FIBER
5 G PROTEIN
Protein and fiber supply more than a third of these calories.

FLATOUT
Original Flatbread
(1 piece, 57 g)
130 CALORIES
2 G FAT (0 G saturated)
310 MG SODIUM
24 G CARBOHYDRATES / **3 G** FIBER
7 G PROTEIN
Not one of Flatout's flatbreads has fewer than 3 grams of fiber.

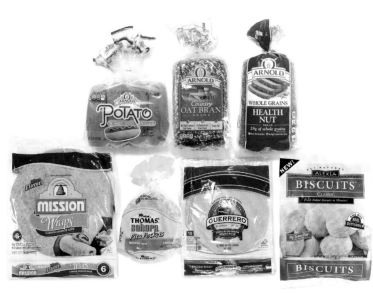

Arnold's Health Nut
(2 slices, 86 g)

240 CALORIES

4 G FAT (0 G saturated)

300 MG SODIUM

42 G CARBOHYDRATES

4 G FIBER

10 G PROTEIN

★

The second, third, and fourth ingredients are enriched flour, water, and sugar, leading to plenty of calories and only a modest amount of fiber.

OTHER PASSES

ARNOLD
Potato Hot Dog Rolls
(1 roll, 76 g)
140 CALORIES
1 G FAT (0 G saturated)
280 MG SODIUM
27 G CARBOHYDRATES / 1 G FIBER
5 G PROTEIN
Like most rolls, these are just pillows of empty carbs.

ARNOLD
Country Oat Bran
(2 slices, 86 g)
220 CALORIES
3 G FAT (0 G saturated)
300 MG SODIUM
40 G CARBOHYDRATES / 2 G FIBER
6 G PROTEIN
Oat bran comes fourth on the ingredients list after refined flour, water, and sugar.

MISSION
Garden Spinach Herb Wraps
(1 wrap, 70 g)
210 CALORIES
5 G FAT (2 G saturated)
440 MG SODIUM
36 G CARBOHYDRATES / 3 G FIBER
6 G PROTEIN
The only spinach here is "spinach powder," which accounts for less than 2 percent of each wrap.

THOMAS'
White Sahara Pita Pockets
(1 pita, 57 g)
160 CALORIES
1.5 G FAT (0 G saturated)
250 MG SODIUM
31 G CARBOHYDRATES / 1 G FIBER
6 G PROTEIN
Switch to a pita with fewer carbs and use the saved calories to double up on hummus!

GUERRERO
Soft Taco Homemade Flour Tortillas
(1 tortilla, 37 g)
130 CALORIES
5 G FAT (2.5 G saturated)
260 MG SODIUM
17 G CARBOHYDRATES / 1 G FIBER
3 G PROTEIN
It takes more than 15 ingredients to construct this tortured tortilla.

ALEXIA
Classic Biscuits
(1 biscuit, 50 g)
170 CALORIES
9 G FAT (5 G saturated)
450 MG SODIUM
20 G CARBOHYDRATES / <1 G FIBER
3 G PROTEIN
Traditional biscuits come sodden with fat, and Alexia's are no different.

GRAINS & NOODLES

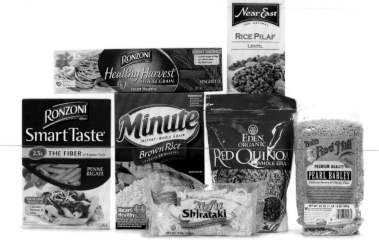

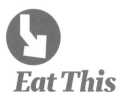

Eat This

Ronzoni Healthy Harvest Whole Grain Spaghetti

(2 oz, 56 g dry)

180 CALORIES

1.5 G FAT (0 G saturated)

39 G CARBOHYDRATES

5 G FIBER

★

Whole-grain pastas are loaded with fiber, and diets rich in fiber are shown to decrease your odds of developing both diabetes and heart disease. You want about 20 grams per day, and this spaghetti has 30 percent of that.

OTHER PICKS

Near East Rice Pilaf Mix Lentil
(¼ cup, 56 g dry)
180 CALORIES
0.5 G FAT (0 G saturated)
650 MG SODIUM
36 G CARBOHYDRATES / **8 G** FIBER
This box contains exactly seven ingredients, and you probably have every one of them in your pantry.

Ronzoni Smart Taste Penne Rigate
(56 g dry)
180 CALORIES
0.5 G FAT (0 G saturated)
39 G CARBOHYDRATES / **5 G** FIBER
Whole-wheat pasta can be a gritty departure from normal noodles, but Smart Taste combines fiber with the taste of white pasta.

Minute Brown Rice
(½ cup, 43 g dry)
150 CALORIES
1.5 G FAT (0 G saturated)
34 G CARBOHYDRATES / **2 G** FIBER
Eating healthy doesn't take more time; it just requires being more strategic in the supermarket.

House Foods Tofu Shirataki Spaghetti
(113 g)
20 CALORIES
1 G FAT (0 G saturated)
6 G CARBOHYDRATES / **4 G** FIBER
These traditional Asian noodles are made from tofu and yam flour. Don't be afraid—they have a neutral flavor that's perfect for dressing up.

Eden Organic Red Quinoa
(¼ cup, 45 g dry)
170 CALORIES
2 G FAT (0 G saturated)
32 G CARBOHYDRATES / **5 G** FIBER
Quinoa contains every amino acid your body needs from food. That's a claim rice can't make.

Bob's Red Mill Pearl Barley
(¼ cup, 50 g dry)
180 CALORIES
1 G FAT (0 G saturated)
39 G CARBOHYDRATES / **8 G** FIBER
Perfect for adding nutritional heft to everyday soups. Try using it as a replacement for noodles in minestrone.

114

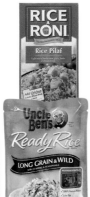

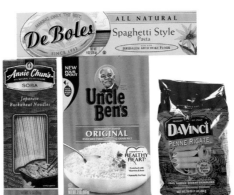

Not That!

DeBoles All Natural Artichoke Spaghetti Style Pasta

(56 g dry)

210 CALORIES

1 G FAT (0 G saturated)

43 G CARBOHYDRATES

1 G FIBER

★

This pasta doesn't have the fiber you're looking for. That means it won't keep you full as long, and you'll be pawing through the fridge for snacks in no time.

OTHER PASSES

RICE-A-RONI
Rice Pilaf
(⅓ cup, 70 g dry)
240 CALORIES
1 G FAT (0 G saturated)
970 MG SODIUM
52 G CARBOHYDRATES / **2 G** FIBER
The first ingredient is white rice, and shortly after it on the list are monosodium glutamate, hydrolyzed corn protein, and chicken fat.

RICESELECT
Orzo
(⅓ cup, 56 g dry)
210 CALORIES
2 G FAT (0 G saturated)
42 G CARBOHYDRATES / **2 G** FIBER
Essentially, these are little nibs of refined pasta. You're far better off using a legitimate whole grain.

UNCLE BEN'S
Ready Rice
Long Grain & Wild
(1 cup cooked)
200 CALORIES
0.5 G FAT (0 G saturated)
42 G CARBOHYDRATES / **1 G** FIBER
This grain performs poorly on the fiber scale, and no rice dish should ever have 650 milligrams of sodium in a serving.

ANNIE CHUN'S
Soba Noodles
(57 g dry)
200 CALORIES
1 G FAT (0 G saturated)
39 G CARBOHYDRATES / **3 G** FIBER
Japanese-style soba noodles tend to carry much more salt than Italian pasta noodles. A single serving of these packs 390 milligrams of sodium.

UNCLE BEN'S
Original Rice
(¼ cup, 47 g dry)
170 CALORIES
0 G FAT
37 G CARBOHYDRATES / **0 G** FIBER
Never eat rice, pasta, or other starchy sides unless they have fiber. Otherwise, they'll spike your blood sugar like a pile of candy.

DAVINCI
Penne Rigate
(56 g dry)
200 CALORIES
1 G FAT (0 G saturated)
41 G CARBOHYDRATES / **2 G** FIBER
Healthier noodles are available in all shapes and sizes, so there's never a reason to settle for one that's high in calories and low in fiber, like this one is.

SAUCES

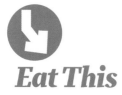

Eat This

La Choy Teriyaki Stir Fry Sauce & Marinade
(1 Tbsp)

10 CALORIES	
0 G FAT	
105 MG SODIUM	
1 G SUGARS	

 ★

The typical teriyaki sauce suffers from two blights: too much sodium and too much sugar. This one avoids both, which makes it by far the best teriyaki in the supermarket.

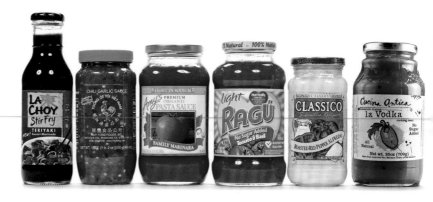

OTHER PICKS

HUY FONG
Chili Garlic Sauce
(1 tsp)
0 CALORIES
0 G FAT
115 MG SODIUM / **<1 G** SUGARS
Chili pepper is the primary ingredient, and it contains not a single gram of added sugar.

AMY'S
Light in Sodium Organic Family Marinara
(½ cup)
80 CALORIES
4.5 G FAT (0.5 G saturated)
290 MG SODIUM / **5 G** SUGARS
Stick with the low-sodium version. Amy's regular marinara has 290 milligrams more sodium.

RAGÚ
Light No Sugar Added Tomato & Basil
(½ cup)
50 CALORIES
0 G FAT (0 G saturated)
320 MG SODIUM / **6 G** SUGARS
Think Italians add sugar to their marinara? Of course not—added sugars mask the naturally sweet flavor of cooked tomatoes.

CLASSICO
Roasted Red Pepper Alfredo
(½ cup)
120 CALORIES
8 G FAT (5 G saturated)
560 MG SODIUM / **4 G** SUGARS
Smart move: The roasted red peppers in this jar displace a heavy load of fatty cream and cheese calories.

CUCINA ANTICA
La Vodka
(½ cup)
50 CALORIES
3.5 G FAT (2.5 G saturated)
220 MG SODIUM
2 G SUGARS
Cucina Antica gets the tomato-to-cream ratio right with this superlative sauce.

Not That!

La Choy Teriyaki Marinade and Sauce

(1 Tbsp)

40 CALORIES

0 G FAT

570 MG SODIUM

8 G SUGARS

★

If you end up with 2 tablespoons of this stuff on your plate, you'll be about to take in almost half your day's sodium and more sugar than you'd find in a scoop of Edy's Slow Churned Double Fudge Brownie Ice Cream.

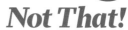

OTHER PASSES

BERTOLLI
Vodka Sauce
(½ cup)
150 CALORIES
9 G FAT (4.5 G saturated)
700 MG SODIUM / **8 G** SUGARS
It's not the vodka you have to worry about, it's the belt-buckling triad of cream, oil, and sugar.

NEWMAN'S OWN
Alfredo
(½ cup)
180 CALORIES
16 G FAT (9 G saturated)
820 MG SODIUM / **2 G** SUGARS
Worse Alfredo sauces exist, but that doesn't make Newman's a winner. One serving packs nearly half a day's sodium and saturated fat.

PREGO
Veggie Smart Smooth and Simple
(½ cup)
70 CALORIES
1.5 G FAT (0 G saturated)
410 MG SODIUM / **9 G** SUGARS
Nice try, Prego, but the vegetable juice concentrates in this jar do more harm than good. Rule of marinara: Keep it simple.

AMY'S ORGANIC
Tomato Basil
(½ cup)
110 CALORIES
6 G FAT (1 G saturated)
580 MG SODIUM / **6 G** SUGARS
We applaud Amy's use of organic tomatoes, but 110 calories is just far too much for a tomato-based pasta sauce.

MAGGI
Sweet Chili Sauce
(1 Tbsp)
35 CALORIES
0 G FAT
250 MG SODIUM / **8 G** SUGARS
The first two ingredients are sugar and water. That not only adds unnecessary calories, but also makes this sauce seem less spicy, meaning you'll need more to achieve the desired effect.

SOUPS

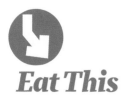

 Eat This

V8 Tomato Herb

(1 cup)

90 CALORIES

0 G FAT

480 MG SODIUM

19 G CARBOHYDRATES

3 G FIBER

3 G PROTEIN

★

Carrots and red peppers are among the primary ingredients in this carton. That's how each serving earns you nearly half of your daily vitamin A requirement.

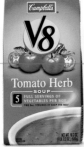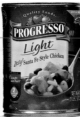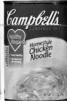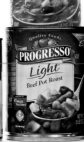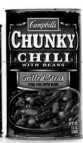

OTHER PICKS

PROGRESSO
Light Zesty! Santa Fe Style Chicken
(1 cup)
80 CALORIES
1 G FAT (0 G saturated)
460 MG SODIUM
10 G CARBOHYDRATES / **2 G** FIBER
5 G PROTEIN
The black beans in this soup bolster the fiber content, plus add a shot of brain-boosting antioxidants.

CAMPBELL'S
Healthy Request Condensed Homestyle Chicken Noodle
(1 cup prepared)
60 CALORIES
1.5 G FAT (0.5 G saturated)
410 MG SODIUM
10 G CARBOHYDRATES / **1 G** FIBER
3 G PROTEIN
Low cal, light sodium.

CAMPBELL'S
Home Style Light Southwestern-Style Vegetable
(1 cup)
60 CALORIES
0 G FAT (0 saturated)
650 MG SODIUM
13 G CARBOHYDRATES / **3 G** FIBER
2 G PROTEIN
One-third of the calories come from fiber.

PROGRESSO
Light Beef Pot Roast
(1 cup)
80 CALORIES
2 G FAT (1 G saturated)
470 MG SODIUM
10 G CARBOHYDRATES / **2 G** FIBER
7 G PROTEIN
There's a bounty of vegetation in this can, and it includes carrots, green beans, potatoes, tomatoes, celery, and peas.

CAMPBELL'S
Chunky Grilled Steak Chili with Beans
(1 cup)
200 CALORIES
3 G FAT (1 G saturated)
870 MG SODIUM
27 G CARBOHYDRATES / **7 G** FIBER
16 G PROTEIN
Campbell's Chunky Chili line is surprisingly lean—not one can tops 240 calories per serving.

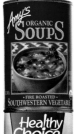
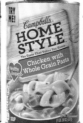
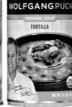
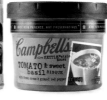
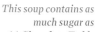

Not That!

Campbell's Slow Kettle Style Soup Tomato & Sweet Basil Bisque

(1 cup)

260 CALORIES	
14 G FAT	(8 G saturated)
750 MG SODIUM	
30 G CARBOHYDRATES	
3 G FIBER	
4 G PROTEIN	

★

This soup contains as much sugar as 66 Chocolate Teddy Graham cookies.

OTHER PASSES

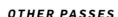

AMY'S
Organic Fire Roasted Southwestern Vegetable
(1 cup)
140 CALORIES
3 G FAT (0 G saturated)
680 MG SODIUM
21 G CARBOHYDRATES / **4 G** FIBER
4 G PROTEIN
We love all of the vegetables, but we don't love the calories.

STAGG
Classic Chili
with Beans
(1 cup)
330 CALORIES
17 G FAT (8 G saturated)
820 MG SODIUM
28 G CARBOHYDRATES / **5 G** FIBER
17 G PROTEIN
Stagg should find a new beef purveyor. The meat in one serving packs 40 percent of your daily saturated fat.

HEALTHY CHOICE
Beef Pot Roast
(1 cup)
100 CALORIES
1 G FAT (0 G saturated)
430 MG SODIUM
18 G CARBOHYDRATES / **3 G** FIBER
6 G PROTEIN
Switch to Progresso's version and save 20 calories per serving.

CAMPBELL'S
Homestyle Healthy Request Chicken
with Whole Grain Pasta
(1 cup)
100 CALORIES
2 G FAT (0.5 G saturated)
410 MG SODIUM
13 G CARBOHYDRATES / **1 G** FIBER
7 G PROTEIN
Where's the fiber?

WOLFGANG PUCK
Organic Signature Tortilla Soup
(1 cup)
140 CALORIES
3.5 G FAT (1 G saturated)
680 MG SODIUM
21 G CARBOHYDRATES / **6 G** FIBER
5 G PROTEIN
Organic, yes, but still loaded with excessive sugar and sodium.

BARS

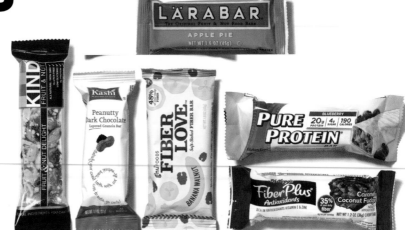

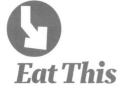

Eat This

KIND Fruit & Nut Delight
(1 bar, 40 g)

200 CALORIES

13 G FAT
(1.5 G saturated)

17 G CARBOHYDRATES

3 G FIBER

9 G SUGARS

6 G PROTEIN

★

Here's a great trick for evaluating a bar. Add the fiber and protein grams together. The total should be equal to or greater than the sugar grams. KIND's mix of real fruit, nuts, and not much else makes it worth an extra 10 calories.

OTHER PICKS

LÄRABAR
Apple Pie
(1 bar, 45 g)
190 CALORIES
10 G FAT (1 G saturated)
5 MG SODIUM
24 G CARBOHYDRATES / **5 G** FIBER
18 G SUGARS / **4 G** PROTEIN
Ordinarily 18 grams is too much sugar, but in Lärabar's case, every single gram comes directly from real fruit.

KASHI
Peanutty Dark Chocolate Layered Granola Bar
(1 bar, 32 g)
130 CALORIES
4.5 G FAT (1 G saturated)
20 G CARBOHYDRATES / **4 G** FIBER
7 G SUGARS / **4 G** PROTEIN
A fiber-and-protein-packed alternative to fix your candy bar cravings.

GNU FOODS
Flavor & Fiber Banana Walnut Bar
(1 bar, 36 g)
130 CALORIES
4 G FAT (3 G saturated)
26 G CARBOHYDRATES / **9 G** FIBER
7 G SUGARS / **2 G** PROTEIN
Gnu builds its fruit-and-nut bars on a base of fiber-rich grains.

PURE PROTEIN
Greek Yogurt Blueberry
(1 bar, 50 g)
190 CALORIES
4.5 G FAT (2.5 G saturated)
19 G CARBOHYDRATES / **2 G** FIBER
4 G SUGARS / **20 G** PROTEIN
This bar's ratio of protein to sugar is as good as you'll find anywhere in the supermarket.

KELLOGG'S
Fiber Plus Antioxidants Caramel Coconut Fudge
(1 bar, 45 g)
140 CALORIES
4 G FAT (0 G saturated)
30 G CARBOHYDRATES / **12 G** FIBER
8 G SUGARS / **4 G** PROTEIN
A hefty dose of fiber to quell your cravings.

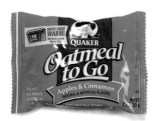

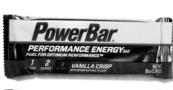

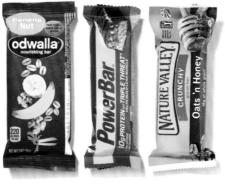

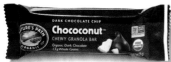

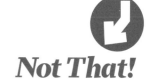

Not That!

Nature Valley Crunchy Oats 'n Honey
(2 bars, 42 g)

---

190 CALORIES

6 G FAT
(0.5 G saturated)

29 G CARBOHYDRATES

2 G FIBER

12 G SUGARS

4 G PROTEIN

★

This bar has twice as much sugar as it does fiber and protein combined. That makes it a great example of the sort of snack you want to avoid.

OTHER PASSES

QUAKER
Oatmeal to Go Apples
and Cinnamon
(1 bar, 60 g)
220 CALORIES
4 G FAT (1 G saturated)
200 MG SODIUM
44 G CARBOHYDRATES / **5 G** FIBER
22 G SUGARS / **4 G** PROTEIN
There's far more sugar, brown sugar, and high-fructose corn syrup than apple.

POWERBAR
Performance Energy Vanilla Crisp
(1 bar, 57 g)
240 CALORIES
3.5 G FAT (0.5 G saturated)
45 G CARBOHYDRATES / **1 G** FIBER
26 G SUGARS / **8 G** PROTEIN
Four kinds of sugar make this "performance" bar sweeter than a Kit Kat.

NATURE'S PATH
Organic Choconut
(1 bar, 35 g)
140 CALORIES
4.5 G FAT (1.5 G saturated)
24 G CARBOHYDRATES / **2 G** FIBER
11 G SUGARS / **2 G** PROTEIN
Sugar, in its various guises, appears five times in this ingredient statement.

ODWALLA
Banana Nut Bar
(1 bar, 56 g)
220 CALORIES
5 G FAT (0.5 G saturated)
39 G CARBOHYDRATES / **5 G** FIBER
17 G SUGARS / **4 G** PROTEIN
Don't be duped by "brown rice syrup," the first ingredient in this bar. It's a euphemism for sugar.

POWERBAR
Triple Threat Caramel Peanut Fusion
(1 bar, 45 g)
230 CALORIES
9 G FAT (4.5 G saturated)
31 G CARBOHYDRATES / **3 G** FIBER
15 G SUGARS / **10 G** PROTEIN
The main components of this "Power" bar are caramel and "chocolate coating."

CRACKERS

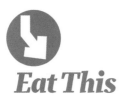

Eat This

Wheat Thins Fiber Selects Garden Vegetable

(15 crackers, 30 g)

120 CALORIES

4 G FAT
(0 G saturated)

240 MG SODIUM

21 G CARBOHYDRATES

5 G FIBER

★

The primary ingredient here is whole-wheat flour, which is precisely what you want. The extra fiber— a form of oat fiber that Nabisco adds to this Fiber Selects line—is just a bonus.

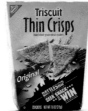

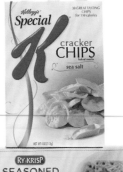

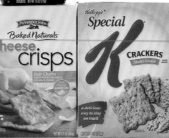

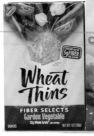

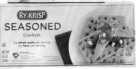

OTHER PICKS

NABISCO
Triscuit Thin Crisps Original
(15 crackers, 30 g)
130 CALORIES
4.5 G FAT (0.5 G saturated)
170 MG SODIUM
21 G CARBOHYDRATES / **3 G** FIBER
You can't beat the purity of this recipe: whole wheat, oil, and salt. Period.

KELLOGG'S
Special K Sea Salt Cracker Chips
(30 crackers, 30 g)
110 CALORIES
2.5 G FAT (0 G saturated)
230 MG SODIUM
23 G CARBOHYDRATES / **3 G** FIBER
Potato starch is used to bolster this cracker chip's fiber content.

PEPPERIDGE FARM
Baked Naturals Cheese Crisps Four Cheese
(20 pieces, 30 g)
140 CALORIES
6 G FAT (1 G saturated)
270 MG SODIUM
19 G CARBOHYDRATES / **1 G** FIBER
A touch of fiber and real cheese save this cracker.

SPECIAL K
Multi-Grain Crackers
(24 crackers, 30 g)
120 CALORIES
3 G FAT (0 G saturated)
220 MG SODIUM
23 G CARBOHYDRATES / **3 G** FIBER
This is as few calories as you can reasonably expect in a serving of whole-grain crackers.

RY-KRISP
Seasoned Crackers
(2 crackers, 14 g)
60 CALORIES
1 G FAT (0 G saturated)
90 MG SODIUM
11 G CARBOHYDRATES / **3 G** FIBER
Prevention of gallstones is among the many benefits of foods high in insoluble fiber.

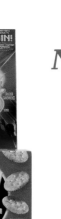

Ritz Roasted Vegetable
(10 crackers, 32 g)

160 CALORIES	
7 G FAT	
(2 G saturated)	
300 MG SODIUM	
20 G CARBOHYDRATES	
0 G FIBER	

★

As the name suggests, this box contains a handful of dehydrated vegetables. The problem is, the main ingredient is still refined flour, and it's bogged down with hydrogenated oils and high-fructose corn syrup.

OTHER PASSES

NABISCO
Wheat Thins Great Plains Multigrain Toasted Chips
(13 pieces, 28 g)
130 CALORIES
5 G FAT (1 G saturated)
230 MG SODIUM
19 G CARBOHYDRATES / **2 G** FIBER
Definitely plain, but not so great.

NABISCO
Ritz Bits Sandwiches Cheese
(13 pieces, 31 g)
160 CALORIES
9 G FAT (3 G saturated)
160 MG SODIUM
18 G CARBOHYDRATES / **0 G** FIBER
Soiled with sugar and partially hydrogenated cottonseed oil.

KEEBLER
Town House Flatbread Crisps Sea Salt & Olive Oil
(16 crackers, 30 g)
140 CALORIES
4 G FAT (0 G saturated)
280 MG SODIUM
22 G CARBOHYDRATES / **<1 G** FIBER
The 4 grams of fat here come from soybean oil.

NABISCO
Wheat Thins Original
(16 crackers, 31 g)
140 CALORIES
5 G FAT (1 G saturated)
230 MG SODIUM
22 G CARBOHYDRATES / **3 G** FIBER
Wheat Thins rely heavily on refined grains, which means less protein and fiber in each serving.

SUNSHINE
Cheez-It Original
(27 crackers, 30 g)
150 CALORIES
8 G FAT (2 G saturated)
230 MG SODIUM
17 G CARBOHYDRATES / **<1 G** FIBER
Cheez-Its' lack of fiber prevents these crackers from having a meaningful impact on hunger. If you're going to snack, do so smartly.

CHIPS

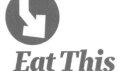

Eat This

Lay's Oven Baked Original Potato Crisps

(18 crisps, 1 oz)

120 CALORIES

2 G FAT
(0 G saturated)

135 MG SODIUM

Baked chips don't rely on oil to crisp up, which means they can get by with far less fat. If you eat just one 1-ounce bag a week, you'll shed more than 2 pounds this year by choosing Lay's Baked! instead of Ruffles Reduced Fat.

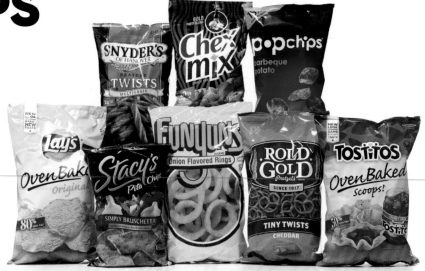

OTHER PICKS

SNYDER'S OF HANOVER
Braided Twists Multigrain
(8 twists, 30 g)
120 CALORIES
2 G FAT (0 G saturated)
160 MG SODIUM
The 3 grams of fiber in each serving make this a respectable snack.

CHEX MIX
Bold Party Blend
(½ cup, 29 g)
120 CALORIES
3.5 G FAT (0.5 G saturated)
200 MG SODIUM
The "bold" blend, surprisingly, is lower in sodium than some of the other Chex mixes.

POPCHIPS
Barbeque Potato
(20 chips, 1 oz)
120 CALORIES
4 G FAT (0 G saturated)
200 MG SODIUM
More crunch than a baked chip, yet less fat than a fried chip.

STACY'S
Pita Chips Simply Bruschetta
(9 chips, 1 oz)
130 CALORIES
5 G FAT (0.5 G saturated)
190 MG SODIUM
Delivers a respectable 3 grams of protein per serving.

Funyuns
(13 rings, 1 oz)
130 CALORIES
6 G FAT (1 G saturated)
280 MG SODIUM
Funyuns inflict surprisingly little damage by novelty snack standards.

ROLD GOLD
Tiny Twists Cheddar
(20 pretzels, 1 oz)
110 CALORIES
1 G FAT (0 G saturated)
490 MG SODIUM
We wish Rold Gold would take it easy with the salt, but you won't find a lower-calorie cheese snack in the snack aisle.

TOSTITOS
Oven Baked Scoops!
(16 chips, 1 oz)
120 CALORIES
3 G FAT (0.5 G saturated)
140 MG SODIUM
This is the healthiest salsa-shoveling device on the shelf.

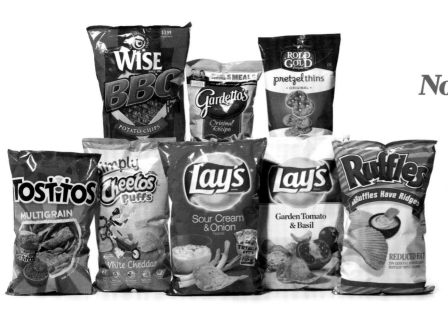

OTHER PASSES

WISE
BBQ Flavored Potato Chips
(15 chips, 1 oz)
150 CALORIES
10 G FAT (3 G saturated)
210 MG SODIUM
This bag contains a bunch of processing junk like monosodium glutamate and artificial colors.

GARDETTO'S
Original Recipe Snack Mix
(½ cup, 32 g)
150 CALORIES
6 G FAT
(1 G saturated, 1 G trans)
300 MG SODIUM
Just one cup of this mix gives you an entire day's worth of artery-clogging trans fats. Avoid at all costs.

ROLD GOLD
Pretzel Thins Original
(14 pretzels, 1 oz)
120 CALORIES
2 G FAT (0 G saturated)
470 MG SODIUM
More sodium than a large order of McDonald's fries.

TOSTITOS
Multigrain
(8 chips, 1 oz)
150 CALORIES
7 G FAT (1 G saturated)
110 MG SODIUM
The "multiple" grains in this bag consist almost entirely of corn.

SIMPLY
Cheetos Puffs White Cheddar
(32 pieces, 1 oz)
150 CALORIES
9 G FAT (1.5 G saturated)
290 MG SODIUM
Being "puffed" doesn't cut down on fat, calories, or sodium.

LAY'S
Sour Cream and Onion Chips
(17 chips, 28 g)
160 CALORIES
10 G FAT (1.5 G saturated)
160 MG SODIUM
Packed with inflammatory omega-6 fatty acids from sunflower and corn oils.

LAY'S
Garden Tomato & Basil Flavored Potato Chips
(15 chips, 1 oz)
160 CALORIES
10 G FAT (1.5 G saturated)
170 MG SODIUM
"Garden" here means little more than tomato powder.

DIPS & SPREADS

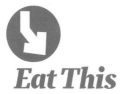

Eat This

Newman's Own Mild Salsa

(2 Tbsp, 32 g)

10 CALORIES

0 G FAT

65 MG SODIUM

★

We balked when Ronald Reagan tried to turn ketchup into a vegetable, but if someone did the same for salsa, a legitimate nutritional superpower, we'd throw our support behind it.

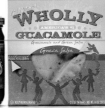
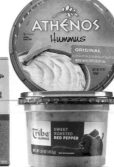

OTHER PICKS

WHOLLY GUACAMOLE
Guaca Salsa
(2 Tbsp, 30 g)

35 CALORIES
3 G FAT (0 G saturated)
110 MG SODIUM

Avocados are the first of only seven ingredients, all of which you likely keep stocked in your kitchen.

ATHENOS
Hummus Original
(2 Tbsp, 27 g)

50 CALORIES
3 G FAT (0 G saturated)
160 MG SODIUM

Made with real olive oil, which lends an authentic flavor and more heart-healthy fats.

TRIBE
Hummus Sweet Roasted Red Peppers
(2 Tbsp, 28 g)

50 CALORIES
3 G FAT (0 G saturated)
125 MG SODIUM

Based on chickpeas and tahini, hummus makes for an incredible vegetable dip and sandwich spread.

DESERT PEPPER
Black Bean Dip Spicy
(2 Tbsp, 31 g)

25 CALORIES
0 G FAT
240 MG SODIUM

This jar contains a trio of nutritional A-listers: black beans, tomatoes, and green bell peppers.

SABRA
Caponata
(2 Tbsp, 28 g)

30 CALORIES
2.5 G FAT (0 G saturated)
140 MG SODIUM

Built from potent Mediterranean produce like eggplants and tomatoes, this dip is perfect for dressing up chicken or fish or spreading on a pita.

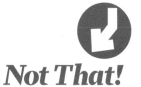

Not That!

Herdez Salsa Casera Mild

(2 Tbsp, 31 g)

5 CALORIES

0 G FAT

240 MG SODIUM

★

Be on the watch for elevated sodium in salsa. Combined with some salty chips, you could easily approach half a day's sodium intake.

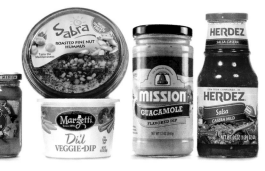

OTHER PASSES

SABRA
Roasted Pine Nut Hummus
(2 Tbsp, 28 g)
80 CALORIES
6 G FAT (1 G saturated)
130 MG SODIUM
Instead of the traditional olive oil, Sabra's ingredient statement lists "soybean and/or canola oil."

SABRA
Babaganoush
(2 Tbsp, 28 g)
70 CALORIES
7 G FAT (1 G saturated)
180 MG SODIUM
Babaganoush traditionally gets its creaminess from tahini and roasted eggplant, but Sabra cheats by loading its version with mayonnaise.

TOSTITOS
Zesty Bean & Cheese Dip Medium
(2 Tbsp, 33 g)
45 CALORIES
2 G FAT (0.5 G saturated)
230 MG SODIUM
Contains more than 25 ingredients, including corn oil, monosodium glutamate, DATEM, and two artificial shades of yellow.

MARZETTI
Dill Veggie Dip
(2 Tbsp, 30 g)
110 CALORIES
12 G FAT (3 G saturated)
170 MG SODIUM
This dip is mostly sour cream. The veggies you see on the package? You'll have to supply those yourself.

MISSION
Guacamole Flavored Dip
(2 Tbsp, 32 g)
30 CALORIES
2 G FAT (1 G saturated)
130 MG SODIUM
"Flavored" is the key word. This imposter is made mostly of water, oil, and cornstarch. Oh, and less than 2 percent real avocado.

DRESSINGS

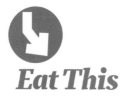

Eat This

Bolthouse Farms Chunky Blue Cheese Yogurt Dressing

(2 Tbsp, 30 g)

---

35 CALORIES

2.5 G FAT
(1 G saturated)

---

135 MG SODIUM

★

Bolthouse Farms casts yogurt as the star in classic flavors such as ranch, honey mustard, Thousand Island, and blue cheese, allowing you to swap out vegetable oil for worthwhile hits of calcium and probiotic bacteria.

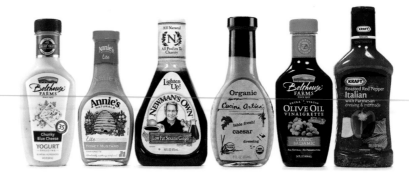

OTHER PICKS

ANNIE'S NATURALS
Lite Honey Mustard Vinaigrette
(2 Tbsp, 31 g)
40 CALORIES
3 G FAT (0 G saturated)
125 MG SODIUM
After water, mustard is the main ingredient, a surprising rarity among honey mustard dressings.

NEWMAN'S OWN
Lite Low Fat Sesame Ginger
(2 Tbsp, 30 g)
35 CALORIES
1.5 G FAT (0 G saturated)
330 MG SODIUM
Relegates oil to a supporting role so that vinegar, soy sauce, and ginger can drive the flavor.

CUCINA ANTICA
Organic Caesar Dressing
(2 Tbsp, 30 g)
80 CALORIES
8 G FAT (1 G saturated)
190 MG SODIUM
A touch of Romano cheese, not an excess of cheap oil, supplies rich flavor for a fraction of the fat.

BOLTHOUSE FARMS
Classic Balsamic Olive Oil Vinaigrette
(2 Tbsp, 30 g)
30 CALORIES
0 G FAT
150 MG SODIUM
The lightest vinaigrette we've ever come across. Just another reason why Bolthouse is one of our favorite producers.

KRAFT
Roasted Red Pepper Italian with Parmesan
(2 Tbsp, 32 g)
40 CALORIES
2 G FAT (0 G saturated)
349 MG SODIUM
The bulk of this bottle is filled with vinegar and tomato puree, a huge improvement over the typical oil-based formula.

Not That!

Kraft Roka Blue Cheese

(2 Tbsp, 29 g)

120 CALORIES

13 G FAT
(2 G saturated)

290 MG SODIUM

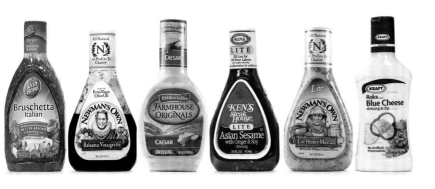

★

Virtually every calorie in this bottle comes from soybean oil, which is a common theme in the dressing aisle. Consider them wasted calories; soybean oil doesn't have the same heart-healthy cachet as olive or canola oil.

OTHER PASSES

WISH-BONE
Bruschetta Italian
(2 Tbsp, 30 ml)
60 CALORIES
5 G FAT (1 G saturated)
340 MG SODIUM
The front label boasts about olive oil, but the ingredient statement reveals that it accounts for less than 2 percent of the recipe.

NEWMAN'S OWN
Balsamic Vinaigrette
(2 Tbsp, 30 g)
90 CALORIES
9 G FAT (1 G saturated)
290 MG SODIUM
Save cash and calories by making your own vinaigrette at home: Mix two parts olive oil with one part balsamic, plus salt and pepper.

HIDDEN VALLEY
Farmhouse Originals Caesar
(2 Tbsp, 30 ml)
120 CALORIES
11 G FAT (1.5 G saturated)
220 MG SODIUM
Hidden in this valley, you'll find MSG and propylene glycol, an ingredient also found in antifreeze. We don't remember those from any farm.

KEN'S STEAK HOUSE
Lite Asian Sesame
with Ginger and Soy
(2 Tbsp, 30 g)
70 CALORIES
4 G FAT (0.5 G saturated)
390 MG SODIUM
After water, sugar is the first ingredient in this bottle, which is why each serving packs 7 grams of the sweet stuff.

NEWMAN'S OWN
Lite Honey Mustard Dressing
(2 Tbsp, 30 g)
70 CALORIES
4 G FAT (0.5 G saturated)
280 MG SODIUM
Keep in mind that "light" is a relative term.

COOKIES

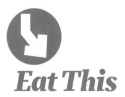

Eat This

Newman's Own Newman-Os Chocolate Crème Filled Chocolate Cookies
(2 cookies, 27 g)

120 CALORIES

5 G FAT (1.5 G saturated)

85 MG SODIUM

10 G SUGARS

Compared with Oreo, Newman takes a moderate approach to oil and sugar.

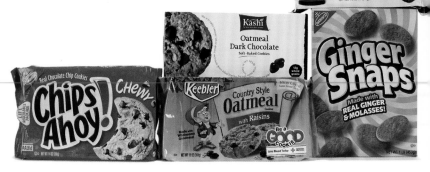

OTHER PICKS

CHIPS AHOY!
Chewy
(2 cookies, 31 g)
140 CALORIES
6 G FAT (3 G saturated)
95 MG SODIUM
12 G SUGARS
This cookie is the best of the Chips Ahoy! line, and a surprisingly low-calorie treat for how indulgent it seems.

KASHI
Oatmeal Dark Chocolate Soft-Baked Cookies
(1 cookie, 30 g)
130 CALORIES
5 G FAT (1.5 G saturated)
65 MG SODIUM
8 G SUGARS
Thanks to oats, rye, barley, and buckwheat, Kashi's cookie has more fiber (4 grams) than a standard slice of whole-wheat bread.

KEEBLER
Country Style Oatmeal Cookies with Raisins
(2 cookies, 28 g)
140 CALORIES
6 G FAT (2 G saturated)
100 MG SODIUM
8 G SUGARS
Raisins will always trump chocolate chips or candy pieces as a cookie mix-in.

NABISCO
Ginger Snaps
(4 cookies, 28 g)
120 CALORIES
2.5 G FAT (0 G saturated)
190 MG SODIUM
11 G SUGARS
Eating a handful of small cookies instead of one regular cookie is a good strategy—it can help you feel like you're eating more than you actually are.

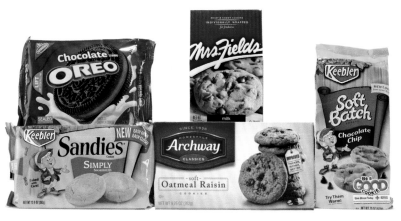

Not That!

Nabisco Chocolate Crème Oreo

(2 cookies, 29 g)

140 CALORIES

6 G FAT (2 G saturated)

100 MG SODIUM

13 G SUGARS

Regular Oreos are even worse—they deliver an extra gram of sugar and 20 extra calories per serving.

OTHER PASSES

KEEBLER
Sandies Simply Shortbread
(2 cookies, 31 g)

160 CALORIES
9 G FAT (4 G saturated)
90 MG SODIUM
7 G SUGARS

We love the low sugar count, but not the heavy deposits of soybean and palm oils.

MRS. FIELDS
Milk Chocolate Chip
(1 cookie, 32 g)

140 CALORIES
7 G FAT (3.5 G saturated)
125 MG SODIUM
12 G SUGARS

The dearth of fiber ensures that this will pass straight through your belly, spike your blood sugar, and convert quickly to flab.

ARCHWAY CLASSICS
Soft Oatmeal Raisin Cookies
(2 cookies, 66 g)

280 CALORIES
9 G FAT (4 G saturated)
170 MG SODIUM
24 G SUGARS

Add just one of these 140-calorie cookies to your daily diet and you'll gain nearly 15 pounds this year.

KEEBLER
Soft Batch Chocolate Chip
(2 cookies, 32 g)

150 CALORIES
7 G FAT (3 G saturated)
110 MG SODIUM
12 G SUGARS

This cookie has more fat, more sodium, and more sugar than the same cookie from Chips Ahoy!

CANDY BARS

Eat This

Pretzel M&M's
(1 bag, 32 g)

150 CALORIES

4.5 G FAT (3 G saturated)

17 G SUGARS

★

This clever spin on M&M's trounces everything else in the candy company's sugary arsenal. The original milk chocolate core has been replaced with pretzel, which is low in calories by confectionary standards. As a result, you trade in a boatload of sugar for a satisfying cookie-like crunch.

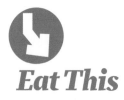

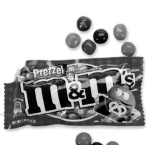

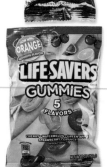

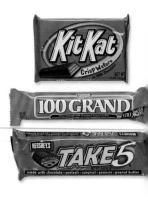

OTHER PICKS

YORK
Peppermint Pattie
(1 patty, 39 g)

140 CALORIES
2.5 G FAT (1.5 G saturated)
25 G SUGARS

For a smaller treat, go with York Miniatures. You can have three for about the same number of calories.

HERSHEY'S
Kit Kat
(1 package, 42 g)

210 CALORIES
11 G FAT (7 G saturated)
21 G SUGARS

The wafer core is light and porous, which saves you calories over the denser bars.

LIFE SAVERS
Gummies
(10 pieces, 42 g)

130 CALORIES
0 G FAT
25 G SUGARS

The secret to the chew: gelatin. Starburst uses the same trick, but spoils it with a strange mix of oils.

NESTLÉ
100 Grand
(1 package, 43 g)

190 CALORIES
8 G FAT (5 G saturated)
22 G SUGARS

This is an Eat This, Not That! Hall of Famer, routinely beating out more common chocolate bars by 80 or more calories.

HERSHEY'S
Take 5
(1 package, 42 g)

210 CALORIES
11 G FAT (5 G saturated)
18 G SUGARS

The pretzel core saves you a boatload of calories.

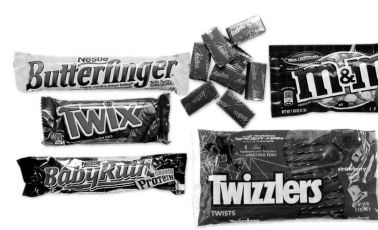

Milk Chocolate M&M's
(1 bag, 48 g)

240 CALORIES

10 G FAT (6 G saturated)

30 G SUGARS

★

M&M's pack in a lot of sugar even by candy-bar standards. This little bag is loaded with more sweetness than two Little Debbie Chocolate Marshmallow Pies.

OTHER PASSES

NESTLÉ
Butterfinger
(1 bar, 60 g)
270 CALORIES
11 G FAT (6 G saturated)
29 G SUGARS
Nobody better lay a finger on this Butterfinger.

ANDES
Thins Crème de Menthe
(8 pieces, 40 g)
220 CALORIES
14 G FAT (13 G saturated)
22 G SUGARS
This is one of the worst candies in the supermarket. The first two ingredients are sugar and partially hydrogenated oil.

MARS
Twix Caramel
(1 package, 51 g)
250 CALORIES
12 G FAT (7 G saturated)
24 G SUGARS
This sticky situation contains nearly as much saturated fat as two Snickers bars.

NESTLÉ
Baby Ruth
(1 bar, 60 g)
280 CALORIES
14 G FAT (8 G saturated)
33 G SUGARS
Together, saturated fat and sugar account for more than 200 of the calories in this package.

TWIZZLERS
Strawberry Twists
(4 pieces, 45 g)
160 CALORIES
0.5 G FAT (0 G saturated)
19 G SUGARS
You could have 40 real strawberries for the same number of calories.

FROZEN BREAKFAST EN[T]

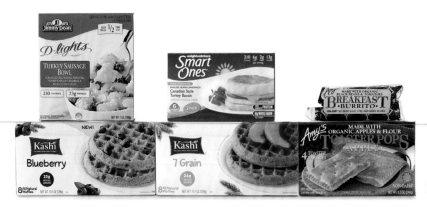

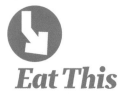

Eat This

Jimmy Dean Delights Turkey Sausage Breakfast Bowl

(1 bowl, 198 g)

240 CALORIES

8 G FAT (3.5 G saturated)

720 MG SODIUM

19 G CARBOHYDRATES

2 G FIBER

22 G PROTEIN

★

An ideal breakfast includes a substantial load of protein, and this bowl has that nailed. Protein accounts for 40 percent of the calories, which increases your odds of making it to lunch without snacking.

OTHER PICKS

**KASHI
Blueberry Waffles**
(2 waffles, 72 g)
150 CALORIES
5 G FAT (0.5 G saturated)
340 MG SODIUM
25 G CARBOHYDRATES / **6 G** FIBER
4 G PROTEIN
Blueberries figure prominently
in these first-rate waffles,
explaining the huge hit of fiber.

**WEIGHT WATCHERS
Smart Ones Smart
Beginnings Canadian
Style Turkey Bacon
English Muffin Sandwich**
(1 sandwich, 113 g)
210 CALORIES
6 G FAT (2.5 G saturated)
510 MG SODIUM
27 G CARBOHYDRATES / **2 G** FIBER
13 G PROTEIN
This is a lean protein machine.

**KASHI
7 Grain Waffles**
(2 waffles, 72 g)
150 CALORIES
5 G FAT (0.5 G saturated)
340 MG SODIUM
25 G CARBOHYDRATES / **7 G** FIBER
4 G PROTEIN
The most fiber-packed waffles
in the freezer.

**AMY'S
Black Beans & Tomatoes
Breakfast Burrito**
(1 burrito, 170 g)
270 CALORIES
8 G FAT (1 G saturated)
540 MG SODIUM
38 G CARBOHYDRATES / **6 G** FIBER
12 G PROTEIN
Black beans are one of
the healthiest foods on the planet.

**AMY'S
Toaster Pops Apple**
(1 pastry, 2.11 oz)
160 CALORIES
3.5 G FAT (0 G saturated)
110 MG SODIUM
29 G CARBOHYDRATES / **2 G** FIBER
4 G PROTEIN
The thinking parent's
smarter Pop Tart.

ÉES

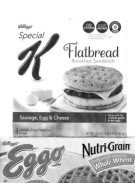
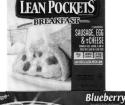
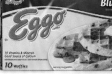

Lean Pockets Sausage, Egg & Cheese Breakfast

(1 piece, 127 g)

270 CALORIES

9 G FAT (4 G saturated)

380 MG SODIUM

37 G CARBOHYDRATES

0 G FIBER

11 G PROTEIN

★

More than 150 of these calories are carbohydrates, which is not how you want to start your day.

OTHER PASSES

EVOL
Egg & Potato Burrito
(1 burrito, 170 g)
330 CALORIES
13 G FAT (5 G saturated)
340 MG SODIUM
43 G CARBOHYDRATES / **2 G** FIBER
11 G PROTEIN
Evol makes some decent burritos, but this isn't one of them. It features more potatoes than eggs.

KELLOGG'S
Special K Flatbread Breakfast Sandwich Sausage, Egg & Cheese
(1 sandwich, 116 g)
240 CALORIES
11 G FAT (4 G saturated)
820 MG SODIUM
20 G CARBOHYDRATES / **3 G** FIBER
14 G PROTEIN
The ingredients list is a novel.

PILLSBURY
Apple Toaster Strudel
(1 pastry, 54 g)
180 CALORIES
7 G FAT (3 G saturated)
180 MG SODIUM
26 G CARBOHYDRATES / **<1 G** FIBER
2 G PROTEIN
This has half the protein and fiber of Amy's version.

KELLOGG'S
Eggo Nutri-Grain Whole Wheat Waffles
(2 waffles, 70 g)
170 CALORIES
6 G FAT (1.5 G saturated)
400 MG SODIUM
26 G CARBOHYDRATES / **3 G** FIBER
5 G PROTEIN
There are better fiber-rich waffles to be had.

KELLOGG'S
Eggo Blueberry Waffles
(2 waffles, 70 g)
180 CALORIES
6 G FAT (1.5 G saturated)
370 MG SODIUM
29 G CARBOHYDRATES / **<1 G** FIBER
4 G PROTEIN
Blueberries are the eleventh ingredient on the list.

FROZEN PIZZAS

Eat This

Kashi Stone-Fired Mushroom Trio & Spinach Thin Crust Pizza

(⅓ pie, 113 g)

150 CALORIES

9 G FAT
(4.5 G saturated)

660 MG SODIUM

28 G CARBOHYDRATES

4 G FIBER

14 G PROTEIN

★

This pie features more pesto than cheese, which means you end up with more monounsaturated fat from olive oil than saturated fat from dairy. That's a healthy swap.

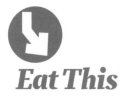

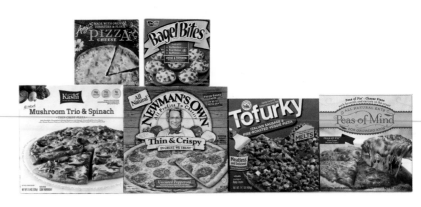

OTHER PICKS

AMY'S
Cheese
(1 pie, 167 g)
420 CALORIES
17 G FAT (6 G saturated)
720 MG SODIUM
49 G CARBOHYDRATES / **3 G** FIBER
18 G PROTEIN
For the rare times when you allow yourself the privilege of eating a whole pizza, this is exactly where you should turn.

BAGEL BITES
Cheese & Pepperoni
(4 pieces, 88 g)
200 CALORIES
6 G FAT (2.5 G saturated)
340 MG SODIUM
28 G CARBOHYDRATES / **2 G** FIBER
7 G PROTEIN
Not a perfect snack, but still decent for a non-diet pizza product.

NEWMAN'S OWN
Thin & Crispy Uncured Pepperoni
(⅓ pie, 125 g)
320 CALORIES
16 G FAT (6 G saturated)
800 MG SODIUM
31 G CARBOHYDRATES / **1 G** FIBER
15 G PROTEIN
Newman's skips the nitrates and nitrites with its pepperoni.

TOFURKY
Italian Sausage & Fire Roasted Veggie
(⅓ pie, 132 g)
270 CALORIES
6 G FAT (1 G saturated)
320 MG SODIUM
40 G CARBOHYDRATES / **5 G** FIBER
13 G PROTEIN
Tofurky's lactose-free "cheese" is made using protein, flour, and oils.

PEAS OF MIND
Cheese
(⅓ pie, 109 g)
240 CALORIES
5 G FAT (2 G saturated)
510 MG SODIUM
36 G CARBOHYDRATES / **2 G** FIBER
11 G PROTEIN
They snuck broccoli and carrots into the crust. Clever devils!

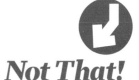

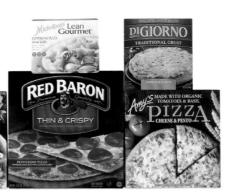

Not That!

Amy's Whole Wheat Crust Cheese & Pesto Pizza

(⅓ pie, 132 g)

---

360 CALORIES

---

18 G FAT
(4 G saturated)

---

680 MG SODIUM

---

37 G CARBOHYDRATES

---

4 G FIBER

---

13 G PROTEIN

★

The crust is the least nutritious part of any pie, and unfortunately, Amy's is just a little bit too thick.

OTHER PASSES

STOUFFER'S
French Bread Sausage & Pepperoni
(2 pieces, 177 g)
460 CALORIES
24 G FAT (8 G saturated)
880 MG SODIUM
43 G CARBOHYDRATES / **4 G** FIBER
17 G PROTEIN
One contains the saturated fat
of 16 Burger King Chicken Tenders.

AMY'S
Roasted Vegetable No Cheese
(⅓ pie, 113 g)
280 CALORIES
9 G FAT (1.5 G saturated)
540 MG SODIUM
42 G CARBOHYDRATES / **3 G** FIBER
7 G PROTEIN
For the lactose intolerant, there are
options closer to the real thing.

MICHELINA'S
Lean Gourmet Pepperoni Pizza Snackers
(11 pieces, 85 g)
200 CALORIES
8 G FAT (1.5 G saturated)
290 MG SODIUM
26 G CARBOHYDRATES / **2 G** FIBER
7 G PROTEIN
Nitrites and soybean oil,
but not much good stuff.

RED BARON
Thin & Crispy Pepperoni Pizza
(⅓ pie, 149 g)
400 CALORIES
19 G FAT (9 G saturated)
1,020 MG SODIUM
41 G CARBOHYDRATES / **2 G** FIBER
15 G PROTEIN
Even the Baron's thin-crust pies
pack too much of the bad stuff.

DIGIORNO
Traditional Crust Four Cheese Pizza
(1 pie, 260 g)
350 CALORIES
15 G FAT (6 G saturated)
590 MG SODIUM
42 G CARBOHYDRATES / **2 G** FIBER
13 G PROTEIN
These personal pies are undone
by thick crusts and excess cheese.

FROZEN PASTA ENTRÉE

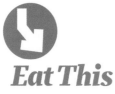

Eat This

Kashi Chicken Pasta Pomodoro

(1 entrée, 283 g)

280 CALORIES

6 G FAT
(1.5 G saturated)

470 MG SODIUM

38 G CARBOHYDRATES

6 G FIBER

19 G PROTEIN

Small savings in everyday choices is the key to sustainable weight loss. A simple savings of 20 calories every day adds up to 2 pounds a year. That's 20 pounds over the course of a decade.

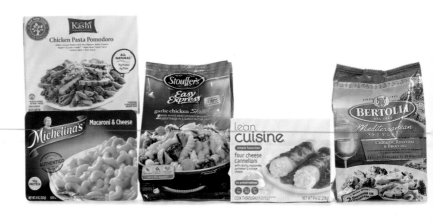

OTHER PICKS

MICHELINA'S
Macaroni & Cheese
(1 package, 213 g)

250 CALORIES
6 G FAT (2.5 G saturated)
500 MG SODIUM
38 G CARBOHYDRATES / **1 G** FIBER
9 G PROTEIN

Defuse the comfort food's flab-producing potential by opting for this light rendition.

STOUFFER'S
Easy Express Garlic Chicken Skillet
(½ package, 326 g)

330 CALORIES
6 G FAT (2.5 G saturated)
990 MG SODIUM
45 G CARBOHYDRATES / **5 G** FIBER
24 G PROTEIN

Budding chefs, take note: The more vegetables you use, the less sauce and pasta you'll need.

LEAN CUISINE
Four Cheese Cannelloni
(1 package, 258 g)

230 CALORIES
6 G FAT (3 G saturated)
690 MG SODIUM
33 G CARBOHYDRATES / **3 G** FIBER
11 G PROTEIN

Swap out white sauce for red sauce and you'll save a few hundred calories per serving every time.

BERTOLLI
Mediterranean Style Chicken, Rigatoni & Broccoli
(½ package, 340 g)

400 CALORIES
16 G FAT (4 G saturated)
860 MG SODIUM
44 G CARBOHYDRATES / **4 G** FIBER
20 G PROTEIN

After pasta, the first two ingredients are broccoli and chicken.

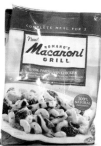
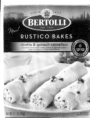
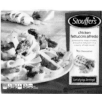
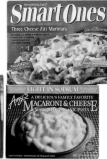

Smart Ones Three Cheese Ziti Marinara

(1 entrée, 255 g)

300 CALORIES	
8 G FAT (3 G saturated)	
510 MG SODIUM	
45 G CARBOHYDRATES	
7 G FIBER	
13 G PROTEIN	

★

Marinara is typically the safest of the pasta sauces, but that rule fails to hold as soon as Smart Ones buries the plate under a rubbery quilt of cheese.

OTHER PASSES

ROMANO'S MACARONI GRILL
Creamy Basil Parmesan Chicken & Pasta
(½ package, 340 g)
470 CALORIES
21 G FAT (12 G saturated)
1,040 MG SODIUM
42 G CARBOHYDRATES / **4 G** FIBER
29 G PROTEIN

Romano takes a heavy-handed approach
with cream, as demonstrated by the exorbitant glut
of saturated fat in this dish.

BERTOLLI
Rustico Bakes Ricotta & Spinach Cannelloni
(1 meal, 314 g)
500 CALORIES
28 G FAT (17 G saturated)
1,290 MG SODIUM
41 G CARBOHYDRATES / **5 G** FIBER
21 G PROTEIN

These noodles are stuffed with cheese and covered with
cream, plus more than half a day's allotment of salt.

STOUFFER'S
Chicken Fettuccini Alfredo
(1 package, 297 g)
570 CALORIES
27 G FAT (7 G saturated)
850 MG SODIUM
55 G CARBOHYDRATES / **5 G** FIBER
26 G PROTEIN

Alfredo sauce contains any of the following:
oil, butter, cheese, cream, and egg yolk.
In other words, it's a full-fat assault.

AMY'S
Light in Sodium Macaroni & Cheese
(1 entrée, 255 g)
400 CALORIES
16 G FAT (10 G saturated)
290 MG SODIUM
47 G CARBOHYDRATES / **3 G** FIBER
16 G PROTEIN

We've seen worse mac out there,
but Amy's packages its pasta as a healthy alternative
to the normal stuff, and we're just not buying it.

FROZEN FISH ENTRÉES

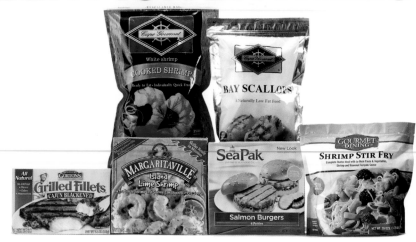

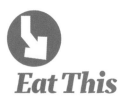

Eat This

Gorton's Grilled Fillets Cajun Blackened

(1 fillet, 101 g)

90 CALORIES

3 G FAT
(0.5 G saturated)

400 MG SODIUM

15 G PROTEIN

The smoky, spicy finesse of a blackening rub can imbue any fillet with massive flavor at no caloric cost. It's easily one of the healthiest ways to prepare meat and fish.

OTHER PICKS

CAPE GOURMET
Cooked Shrimp
(3 oz)
50 CALORIES
0.5 G FAT
330 MG SODIUM / **10 G** PROTEIN
Unadulterated shrimp are among the leanest sources of protein on the planet.

CAPE GOURMET
Bay Scallops
(4 oz)
150 CALORIES
1 G FAT (0 G saturated)
155 MG SODIUM / **29 G** PROTEIN
Scallops are teeming with the amino acid tryptophan, which bolsters feelings of well-being and helps regulate the sleep cycle.

MARGARITAVILLE
Island Lime Shrimp
(6 shrimp, 4 oz)
240 CALORIES
11 G FAT (3 G saturated)
330 MG SODIUM / **12 G** PROTEIN
These shrimp have also been tossed in butter. The difference is quantity; here it's a light bath, but in SeaPak's scampi it's a tidal wave.

SEAPAK
Salmon Burgers
(1 burger, 91 g)
110 CALORIES
5 G FAT (1 G saturated)
340 MG SODIUM / **16 G** PROTEIN
Toss this on the grill, then sandwich it between a toasted bun with arugula, grilled onions, and Greek yogurt spiked with olive oil, garlic, and fresh dill.

GOURMET DINING
Shrimp Stir Fry
(¼ package, 198 g)
200 CALORIES
1 G FAT (0 G saturated)
640 MG SODIUM / **12 G** PROTEIN
American interpretations of Asian cuisine tend to be high in sodium, but this solid blend of fiber and protein more than makes up for it.

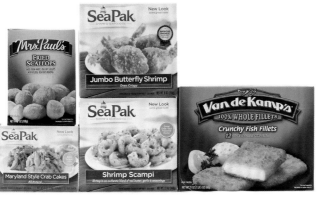

Not That!

Van de Kamp's Crunchy Fish Fillets

(2 fillets, 99 g)

230 CALORIES

13 G FAT
(4.5 G saturated)

440 MG SODIUM

8 G PROTEIN

★

You know what makes the breading crunchy? The same thing that makes it 150 percent more caloric and 267 percent fattier: oil.

OTHER PASSES

P.F. CHANG'S
**Home Menu
Shrimp Lo Mein**
(½ package, 312 g)
390 CALORIES
12 G FAT (1.5 G saturated)
740 MG SODIUM / **16 G** PROTEIN
Chang's sauce is polluted
with three kinds of oil.

MRS. PAUL'S
Fried Scallops
(13 scallops)
260 CALORIES
11 G FAT (4 G saturated)
700 MG SODIUM / **12 G** PROTEIN
Scallops are among the sea's
greatest gifts to man. Spoiling them
with the fryer treatment is an
abomination. You end up with
more calories from fat than protein.

SEAPAK
**Maryland Style
Crab Cakes**
(1 crab cake with 1 oz sauce, 113 g)
240 CALORIES
13 G FAT (1.5 G saturated)
830 MG SODIUM / **11 G** PROTEIN
These crab cakes deliver more
starchy filler than actual shellfish.
Somewhere, a Marylander is
shaking his head.

SEAPAK
Jumbo Butterfly Shrimp
(4 shrimp, 84 g)
230 CALORIES
11 G FAT (2 G saturated)
480 MG SODIUM / **10 G** PROTEIN
Each shrimp delivers more than
50 calories, and nearly half of that
comes from unnecessary fats.

SEAPAK
Shrimp Scampi
(6 shrimp, 113 g)
340 CALORIES
31 G FAT (12 G saturated)
480 MG SODIUM / **12 G** PROTEIN
Shrimp are essentially pure protein,
so it's puzzling to find that
protein accounts for just 13 percent
of this entrée's calories.

FROZEN CHICKEN ENTR

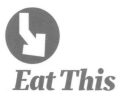

Eat This

Evol Bowls Teriyaki Chicken

(1 bowl, 255 g)

260 CALORIES

3 G FAT
(0 G saturated)

560 MG SODIUM

43 G CARBOHYDRATES

3 G FIBER

14 G PROTEIN

Evol's teriyaki bowl is made with brown rice, free-range chicken, and enough produce to meet 90 percent of your day's vitamin A needs.

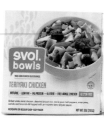
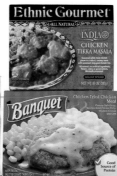
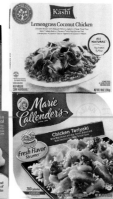
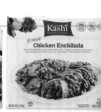

OTHER PICKS

ETHNIC GOURMET
Chicken Tikka Masala
(1 package, 283 g)
260 CALORIES
6 G FAT (2 G saturated)
680 MG SODIUM
32 G CARBOHYDRATES / **3 G** FIBER
19 G PROTEIN
The sauce is created with fat-free yogurt, for a low-calorie creaminess.

BANQUET
Chicken Fried Chicken Meal
(1 entrée, 286 g)
350 CALORIES
17 G FAT (4 G saturated)
930 MG SODIUM
35 G CARBOHYDRATES / **5 G** FIBER
12 G PROTEIN
Thinner breading and better sides save you 90 calories over Banquet's "premium" version.

KASHI
Lemongrass Coconut Chicken
(1 entrée, 283 g)
300 CALORIES
8 G FAT (4 G saturated)
680 MG SODIUM
38 G CARBOHYDRATES / **7 G** FIBER
18 G PROTEIN
Instead of the standard white rice, this meal rests on a blend of oats, wheat, and quinoa.

MARIE CALLENDER'S
Fresh Flavor Steamer Chicken Teriyaki
(1 meal, 283 g)
280 CALORIES
3.5 G FAT (1 G saturated)
890 MG SODIUM
44 G CARBOHYDRATES / **3 G** FIBER
17 G PROTEIN
The wealth of veggies keeps the calories low.

KASHI
Chicken Enchilada
(1 entrée)
280 CALORIES
9 G FAT (2.5 G saturated)
620 MG SODIUM
6 G FIBER
12 G PROTEIN
Kashi's blend of whole grains makes these corn tortillas surprisingly healthy.

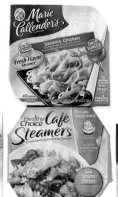
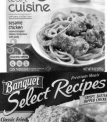
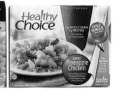

Not That!

Healthy Choice Pineapple Chicken

(1 entrée, 280 g)

300 CALORIES	
5 G FAT (1 G saturated)	
510 MG SODIUM	
46 G CARBOHYDRATES	
5 G FIBER	
18 G PROTEIN	

★

This bowl contains more sugar than protein—19 grams of sugar, in fact, more than you'd find in a scoop of Breyers Chocolate Ice Cream.

OTHER PASSES

EVOL
Chicken Enchilada Bake
(1 bowl, 255 g)
380 CALORIES
13 G FAT (6 G saturated)
630 MG SODIUM
46 G CARBOHYDRATES / **6 G** FIBER
21 G PROTEIN
Make this kind of simple mistake once a day, and that 120 calories adds up to 11 pounds a year.

MARIE CALLENDER'S
Fresh Flavor Steamer Sesame Chicken
(1 meal, 291 g)
400 CALORIES
12 G FAT (2 G saturated)
710 MG SODIUM
54 G CARBOHYDRATES / **5 G** FIBER
18 G PROTEIN
A chicken dish shouldn't be a festival of fat and carbohydrates.

HEALTHY CHOICE
Café Steamers Sweet Sesame Chicken
(1 meal, 276 g)
280 CALORIES
7 G FAT (1.5 G saturated)
520 MG SODIUM
31 G CARBOHYDRATES / **5 G** FIBER
21 G PROTEIN
Packs as much sugar as a two-pack of Twix Peanut Butter.

LEAN CUISINE
Sesame Chicken
(1 package, 255 g)
330 CALORIES
9 G FAT (1 G saturated)
650 MG SODIUM
47 G CARBOHYDRATES / **2 G** FIBER
16 G PROTEIN
There's nothing lean about breaded chicken tossed with 14 grams of sugar.

BANQUET
Select Recipes Classic Fried Chicken Meal
(1 entrée, 228 g)
440 CALORIES
26 G FAT
(6 G saturated, 1.5 G trans)
1,140 MG SODIUM
30 G CARBOHYDRATES / **4 G** FIBER
22 G PROTEIN
Never settle for a frozen dinner with trans fats.

143

FROZEN BEEF ENTRÉES

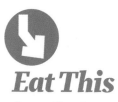

Eat This

Stouffer's Homestyle Classics Beef Pot Roast

(1 entrée, 251 g)

320 CALORIES

8 G FAT
(3 G saturated)

1,570 MG SODIUM

41 G CARBOHYDRATES

8 G FIBER

20 G PROTEIN

★

In the world of frozen entrées, there's always some sacrifice involved. In this case, we'll take the elevated salt count rather than the trans fats—and double our fiber and protein in the process.

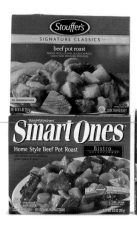

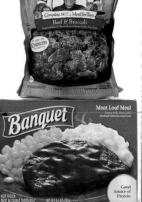

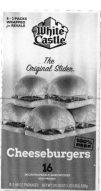

OTHER PICKS

SMART ONES
Home Style Beef Pot Roast
(1 meal, 255 g)
190 CALORIES
6 G FAT (2.5 G saturated)
590 MG SODIUM
18 G CARBOHYDRATES / **3 G** FIBER
16 G PROTEIN
Most protein bars can't deliver this dose for so few calories. Tack on 3 grams of fiber and you have an amazing 190-calorie package.

NEWMAN'S OWN
Beef & Broccoli Complete Skillet Meal
(½ package, 250 g)
250 CALORIES
10 G FAT (3 G saturated)
800 MG SODIUM
22 G CARBOHYDRATES / **5 G** FIBER
19 G PROTEIN
The first ingredient in this bag is broccoli. In the cost-conscious world of processed foods, that's exceedingly rare.

BANQUET
Meat Loaf Meal
(1 meal, 269 g)
280 CALORIES
13 G FAT (5 G saturated)
1,000 MG SODIUM
28 G CARBOHYDRATES / **4 G** FIBER
12 G PROTEIN
When it comes to delivering comfort dishes for a reasonable number of calories, Banquet's regular line of entrées is among the best in the freezer.

WHITE CASTLE
Microwaveable Cheeseburgers
(2 burgers, 104 g)
310 CALORIES
17 G FAT (8 G saturated)
600 MG SODIUM
26 G CARBOHYDRATES / **1 G** FIBER
14 G PROTEIN
With decent at-home nutritionals, Harold and Kumar have less to worry about than ever.

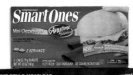
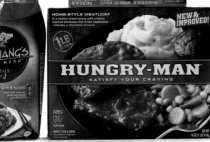
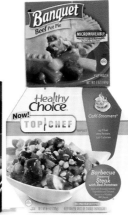

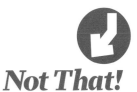

OTHER PASSES

P.F. CHANG'S
Home Menu Beef with Broccoli
(½ package, 312 g)
360 CALORIES
17 G FAT (2.5 G saturated)
1,020 MG SODIUM
30 G CARBOHYDRATES / **5 G** FIBER
22 G PROTEIN
Chang's bagged meals suffer from the same sodium
saturation that plagues its restaurant fare.

SMART ONES
Anytime Selections Mini Cheeseburgers
(2 mini-burgers, 140 g)
380 CALORIES
16 G FAT (6 G saturated)
720 MG SODIUM
42 G CARBOHYDRATES / **6 G** FIBER
18 G PROTEIN
There's a lot of bun around these burgers,
with nearly twice the carbs as White Castle.

HUNGRY-MAN
Home-Style Meatloaf
(1 package, 454 g)
660 CALORIES
35 G FAT (12 G saturated)
1,660 MG SODIUM
61 G CARBOHYDRATES / **5 G** FIBER
26 G PROTEIN
Word of advice to the calorie conscious:
Purge Hungry-Man from your freezer for good. This is
consistently the worst brand in the frozen-foods aisle.

HEALTHY CHOICE
Café Steamers Barbecue Seasoned Steak with Red Potatoes
(1 meal, 269 g)
260 CALORIES
3.5 G FAT (1 G saturated)
470 MG SODIUM
39 G CARBOHYDRATES / **6 G** FIBER
17 G PROTEIN
More fat, calories, and sugar
than the Smart Ones pot roast.

FROZEN SIDES, SNACK.

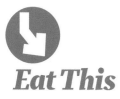

Eat This

Ore-Ida Steak Fries

(7 fries, 84 g)

110 CALORIES

3 G FAT
(0.5 G saturated)

290 MG SODIUM

19 G CARBOHYDRATES

2 G PROTEIN

★

A serving of these hulking spuds contains fewer than half the calories you'd find in the average medium order of fast-food fries.

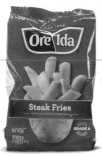

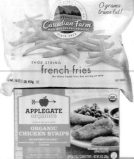

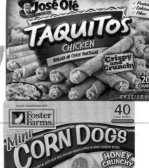

OTHER PICKS

CASCADIAN FARM
Shoe String French Fries
(3 oz, 85 g)
110 CALORIES
5 G FAT (1 G saturated)
10 MG SODIUM
17 G CARBOHYDRATES
2 G PROTEIN
Cascadian Farm tosses these fries
in apple juice, the sugar from which
caramelizes into a crisp, golden crust.

APPLEGATE ORGANICS
Organic Chicken Strips
(3 strips, 84 g)
170 CALORIES
8 G FAT (1 G saturated)
350 MG SODIUM
12 G CARBOHYDRATES
12 G PROTEIN
The relatively light breading makes
Applegate's strips less fatty than the competition's.

JOSÉ OLÉ
Chicken Taquitos Rolled in Corn Tortillas
(3 pieces, 85 g)
200 CALORIES
8 G FAT (1.5 G saturated)
390 MG SODIUM
26 G CARBOHYDRATES
7 G PROTEIN
These taquitos win by virtue of their little corn sleeping
bags, which are lower in fat than flour tortillas.

FOSTER FARMS
Mini Corn Dogs Honey Crunchy
(4 dogs, 76 g)
210 CALORIES
12 G FAT (3.5 G saturated)
490 MG SODIUM
18 G CARBOHYDRATES
7 G PROTEIN
At only 53 calories per dog,
the damage potential here is relatively low.

APPETIZERS

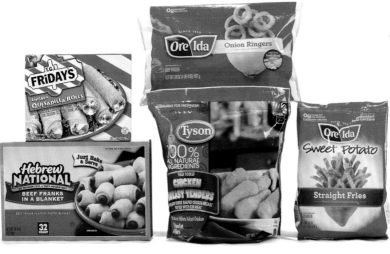

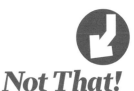

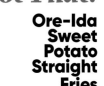

Not That!

Ore-Ida Sweet Potato Straight Fries
(22 fries, 84 g)

160 CALORIES

8 G FAT
(0.5 G saturated)

160 MG SODIUM

21 G CARBOHYDRATES

1 G PROTEIN

★

A raw sweet potato has more fiber and vitamin A than a raw russet potato, but once the food industry starts plowing fat into the produce, all bets are off.

OTHER PASSES

T.G.I. FRIDAY'S
Chicken Quesadilla Rolls
(2 pieces, 83 g)

230 CALORIES
10 G FAT (3 G saturated, 1 G trans)
470 MG SODIUM
27 G CARBOHYDRATES
9 G PROTEIN

Frozen flour tortillas are little trans-fat delivery systems.

HEBREW NATIONAL
Beef Franks in a Blanket
(5 pieces, 81 g)

300 CALORIES
24 G FAT (8 G saturated, 3 G trans)
680 MG SODIUM
12 G CARBOHYDRATES
8 G PROTEIN

You shouldn't consume this much trans fat in an entire day, let alone from a snack.

ORE-IDA
Onion Ringers
(3 pieces, 81 g)

180 CALORIES
10 G FAT (2 G saturated)
160 MG SODIUM
21 G CARBOHYDRATES
2 G PROTEIN

Each ring harbors more than 3 grams of fat.
Fries are almost always the better choice.

TYSON
Chicken Breast Tenders
(4 pieces, 80 g)

190 CALORIES
12 G FAT (2.5 G saturated)
420 MG SODIUM
12 G CARBOHYDRATES
9 G PROTEIN

There's a big difference between "organic," a regulated term, and "natural," which means nothing. In this case, that difference is worth an extra dose of fat and sodium.

ICE CREAMS

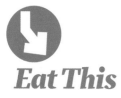

Eat This

Breyers Black Raspberry Chocolate

(½ cup, 67 g)

140 CALORIES

4 G FAT
(3 G saturated)

16 G SUGARS

The secret to a low-calorie ice cream is simple: Lead off with something lighter than cream. This one uses regular milk first and cream last.

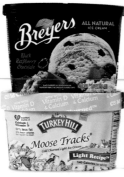
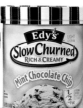
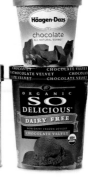
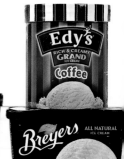

OTHER PICKS

TURKEY HILL
Light Recipe Moose Tracks
(½ cup, 61 g)
140 CALORIES
6 G FAT (2.5 G saturated)
15 G SUGARS
Swirled ice cream flecked with chocolate peanut butter cups— you won't find a more decadent dessert with fewer calories.

EDY'S
Slow Churned Mint Chocolate Chip
(½ cup, 60 g)
120 CALORIES
4.5 G FAT (3 G saturated)
35 MG SODIUM
13 G SUGARS
Edy's Slow Churned line leans more heavily on milk than cream, which keeps the calories in check.

HÄAGEN-DAZS
Chocolate Sorbet
(½ cup, 105 g)
130 CALORIES
0.5 G FAT (0 G saturated)
21 G SUGARS
One of the few Häagen-Dazs products that we can actually stand behind.

SO DELICIOUS
Chocolate Velvet
(½ cup, 81 g)
130 CALORIES
3.5 G FAT (0.5 G saturated)
14 G SUGARS
So Delicious cuts the fat without needing to make up for it with an extra hit of sugar.

EDY'S
Rich & Creamy Grand Coffee
(½ cup, 65 g)
140 CALORIES
7 G FAT (4 G saturated)
13 G SUGARS
Careful—it's made with real coffee, so it's not the best choice right before bed.

BREYERS
Natural Vanilla
(½ cup, 66 g)
130 CALORIES
7 G FAT (4 G saturated)
14 G SUGARS
Breyers Natural has earned our allegiance for both its low-calorie concoctions and the simplicity of its ingredient statements.

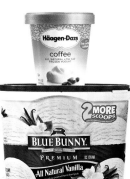
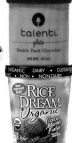
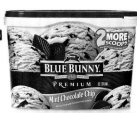
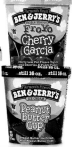

Ben & Jerry's FroYo Cherry Garcia Frozen Yogurt
(½ cup, 108 g)

200 CALORIES

3 G FAT
(2 G saturated)

27 G SUGARS

★

You buy frozen yogurt thinking you're doing your body a favor, only to find out it's worse than three-quarters of the full-fat ice creams in the freezer. Thanks, Ben & Jerry's.

OTHER PASSES

HÄAGEN-DAZS
Low Fat Frozen Yogurt Coffee
(½ cup, 102 g)
180 CALORIES
2.5 G FAT (1 G saturated)
21 G SUGARS
Leave it to Häagen-Dazs to find a way to mess up frozen yogurt.

BLUE BUNNY
Premium All Natural Vanilla
(½ cup, 69 g)
150 CALORIES
9 G FAT (5 G saturated)
16 G SUGARS
The All Natural line is the worst among the many Blue Bunny vanilla ice creams.

TALENTI
Double Dark Chocolate
(½ cup, 101 g)
210 CALORIES
10 G FAT (6 G saturated)
25 G SUGARS
Another player in the "premium" ice cream world, another tub overloaded with saturated fat and sugar.

RICE DREAM
Organic Cocoa Marble Fudge
(½ cup, 90 g)
170 CALORIES
6 G FAT (0.5 G saturated)
17 G SUGARS
Rice Dream adds vegetable oils to create a high-cal approximation of ice cream.

BLUE BUNNY
Mint Chocolate Chip
(½ cup, 67 g)
160 CALORIES
8 G FAT (6 G saturated)
15 G SUGARS
Not terrible, but just north of the calorie and fat counts you want in your ice cream.

BEN & JERRY'S
Peanut Butter Cup
(½ cup, 112 g)
350 CALORIES
24 G FAT (13 G saturated)
25 G SUGARS
Eat two scoops of this and you'll take in more calories than you would with a McDonald's McDouble with a small side of french fries.

FROZEN TREATS

Eat This

Snickers Ice Cream Bar

(1 bar, 49 g)

180 CALORIES

11 G FAT
(6 G saturated)

15 G SUGARS

★

As decadent as it may seem, the Snickers Ice Cream Bar has less fat, sugar, and total calories than an actual Snickers candy bar.

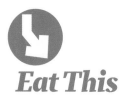

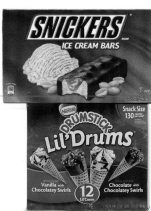

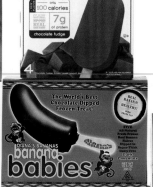

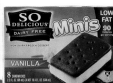

OTHER PICKS

NESTLÉ
Drumstick Lil' Drums Vanilla
with Chocolatey Swirls
(1 cone, 43 g)
110 CALORIES
5 G FAT (3.5 G saturated)
10 G SUGARS
The perfect portion for an after-dinner indulgence.

YASSO
Frozen Greek Yogurt
Chocolate Fudge Bar
(1 bar, 70 g)
100 CALORIES
0 G FAT (0 G saturated)
13 G SUGARS
A classy upgrade to the standard Fudgsicle,
this frozen treat delivers 7 grams of belly-filling protein.

DIANA'S BANANAS
Banana Babies Dark Chocolate
(1 piece, 60 g)
130 CALORIES
6 G FAT (3.5 G saturated)
14 G SUGARS
Banana, chocolate, and peanut oil.
You don't find a frozen treat with a simpler recipe.

SO DELICIOUS
Minis Vanilla
(1 sandwich, 40 g)
90 CALORIES
2 G FAT (0.5 G saturated)
8 G SUGARS
Low in sugar and overall calories, this is a good treat
to keep in mind even if you're not lactose intolerant.

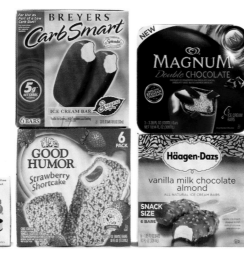

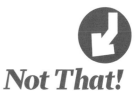

Not That!

Magnum Double Chocolate

(1 bar, 83 g)

340 CALORIES

21 G FAT
(15 G saturated)

29 G SUGARS

★

If the Magnum is your go-to dessert, you could swap in the Snickers each night and you'd save more than 16 pounds in a year!

OTHER PASSES

TOFUTTI
Cuties Vanilla
(1 sandwich, 38 g)
130 CALORIES
6 G FAT (1 G saturated)
17 G CARBOHYDRATES
9 G SUGARS
Made mostly of sugar, corn syrup solids, and vegetable oils. Tofu plays a mere supporting role.

BREYERS
CarbSmart Ice Cream Bar Vanilla
(1 bar, 58 g)
180 CALORIES
14 G FAT (10 G saturated)
6 G SUGARS
Sure, it's "carb smart," but it's also sat-fat dumb.

GOOD HUMOR
Strawberry Shortcake
(1 bar, 83 g)
230 CALORIES
10 G FAT (3.5 G saturated)
17 G SUGARS
This bar does contain real strawberries, but it contains even more sugar, corn syrup, palm oil, and food coloring.

HÄAGEN-DAZS
Vanilla Milk Chocolate Almond Snack Size
(1 bar, 52 g)
195 CALORIES
24.5 G FAT (7 G saturated)
11.5 G SUGARS
Cream is the first ingredient, which is how it packs 40 percent of your day's saturated fat into each bar.

JUICES

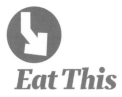

Eat This

Lakewood Organic Lemonade
(8 fl oz)

80 CALORIES

0 G FAT

16 G SUGARS

This drink is sweetened with grape juice instead of sugar.

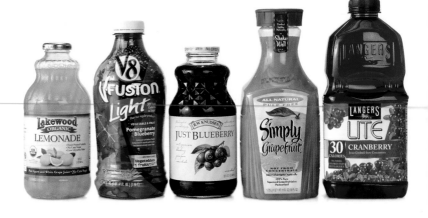

OTHER PICKS

V8
V-Fusion Light Pomegranate Blueberry
(8 fl oz)
50 CALORIES
0 G FAT
10 G SUGARS
Every calorie in this bottle comes from the blend of sweet potatoes, carrots, apples, pomegranates, and blueberries.

R.W. KNUDSEN
Just Blueberry
(8 fl oz)
100 CALORIES
0 G FAT
19 G SUGARS
Blueberries are bursting with brain-boosting antioxidants, and R.W. Knudsen's juice is the only one to give you 100 percent blueberries.

SIMPLY
Grapefruit
(8 fl oz)
100 CALORIES
0 G FAT
25 G SUGARS
Grapefruit is the most underrated juice in the cooler. It's delicious, it's naturally low in sugar, and it delivers a dose of cancer-fighting lycopene.

LANGERS
Lite Cranberry
(8 fl oz)
30 CALORIES
0 G FAT
8 G SUGARS
Cranberries make for a tart juice, which is why you routinely see 15 or more grams of sugar added to each serving. Langers Lite keeps it simple.

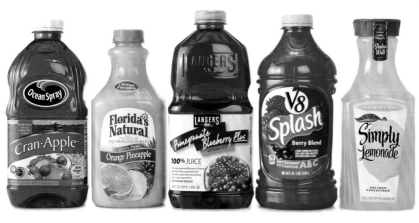

Not That!

Simply Lemonade

(8 fl oz)

120 CALORIES

0 G FAT

28 G SUGARS

★

*Contains only
11 percent juice.
The rest of the
bottle is pure
sugar water. Most
lemonades follow
the same disap-
pointing formula.*

OTHER PASSES

OCEAN SPRAY
Cran-Apple
(8 fl oz)

120 CALORIES
0 G FAT
31 G SUGARS

This bottle, like so many in Ocean Spray's lineup,
contains only 15 percent juice.
Water and sugar are the first two ingredients.

FLORIDA'S NATURAL
100% Pure Orange Pineapple
(8 fl oz)

130 CALORIES
0 G FAT
30 G SUGARS

It's hard to find fault with 100 percent juice products,
but blends like this tend to pack in too much sugar.

LANGERS
Pomegranate Blueberry Plus
(8 fl oz)

140 CALORIES
0 G FAT
30 G SUGARS

There's more sugar in this bottle than
there are blueberries or pomegranates.

V8 SPLASH
Berry Blend
(8 fl oz)

70 CALORIES
0 G FAT
16 G SUGARS

Splash is unfit to carry the V8 brand name.
It's made with artificial colors, high-fructose corn syrup,
and a pathetic 5 percent juice.

TEAS & FLAVORED WA

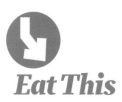

Eat This

Honest Tea Community Green Tea

(16 fl oz)

34 CALORIES

0 G FAT

10 G SUGARS

 ★

High in antioxidants and low in sugar, Honest Tea is one of the most reliable brands in any cooler.

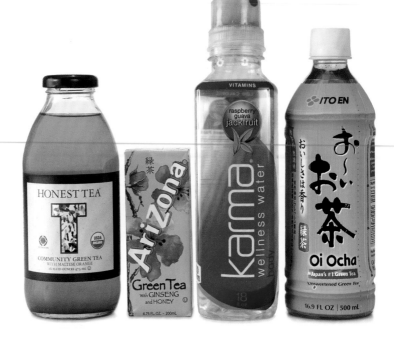

OTHER PICKS

ARIZONA
Green Tea
with Ginseng and Honey
(8 fl oz)

70 CALORIES

0 G FAT

17 G SUGARS

This is one of the few AriZona drinks worth purchasing. The generous size and better ingredients list gives it the narrow edge over Ssips.

KARMA
Wellness Water
Raspberry
Guava Jackfruit
(18 fl oz)

20 CALORIES

0 G FAT

2 G SUGARS

Pushing the cap releases a vitamin powder lightly sweetened with stevia and cane sugar. Makers claim this mixing method ensures potency. We just like the low sugar count.

ITO EN
Oi Ocha
Unsweetened Green Tea
(16.9 fl oz)

0 CALORIES

0 G FAT

0 G SUGARS

Researchers believe green tea plays a prominent role in the long life spans of the Japanese. ITO EN is the most popular tea in Japan.

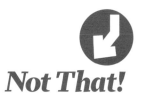

Not That!

Tazo Organic Iced Green Tea

(14 fl oz)

120 CALORIES

0 G FAT

30 G SUGARS

★

A lot of things that are organic aren't necessarily good for you, and sugar is one of them.

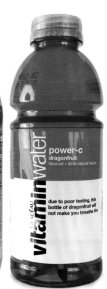

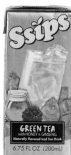

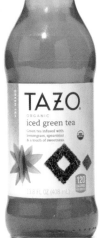

OTHER PASSES

SNAPPLE
Green Tea
(16 fl oz)
120 CALORIES
0 G FAT
30 G SUGARS
Catechins found in green tea can boost metabolism, but whatever metabolic boost you find in this bottle is more than offset by the sugar rush.

VITAMINWATER
Power-C Dragonfruit Flavored
(20 fl oz)
120 CALORIES
0 G FAT
31 G SUGARS
Getting your daily dose of vitamin C shouldn't cost you the sugar equivalent of 13 Jolly Ranchers.

SSIPS
Green Tea
with Honey & Ginseng
(6.75 fl oz)
60 CALORIES
0 G FAT
12 G SUGARS
The honey in the name is just a diversionary tactic. Much of the sweetness here comes from high-fructose corn syrup, which is the second ingredient on the list. Either way, skip it.

MIXERS

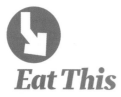

Eat This

Stirrings Simple Cosmopolitan Mix

(3 fl oz)

60 CALORIES

0 G FAT

16 G SUGARS

★

Made with real cranberry and key lime juices—a rarity in the world of mixers.

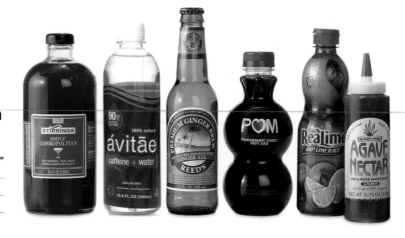

OTHER PICKS

ÁVITAE
Caffeine + Water
(16.9 fl oz)

0 CALORIES
0 G FAT
0 G SUGARS

This club soda will give you the caffeine boost of Red Bull, just without all the sugar.

REED'S
Premium Ginger Brew
(12 fl oz)

145 CALORIES
0 G FAT
37.4 G SUGARS

Ginger beer is made with a larger dose of ginger than ginger ale, which means more of a kick and more of ginger's anti-inflammatory properties.

POM
Wonderful Pomegranate Cherry
100% Juice
(4 fl oz)

75 CALORIES
0 G FAT
14.5 G SUGARS

These are natural sugars, which means you get nutrients, too.

REALIME
100% Lime Juice
(3 Tbsp)
MADHAVA Agave Nectar
(1 Tbsp)

60 CALORIES
0 G FAT
15 G SUGARS

This is how real margaritas are made, with fresh lime juice and a hint of sugar.

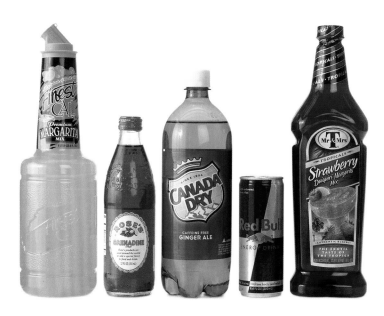

Mr and Mrs T Strawberry Daiquiri-Margarita Mix
(4 fl oz)

---

190 CALORIES

0 G FAT

44 G SUGARS

★

Mostly high-fructose corn syrup and food coloring—enough to spoil any good drink.

OTHER PASSES

FINEST CALL
Premium Margarita Mix
(4 fl oz)
160 CALORIES
0 G FAT
38 G SUGARS
Real margaritas don't contain corn-based sweeteners or artificial colors. Consider this the crutch of the amateur.

ROSE'S
Grenadine
(2 Tbsp)
80 CALORIES
0 G FAT
20 G SUGARS
Looks fruity. Tastes fruity. Yet in truth, there's not a shred of fruit in this syrupy cocktail staple.

CANADA DRY
Ginger Ale
(12 fl oz)
138 CALORIES
0 G FAT
36 G SUGARS
Better for you than 7Up or Sprite because Canada Dry also contains real ginger. Still, we prefer the stronger stuff.

Red Bull
(8.4 fl oz)
110 CALORIES
0 G FAT
27 G SUGARS
Be cautious when mixing alcohol with energy drinks. Research has shown people drinking both tend to underestimate their level of intoxication.

BEERS

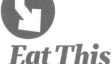

Eat This

Guinness Draught

(11.2 fl oz)

125 CALORIES

10 G CARBS

4% ALCOHOL

★

For our money, Guinness Draught has the best flavor-to-calorie ratio in the cooler.

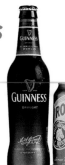
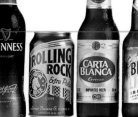
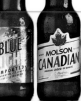

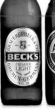
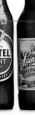

OTHER PICKS

Rolling Rock
(12 fl oz)
130 CALORIES
9.8 G CARBS
4.5% ALCOHOL
A first-rate session beer: crisp, refreshing, and surprisingly gentle in the calorie and carb departments.

Carta Blanca
(12 fl oz)
128 CALORIES
11 G CARBS
4% ALCOHOL
Perfect for a Michelada, one of Mexico's most popular drinks: Combine in a glass with a squeeze of lime, a dash of Worcestershire, and a few hits of hot sauce.

Labatt Blue Light
(11.5 fl oz)
108 CALORIES
8 G CARBS
4% ALCOHOL
Both Labatt and Michelob deliver more robustly flavored light beers. Labatt just does so for fewer calories.

Molson Canadian
(12 fl oz)
148 CALORIES
11 G CARBS
5% ALCOHOL
In the North American showdown, Canada wins out by a 45-calorie margin.

Keystone Premium
(12 fl oz)
111 CALORIES
5.8 G CARBS
4.4% ALCOHOL
Make this swap with a six-pack a week and you'll save more than 3 pounds a year.

Beck's Premier Light
(12 fl oz)
64 CALORIES
3.9 G CARBS
3.2% ALCOHOL
Among the lightest beers in the world, Beck's surprises by actually tasting like, well, beer.

Amstel Light
(12 fl oz)
95 CALORIES
5 G CARBS
3.5% ALCOHOL
One of our favorite light beers, precisely because it doesn't taste like one.

Leinenkugel's Honey Weiss
(12 fl oz)
149 CALORIES
12 G CARBS
4.9% ALCOHOL
Honey- and fruit-based beers tend to come with high calorie counts, so choose your weapon wisely.

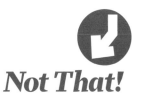

Guinness Extra Stout

(12 fl oz)

176 CALORIES

14 G CARBS

6% ALCOHOL

★

Mix up these two popular Guinness varieties and it could cost you 10 pounds or more over the course of a year if you drink just one a day.

OTHER PASSES

Michelob Honey Lager
(12 fl oz)
174 CALORIES
18.1 G CARBS
4.9% ALCOHOL
One of the most carb-heavy beers you'll find in the cooler.

Bass
(12 fl oz)
156 CALORIES
12 G CARBS
5.1% ALCOHOL
English-style ales tend to pack on the calories, and Bass, among the most famous of all ales, is no exception.

Bud Light
(12 fl oz)
110 CALORIES
7 G CARBS
4.2% ALCOHOL
In the world of light beers, you can choose a more robust-tasting beer than this version for roughly the same or fewer calories.

Pabst Blue Ribbon
(12 fl oz)
144 CALORIES
13 G CARBS
4.7% ALCOHOL
PBR has become a throwback favorite of the hipster crowd in recent years, which doesn't bode well for the bellies of America's young drinkers.

Budweiser Black Crown
(12 fl oz)
165 CALORIES
10 G CARBS
6% ALCOHOL
We appreciate Bud's desire to deliver a beer with a more assertive flavor, but this one packs more calories than 4 Hebrew National Hot Dogs.

Michelob Light
(12 fl oz)
123 CALORIES
9 G CARBS
4.1% ALCOHOL
The heaviest light beer in the cooler. A bottle of Guinness Draught has just 2 calories more.

Corona Extra
(12 fl oz)
148 CALORIES
14 G CARBS
4.6% ALCOHOL
For a beer that doesn't taste like much, it sure comes with plenty of calories.

Heineken
(12 fl oz)
135 CALORIES
10 G CARBS
5% ALCOHOL
It's one of the world's best-selling beers, but for 135 calories a can, we'd expect a lot more flavor.

CHAPTER 3

THE BEST

MEATS

AND

POULTRY

IT'S NO WONDER high-protein diets are the only thing more frequently Googled than the Kardashians these days: Eating a diet rich in protein boosts post-meal calorie burn by as much as 35 percent. This essential nutrient also builds healthy bones and muscle, providing your body with long-lasting energy. And protein-packed foods like beef, pork, and poultry just so happen to contain all nine essential amino acids—the ones your body can't produce on its own. The only problem? Load up on the wrong protein sources—especially highly processed meats—and you could be setting yourself up for serious ailments like high blood pressure, colon cancer, and cardiovascular disease, just to name a few. Not all animal proteins are created equal, so we're separating the filet mignon from the gristle and bringing you the healthiest meat and poultry picks.

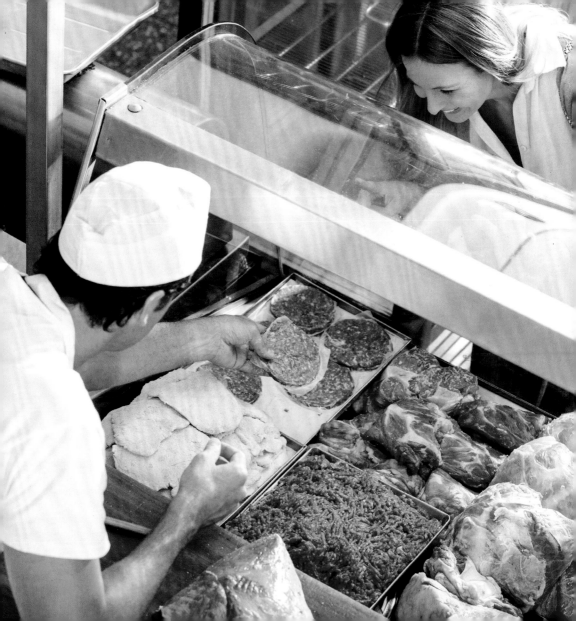

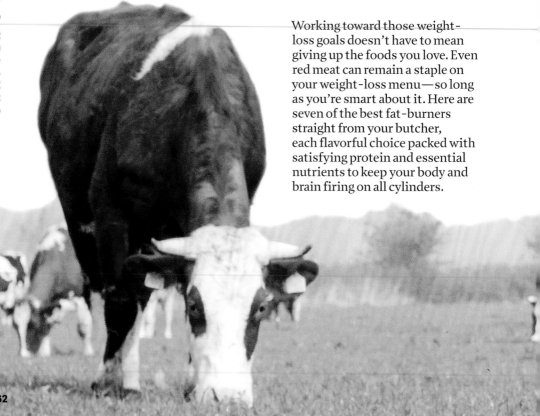

BEST MEATS FOR WEIGHT LOSS

Working toward those weight-loss goals doesn't have to mean giving up the foods you love. Even red meat can remain a staple on your weight-loss menu—so long as you're smart about it. Here are seven of the best fat-burners straight from your butcher, each flavorful choice packed with satisfying protein and essential nutrients to keep your body and brain firing on all cylinders.

1/ GRASS-FED BEEF

Red meat can be part of a healthy diet and even help you lose weight. Aside from delivering amino acids that increase satiety, speed up metabolism, and build lean muscle, beef contains healthy doses of iron, zinc, niacin, selenium, vitamin E, and B vitamins—nutrients that support blood formation as well as brain and nervous system function. When it comes to steak or burgers, always go grass-fed. It may ding your wallet, but it'll also define your abs. Grass-fed beef is naturally leaner and has fewer calories than conventional meat: A lean 7-ounce conventional strip steak has 410 calories and 16 grams of fat. But a 7-ounce grass-fed strip steak has only 250 calories and under 6 grams of fat. Studies show that grass-fed meat also contains higher levels of omega-3 fatty acids, which have been shown to reduce the risk of heart disease.

NUTRITION FACTS
PER 7-OZ SERVING

250 CALORIES

5.8 G FAT (2.2 G saturated)

139 MG CHOLINE

49.4 G PROTEIN

44.9 MG OMEGA-3S

Eat This!

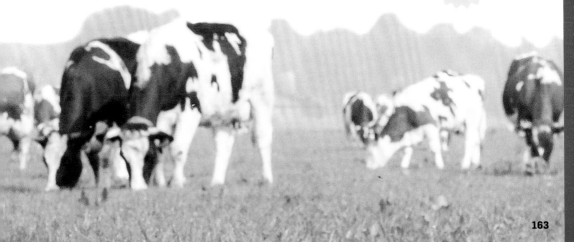

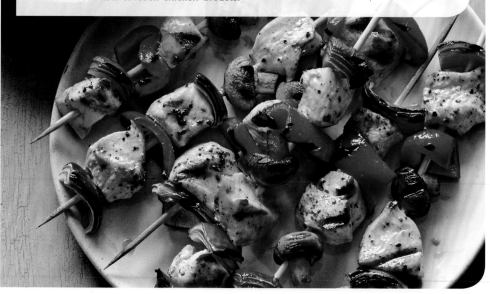

2/ **CHICKEN**

Eat This!

The bird's the word when it comes to weight loss: A 3-ounce chicken breast serving is just 145 calories, yet packs 17.4 grams of muscle-boosting protein. And it's easy to see why this poultry is so popular: It's affordable, easy to prepare, and lower in fat than many other types of meat. Although dark meat contains slightly more fat than white meat (15 grams versus 7), it's this extra fat that provides its juicy texture and rich flavor. Both white and dark meat chicken are excellent sources of protein, niacin, phosphorous, B_6, B_{12}, vitamin D, calcium, iron, and zinc—just be sure to go skinless!

⤷ Amp up the flavor in your chicken dishes with these pro tips: eatthis.com/how-to-cook-chicken-breasts.

NUTRITION FACTS

PER 3-OZ SERVING

144.6 CALORIES

7.8 G FAT (2.1 G saturated)

56.4 MG CHOLINE

17.4 G PROTEIN

100.8 MG OMEGA-3S

3/ Turkey

■ Lean and protein-rich, this bird deserves a regular place on your table (not just on Thanksgiving!). A 4-ounce turkey burger patty has just 151 calories, but packs 33.6 grams of filling protein and only 8 grams of fat. Additionally, turkey is rich in DHA omega-3 acids— 22.4 mg per serving—which has been shown to boost brain function, improve your mood, and turn off fat genes, preventing fat cells from growing in size. Just make sure you gobble up white meat only; dark contains too much fat.

NUTRITION FACTS
PER 4-OZ SERVING

151.2 CALORIES

0.8 G FAT (0.4 G saturated)

94.4 MG CHOLINE

33.6 G PROTEIN

22.4 MG OMEGA-3S

4/ Buffalo and Bison

■ While grass-fed beef is an excellent choice, bison's profile has been rising in recent years, and for good reason: It has half the fat of and fewer calories than beef. According to the USDA, while a 90%-lean hamburger may average 10 grams of fat, a comparatively sized buffalo burger rings in at 2 grams of fat with 24 grams of protein, making it one of the leanest meats around. Taking a chance on this unexpected meat also yields two healthy bonuses: In just one serving you'll get a full day's allowance of vitamin B_{12}, which can boost energy and help shut down the genes responsible for insulin resistance and the formation of fat cells; additionally, since bison are naturally grass-fed, you can confidently down your burger knowing it's free of the hormones and pollutants than can manifest themselves in your belly fat.

NUTRITION FACTS
PER 3-OZ SERVING

122 CALORIES

2.1 G FAT (0.8 G saturated)

97.6 MG CHOLINE

24.2 G PROTEIN

34 MG OMEGA-3S

5/ Ostrich

■ Lower that eyebrow you're raising. Ostrich meat is a rising star of the poultry world. While it's technically red and has the rich taste of beef, it has less fat than turkey or chicken—just 6 grams in a 3-ounce serving. Plus, one serving has 200 percent of the daily recommended allowance of vitamin B$_{12}$. This exotic meat can also help whittle your middle: Ostrich contains 55.8 milligrams of choline, a nutrient that aids fat loss. And it's not as hard to find as it sounds—ostrich is increasingly available in supermarkets around the country.

NUTRITION FACTS
PER 3-OZ SERVING

149 CALORIES

6 G FAT (1.5 G saturated)

55.8 MG CHOLINE

22.2 G PROTEIN

38.2 MG OMEGA-3S

6/ Pork Tenderloin

■ A longtime enemy of doctors and dieters, pork is increasingly being embraced as a healthy option in recent years—as long as you choose the right cut. Your best bet is tenderloin: A 3-ounce serving has slightly less fat than a skinless chicken breast, but packs 16.8 grams of protein and 65.4 milligrams of choline (in the latter case, about half what you'd get in a large egg). Don't believe you can eat pork without looking a little porky, too? In a study published in the journal *Nutrients,* scientists asked 144 overweight people to eat a diet rich in fresh lean pork. After three months, the group saw a significant reduction in waist size, BMI, and belly fat, with no reduction in muscle mass! They speculate that the amino acid profile of pork protein may contribute to greater fat burning.

NUTRITION FACTS
PER 3-OZ SERVING

91.5 CALORIES

2.7 G FAT (0.9 G saturated)

65.4 MG CHOLINE

16.8 G PROTEIN

11.7 MG OMEGA-3S

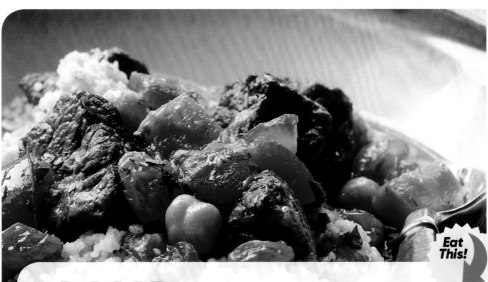

Eat This!

7/ LAMB

Craving better zzzs? Don't count sheep, eat lamb! Lamb is one of the highest sources of tryptophan, an amino acid found in most meats, that has powerful sleep-inducing effects. A recent study among insomniacs found that just ¼ gram—about what you'll find in 3 ounces of lean meat—was enough to significantly increase hours of deep sleep. And that can translate into an easy slim-down. Pair your tryptophan-rich lamb with a carbohydrate-rich food like brown rice (also high in sleep-supporting magnesium and vitamins B_3 and B_6) to enhance the snoozing effects. And when shopping for lamb, follow similar health guidelines as you do for beef—look for cuts labeled "lean" that have little visible fat on them. Lamb chops, legs, and roasts tend to be healthier than blade or ground lamb.

NUTRITION FACTS

PER 3-OZ SERVING

187.2 CALORIES

7.5 G FAT
(2.7 G saturated)

108.6 MG CHOLINE

28.2 G PROTEIN

100.8 MG OMEGA-3S

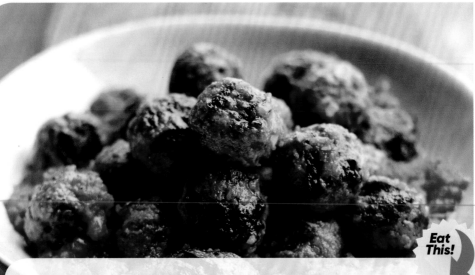

Eat This!

8/ GROUND BEEF

Going ground? Limit weekly consumption to roughly 3 ounces. Consuming fat in excess, healthy or not, results in one thing: flab. Ground beef is sold with 5 to 30 percent fat, giving you the option to choose from 80 to 95 percent lean varieties. However, the leaner the cut, the lower the vitamin and mineral content. We recommend going for 90 percent lean, which yields 182 calories, 9 grams of fat, and up to 23 grams of protein per 3-ounce serving. And for sure, go for grass-fed. It's naturally lower in calories and fat than grain-fed beef, but contains more heart-healthy omega-3s, less saturated fat, and as much as four times the vitamin E.

↘ Beef up your recipe repertoire: eatthis.com/healthy-ground-beef-recipes.

NUTRITION FACTS

PER 3-OZ SERVING OF 90%-LEAN MEAT

182 CALORIES

9.4 G FAT
(3.7 G saturated)

73 MG CHOLINE

22.6 G PROTEIN

34.8 OMEGA-3S

5 Best Cuts of Beef

Stick to these leaner, healthier cuts of steak and watch those pounds melt away.

1. Sirloin Tip Side Steak → We've written about this great cut before, but in case you missed our post on what to eat for flat abs, you should know that steak can be a part of a balanced diet—really!

If you're looking to lose weight, choosing a leaner cut like sirloin tip side steak can help—it has significantly less fat and saturated fat than some other popular steak cuts, like rib eye, but still packs plenty of protein to keep you full and satisfied. It's even been shown that lean meat like this steak can have a thermogenic effect, meaning some of the calories in that lean meat are actually burned off while your body digests.

2. Top Round Steak → Another lean steak cut, top round is a great option when you're craving red meat but still want to make a smart, healthful choice. It's lean (only about 3 grams of fat per 3-ounce cooked serving, according to the USDA), but still flavorful—and, even better, it tends to be more tender than some other lean cuts of beef, so you don't need to marinate it or do a lot of prep work prior to cooking.

3. Eye of Round Steak → Another steak cut that contains less fat and saturated fat than more popular picks. Eye of round, though, can be a little tougher than the two options above, so marinate it for optimal flavor. If you're going to go this route, choose oils with good-for-you fats, like olive oil, and something less caloric to complement it, like lemon juice or vinegar, that will boost the overall flavor of the meat and help tenderize it.

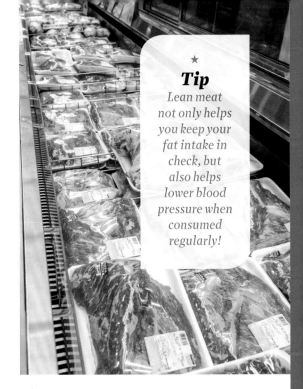

★
Tip
Lean meat not only helps you keep your fat intake in check, but also helps lower blood pressure when consumed regularly!

4. Bottom Round Steak → Much like the steaks already listed, a 3-ounce portion of bottom round is lean (a cooked portion contains about 8 grams of fat, according to the USDA). It can also be a little on the tougher side, since it comes from the posterior part of the cow. Marinate and prepare it as you would an eye of round for best flavor and tenderness.

5. Filet Mignon → Go for a pricier cut of meat if you can afford to do so. Filet mignon is the leanest choice, but also the most expensive. So, it may not be an everyday option, but as a special-occasion meal, it's a great way to indulge without expanding your waistline.

MEATLESS MEAL MAKERS

If you're vegetarian or vegan, or just want
to cut back on meat from time to time,
here are some healthy—and
protein-packed—meatless alternatives
so good you won't miss the real thing.

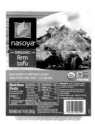

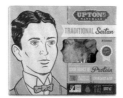

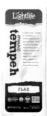

Eat This!

TOFU
Nasoya Organic Firm TofuPlus

PER 3-OZ SERVING

70 CALORIES

3 G FAT (0 G saturated)

0 MG SODIUM

2 G CARBS

7 G PROTEIN

▧ Going vegetarian often increases your risk of B$_{12}$, calcium, and iron deficiency. But thanks to Nasoya's Tofu-Plus line, filling in nutritional gaps has never been easier. A mere 3-ounce serving of the stuff provides 20 percent of the day's calcium and B$_{12}$, 6 percent of the day's bicep-building iron, and 14 percent of your recommended pro-tein intake. Firm tofu is best enjoyed roasted, grilled, stewed, or sautéed—and eaten in moderation.

SEITAN
Upton's Naturals Traditional Seitan

PER 2-OZ SERVING

100 CALORIES

1.5 G FAT (0 G saturated)

264 MG SODIUM

7 G CARBS

15 G PROTEIN

▧ If you're wary of eating too much soy, seitan (pronounced SAY-tan) is a solid alternative. It's derived from wheat gluten and is a great source of protein. Though there are a number of seitan options on supermarket shelves, we're partial to Upton's because of its short and straightforward ingredient list. They use a blend of wheat gluten, whole-wheat flour, water, garlic, sea salt, onion, and soy sauce. To prepare it, simply pan fry with a small amount of oil and throw into stir-fries, stews, or sandwiches.

TEMPEH
Lightlife Organic Flax Tempeh

PER 3-OZ SERVING

160 CALORIES

7 G FAT (1 G saturated)

10 MG SODIUM

9 G CARBS

15 G PROTEIN

▧ Unlike tofu, which is made from soybean curd, tempeh is made from fermented whole soybeans and, there-fore, is less processed (read: has fewer phytoestrogens) and is more protein-packed than its spongy cousin. We're fans of Lightlife's Flax Tempeh (comprised of soybeans, mood-boosting flaxseeds, and brown rice) because it has 15 percent of the day's iron and a whopping 15 grams of satiating protein. Try it diced in a curry or grilled like a steak.

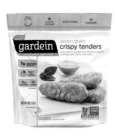

NUGGET ALTERNATIVE

Gardein Seven Grain Crispy Tenders

PER 3-PIECE SERVING

150 CALORIES

6.8 G FAT (0 G saturated)

360 MG SODIUM

12 G CARBS

12 G PROTEIN

■ Craving something fried but don't want to throw your diet off track? Heat up a trio of Gardein Seven Grain Crispy Tenders. With a mere 150 calories and an impressive 12 grams of satiating protein (from whole-food ingredients like amaranth, quinoa, wheat gluten, and pea protein, no less), these nuggets are sure to kick any fast-food craving to the curb. Keep them in the freezer and stock some organic ketchup in your fridge, so you're prepared for a snack craving anytime, day or night.

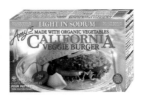

VEGGIE BURGER

Amy's Light in Sodium California Veggie Burger

PER PATTY

110 CALORIES

4 G FAT (0 G saturated)

250 MG SODIUM

16 G CARBS

5 G PROTEIN

■ Veg out on this meatless marvel! Amy's veggie burger is packed with organic ingredients like mushrooms, onions, bulgur, celery, carrots, oats, and walnuts. If you're ever craving a comforting bowl of mushroom risotto, save yourself the unnecessary calories and fat by grilling this veggie burger instead. The patty is rife with umami, garlicky notes that only taste sinful, and the flavor profile remains authentic to the ingredients.

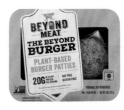

"MEAT-LIKE" BURGER

Beyond Meat Beyond Burger

PER PATTY

290 CALORIES

22 G FAT (5 G saturated)

450 MG SODIUM

6 G CARBS

20 G PROTEIN

■ If you appreciate a beef-like appearance, taste, and texture, this is the burger for you. You'll find these rounds (comprised of non-GMO ingredients) in the meat section. When cooked, it's hard to tell apart from ground beef; it's juicy with a strikingly meat-like flavor. It even "bleeds" (chalk that up to beet juice)—plus packs more than twice the iron and nearly half the saturated fat of an 80%-lean beef burger.

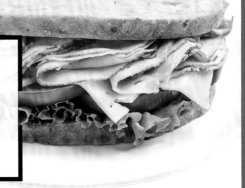

DELI MEATS DECODED

Brown-bagging it at lunch isn't always healthier, especially if you're tucking into a sandwich full of not-so-healthy deli meats. Many of your favorite sliced meats are pumped with harmful preservatives, additives, nitrates, and heaps of sodium—a known contributor to hypertension, heart disease, and a major belly bloater. However, not all those deli cuts should leave you cold: Though there are countless meats you'd be better off avoiding, there are also plenty of healthy options out there if you know where to look.

Roasted Turkey

Applegate Naturals Roasted Turkey Breast

PER 2 OZ (56 G)

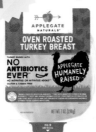

50 CALORIES

0 G FAT
(0 G saturated)

360 MG SODIUM

0 G CARBS

12 G PROTEIN

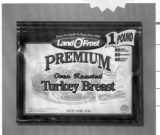

Land O'Frost Premium Oven Roasted Turkey Breast

PER 4 SLICES (50 G)

80 CALORIES

5 G FAT
(1 G saturated)

550 MG SODIUM

1 G CARBS

8 G PROTEIN

Honey-Baked Ham

Applegate Naturals Uncured Honey Ham

PER 2 OZ (56 G)

70 CALORIES

1.5 G FAT
(0.5 G saturated)

450 MG SODIUM

3 G CARBS

10 G PROTEIN

Eat This!

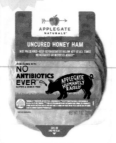

Not That!

Oscar Mayer Deli Fresh Honey Ham

PER 2 OZ (56 G)

60 CALORIES

1.5 G FAT
(0.5 G saturated)

510 MG SODIUM

2 G CARBS

9 G PROTEIN

Roast Beef

Applegate Organics Roast Beef

PER 2 OZ (56 G)

80 CALORIES

3 G FAT
(1 G saturated)

320 MG SODIUM

0 G CARBS

12 G PROTEIN

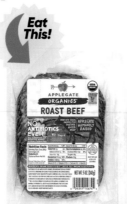

Eat This!

Not That!

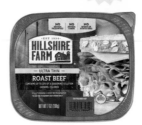

Hillshire Farm Deli Select Ultra Thin Sliced Roast Beef

PER 2 OZ (56 G)

70 CALORIES

3 G FAT
(1 G saturated)

550 MG SODIUM

1 G CARBS

11 G PROTEIN

Rotisserie-Style Chicken

Hormel Natural Choice Rotisserie-Style Deli Chicken Breast

Eat This!

PER 2 OZ (56 G)

50 CALORIES

1 G FAT
(0 G saturated)

470 MG SODIUM

0 G CARBS

11 G PROTEIN

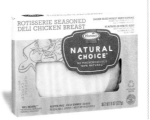

Not That!

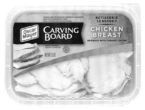

Oscar Mayer Carving Board Rotisserie Seasoned Chicken Breast

PER 2 OZ (56 G)

60 CALORIES

1 G FAT
(0 G saturated)

470 MG SODIUM

0 G CARBS

12 G PROTEIN

Bologna

Saag's German Brand Bologna

PER 1 OZ (28 G)

70 CALORIES

7.5 G FAT
(2.5 G saturated)

210 MG SODIUM

2 G CARBS

3.5 G PROTEIN

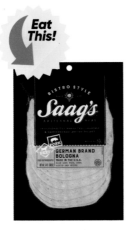

Eat This!

Not That!

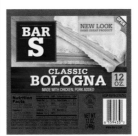

Bar-S Classic Bologna

PER 1 SLICE (32 G)

90 CALORIES

7 G FAT
(2 G saturated)

360 MG SODIUM

2 G CARBS

4 G PROTEIN

Salami

Applegate Naturals Uncured Genoa Salami

PER 1 OZ (28 G)

100 CALORIES

7 G FAT
(3 G saturated)

480 MG SODIUM

0 G CARBS

8 G PROTEIN

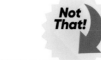

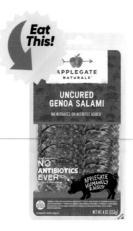

Eat This!

Not That!

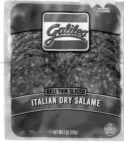

Gallo and Galileo Salame

PER 1 OZ (28 G)

110 CALORIES

9 G FAT
(3 G saturated)

480 MG SODIUM

1 G CARBS

6 G PROTEIN

Pastrami

Saag's Pastrami

PER 2 OZ (56 G)

80 CALORIES

3 G FAT
(1 G saturated)

560 MG SODIUM

0 G CARBS

12 G PROTEIN

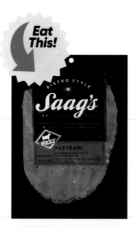

Eat This!

Not That!

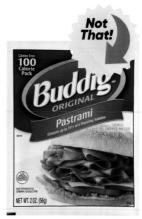

Buddig Original Pastrami

PER 2 OZ (56 G)

100 CALORIES

7 G FAT
(3 G saturated)

600 MG SODIUM

1 G CARBS

9 G PROTEIN

Pepperoni

Applegate Naturals Uncured Mini Pork Pepperoni

PER 1 OZ (28 G)

50 CALORIES

3.5 G FAT
(1.5 G saturated)

350 MG SODIUM

0 G CARBS

3 G PROTEIN

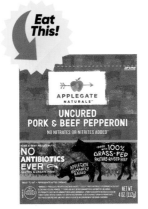

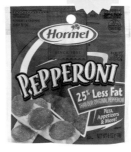

Hormel Pepperoni— 25% Less Fat

PER 1.1 OZ (30 G)

120 CALORIES

10 G FAT
(3.5 G saturated)

610 MG SODIUM

0 G CARBS

7 G PROTEIN

Meat Alternatives

Tofurky Oven Roasted Deli Slices

PER 5 SLICES (52 G)

100 CALORIES

3 G FAT
(0 G saturated)

300 MG SODIUM

6 G CARBS

13 G PROTEIN

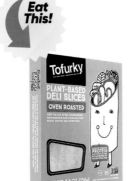

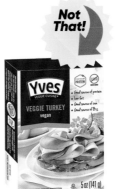

Yves Veggie Deli Turkey Slices

PER 4 SLICES (50 G)

100 CALORIES

1.5 G FAT
(0 G saturated)

340 MG SODIUM

5 G CARBS

16 G PROTEIN

CHAPTER 4

THE BEST (& WORST)

SEAFOOD

THERE'S NOTHING FISHY about the health benefits attributed to your favorite seafood. Health experts have long touted the nutritional benefits of fish, like their heart-healthy omega-3 fatty acids, high-quality protein, metabolism-friendly selenium, energy-boosting B_{12}, and inflammation-fighting vitamin D.

However, it can be tricky to balance your healthy eating ambitions with concerns about everything from mercury levels to heart-healthiness to sustainability. With that in mind, we've ranked the most popular seafood items out there, making it easier than ever to determine which ones are a real catch and which ones you'd be better off throwing back.

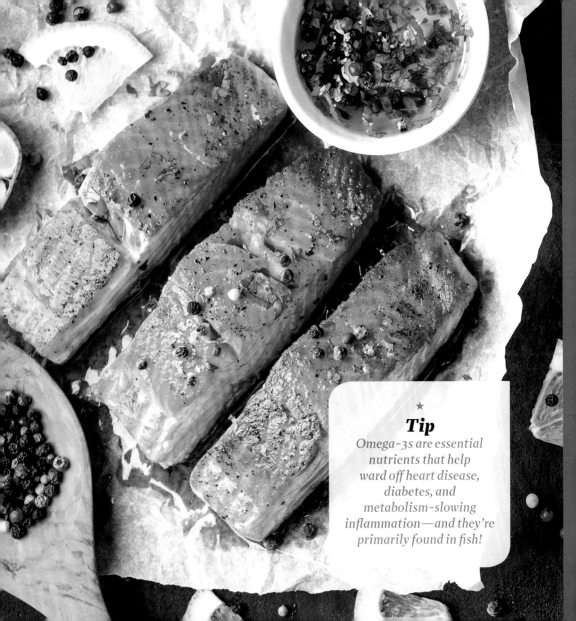

★

Tip

Omega-3s are essential nutrients that help ward off heart disease, diabetes, and metabolism-slowing inflammation—and they're primarily found in fish!

THE MOST NUTRITIOUS & SAFEST SEAFOOD

Eat This ↘

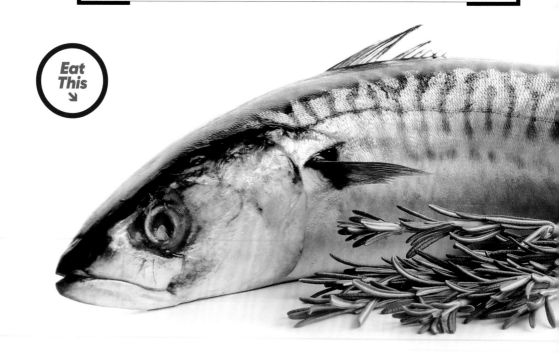

In order to make the best list, these treats from the sea had to have moderate levels of mercury or better (fewer than 350 ppb), be a good source of protein, and have no less than 200 milligrams of omega-3s. In other words, these fish and seafood varieties are actually worth your time and money—and won't make you sick in exchange for their nutrients.

1/ATLANTIC MACKEREL

Listed on Seafood Watch's "Super Green List," this best fish to eat is a triple treat: it's low in mercury, provides almost eight times the recommended omega-3 intake per day, and is classified as a Seafood Watch "Best Choice" in terms of sustainability. Just watch out for canned mackerel, which can have mercury levels up to 586 ppb.

NUTRITION FACTS

PER 3-OZ SERVING

174 CALORIES

11.8 G FAT (2.8 G saturated)

76 MG SODIUM

15.8 G PROTEIN

1,954 MG OMEGA-3S

45 MERCURY LEVELS (PARTS PER BILLION)

Eat This!

2/ Pink Salmon

■ Pink salmon, also known as humpback salmon because of the male's distinctive humpback that occurs during their spawning phase, is native to the cold waters of the Pacific and Arctic Oceans. If eating muscle-building protein and heart-healthy omega-3 levels isn't for you, you can also chow down on this fish's roe, which is a common source for caviar.

NUTRITION FACTS

PER 3-OZ SERVING

108 CALORIES

3.5 G FAT (0.7 G saturated)

64 MG SODIUM

17.4 G PROTEIN

438 MG OMEGA-3S

37 MERCURY LEVELS (PARTS PER BILLION)

3/ Atlantic and Pacific Halibut

■ This meaty white fish's mild flavor makes it immensely versatile. Besides being low-cal, it's also filling—making it a great weight-loss food. Research attributes the satiating factor of white fish like halibut to its impressive protein content and influence on serotonin, one of the key hormones responsible for regulating appetite. Try eating more Pacific than Atlantic fish since the Atlantic halibut population is dwindling.

NUTRITION FACTS

PER 3-OZ SERVING

186 CALORIES

2.7 G FAT (0.6 G saturated)

139 MG SODIUM

37.9 G PROTEIN

396 MG OMEGA-3S

261 MERCURY LEVELS (PARTS PER BILLION)

4/ Canned Sardines in Oil

■ Despite their diminutive size, sardines pack a nutritional punch: a mere 3 ounces provides 12 percent of your recommended daily intake of vitamin D and 64 percent of selenium, a mineral that plays a key role in metabolism, immunity, and reproductive health. Canned versions are known to be high in sodium, so be sure to consume them in moderation or look for low-sodium versions.

NUTRITION FACTS

PER 3-OZ SERVING

177 CALORIES

9.7 G FAT (1.3 G saturated)

261 MG SODIUM

21 G PROTEIN

835 MG OMEGA-3S

79 MERCURY LEVELS (PARTS PER BILLION)

5/ Alaskan Pollock

■ Despite their shared name, Atlantic pollock are larger and darker than the Alaskan pollock, which is actually a different species. Another big difference? The Atlantic fish has a much higher omega-3 content. Its mild flavor and delicate texture make it extremely versatile, so feel free to dress it up however you'd like!

NUTRITION FACTS

PER 3-OZ SERVING

78 CALORIES

0.8 G FAT (0.1 G saturated)

73 MG SODIUM

16.5 G PROTEIN

358 MG OMEGA-3S

160 MERCURY LEVELS (PARTS PER BILLION)

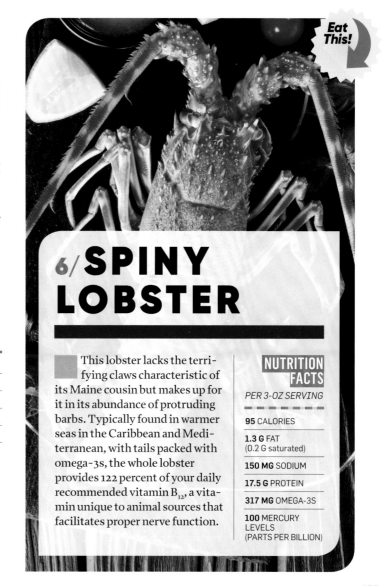

Eat This!

6/ SPINY LOBSTER

■ This lobster lacks the terrifying claws characteristic of its Maine cousin but makes up for it in its abundance of protruding barbs. Typically found in warmer seas in the Caribbean and Mediterranean, with tails packed with omega-3s, the whole lobster provides 122 percent of your daily recommended vitamin B_{12}, a vitamin unique to animal sources that facilitates proper nerve function.

NUTRITION FACTS

PER 3-OZ SERVING

95 CALORIES

1.3 G FAT (0.2 G saturated)

150 MG SODIUM

17.5 G PROTEIN

317 MG OMEGA-3S

100 MERCURY LEVELS (PARTS PER BILLION)

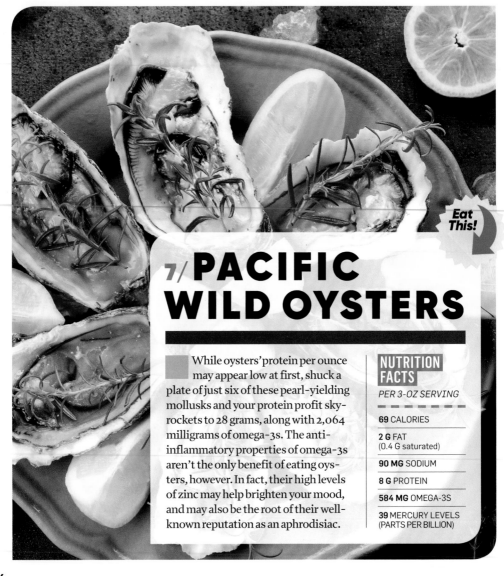

Eat This!

7/ PACIFIC WILD OYSTERS

While oysters' protein per ounce may appear low at first, shuck a plate of just six of these pearl-yielding mollusks and your protein profit sky-rockets to 28 grams, along with 2,064 milligrams of omega-3s. The anti-inflammatory properties of omega-3s aren't the only benefit of eating oysters, however. In fact, their high levels of zinc may help brighten your mood, and may also be the root of their well-known reputation as an aphrodisiac.

NUTRITION FACTS

PER 3-OZ SERVING

69 CALORIES

2 G FAT
(0.4 G saturated)

90 MG SODIUM

8 G PROTEIN

584 MG OMEGA-3S

39 MERCURY LEVELS
(PARTS PER BILLION)

8/ European Anchovy

■ You may already use it in your Caesar salad dressings, but anchovies' high omega-3 levels— five times your recommended daily intake—might give you reason to find more ways to introduce this power food into your cooking arsenal.

NUTRITION FACTS

PER 3-OZ SERVING

111 CALORIES

4.1 G FAT (1.1 G saturated)

88 MG SODIUM

17.3 G PROTEIN

1,231 MG OMEGA-3S

103 MERCURY LEVELS (PARTS PER BILLION)

9/ Atlantic Herring

■ Herring is the super-food of the sea. Besides being one of this list's top three sources of omega-3s per ounce, it's also one of the best sources of vitamin B_{12}— over 160 percent RDI per ounce—and vitamin D—11 percent RDI per ounce. To cook, grill herring and dress with a mixture of mustard, lemon juice, and its own oil for a dinner packed with protein and healthy fats. Serve with a side of sautéed kale and quinoa to round out your plate.

NUTRITION FACTS

PER 3-OZ SERVING

134 CALORIES

7.7 G FAT (1.7 G saturated)

76 MG SODIUM

15.3 G PROTEIN

56% RDA SELENIUM

484% RDA VITAMIN B_{12}

1,336 MG OMEGA-3S

43 MERCURY LEVELS (PARTS PER BILLION)

10/ Sockeye Salmon

■ Sockeye salmon is a much deeper red than other salmon species because it noshes on krill, a type of small shrimp. Besides being a great source of omega-3s, a 3-ounce portion ranks as your seventh best source of vitamin D, with 112 percent of your recommended intake. This sun vitamin is rarely found in food but is important in warding off breast and prostate cancer, as well as boosting heart health.

NUTRITION FACTS

PER 3-OZ SERVING

111 CALORIES

4 G FAT (0.7 G saturated)

66 MG SODIUM

18.9 G PROTEIN

613 MG OMEGA-3S

39 MERCURY LEVELS (PARTS PER BILLION)

11/ Bluefish

■ These fish are strong and aggressive, which is why lifeguards are taught to remove swimmers from the water when they see any signs of bluefish feeding frenzies. During these frenzies, bluefish will continue to attack and eat anything in their way even after they've had their fill. This overeating is most likely the reason that bluefish have a fairly high mercury level. So be sure to consume this fish in moderation—but when you do, you'll still get a great source of omega-3s and filling protein.

NUTRITION FACTS
PER 3-OZ SERVING

105 CALORIES

3.6 G FAT (0.8 G saturated)

51 MG SODIUM

17 G PROTEIN

655 MG OMEGA-3S

350 MERCURY LEVELS (PARTS PER BILLION)

12/ Wild Rainbow Trout

■ Following a rainbow can lead you to a pot of gold—at least when it comes to your health. While wild rainbow trout are loaded with omega-3s and lean protein, because of moderate PCB contamination due to their lake habitats, the Environmental Defense Fund (EDF) recommends kids limit consumption of this tasty trout to two to three meals a month, depending on their age.

NUTRITION FACTS
PER 3-OZ SERVING

101 CALORIES

2.9 G FAT (0.6 G saturated)

26 MG SODIUM

17.4 G PROTEIN

499 MG OMEGA-3S

344 MERCURY LEVELS (PARTS PER BILLION)

13/ Squid

■ Technically, and quite surprisingly, a squid is a type of mollusk: the same family as mussels and clams. This is because squid used to have a shell just like these other shellfish, but over time, it became thinner and more cartilage-like. However, shell or not, squid should still earn a place on your plate: It's so high in omega-3s that it's a source of omega-3 supplement oil.

NUTRITION FACTS
PER 3-OZ SERVING

78 CALORIES

1.2 G FAT (0.3 G saturated)

37 MG SODIUM

13.2 G PROTEIN

415 MG OMEGA-3S

44 MERCURY LEVELS (PARTS PER BILLION)

14/ Mussels

■ Farmed or wild, mussels are a great source of protein and omega-3s, and a super source of vitamin B_{12} with 170 percent of your daily recommended intake per 3 ounces (which is equivalent to only five mussels—way fewer than you'll get in any classic mussel dish). And while other farmed seafood gets a bad rap, as it turns out, farmed mussels are raised in an environmentally responsible manner that may actually improve the surrounding marine environment.

NUTRITION FACTS
PER 3-OZ SERVING

73 CALORIES

1.9 G FAT (0.4 G saturated)

243 MG SODIUM

10.1 G PROTEIN

375 MG OMEGA-3S

28 MERCURY LEVELS
(PARTS PER BILLION)

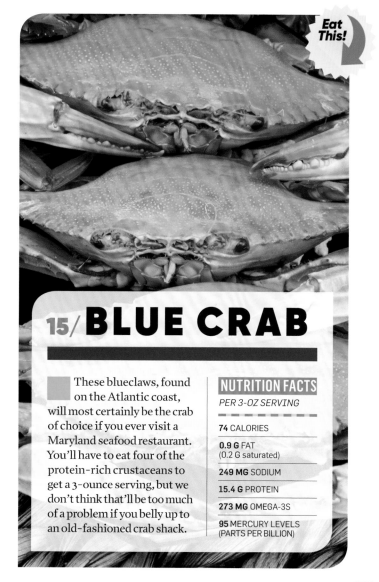

Eat This!

15/ BLUE CRAB

■ These blueclaws, found on the Atlantic coast, will most certainly be the crab of choice if you ever visit a Maryland seafood restaurant. You'll have to eat four of the protein-rich crustaceans to get a 3-ounce serving, but we don't think that'll be too much of a problem if you belly up to an old-fashioned crab shack.

NUTRITION FACTS
PER 3-OZ SERVING

74 CALORIES

0.9 G FAT
(0.2 G saturated)

249 MG SODIUM

15.4 G PROTEIN

273 MG OMEGA-3S

95 MERCURY LEVELS
(PARTS PER BILLION)

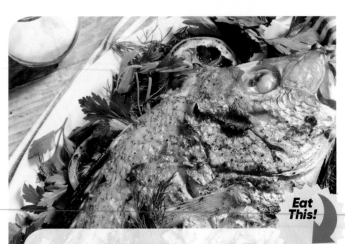

Eat This!

16/ GREY AND RED SNAPPER

The red snapper is one of the Gulf of Mexico's signature fish, and for many commercial fishermen, it's their primary source of profit. In fact, back in 2011, gulf fishermen harvested 3.6 million pounds of red snapper that were valued at $11.4 million. We're definitely on board with its popularity—the fish is a great source of lean protein to help build muscle, boost your metabolism, and increase feelings of fullness.

NUTRITION FACTS

PER 3-OZ SERVING

85 CALORIES

1.1 G FAT
(0.2 G saturated)

54 MG SODIUM

17.4 G PROTEIN

264 MG OMEGA-3S

230 MERCURY LEVELS (PARTS PER BILLION)

17/ Wild Striped Bass

Stripers have longevity on their side, with many living to over 30 years of age. Their long life may increase their levels of mercury, which accounts for the 295 ppb count in every 3-ounce serving. It's also a reason for their large size—the world record for striped bass is over 81 pounds! And all that meat is packed with omega-3s and vitamin B_{12}.

NUTRITION FACTS

PER 3-OZ SERVING

82 CALORIES

2 G FAT (0.4 G saturated)

59 MG SODIUM

15 G PROTEIN

641 MG OMEGA-3S

295 MERCURY LEVELS (PARTS PER BILLION)

18/ Black Sea Bass

■ Inhabiting the eastern coast from Maine to Florida, this petite fish is low in calories and fat, is a good source of selenium, and contains a healthy helping of omega-3 fatty acids. Besides finding it in restaurants, the black sea bass is also a popular recreational catch. Chilean sea bass, however, shouldn't be consumed as often, as its mercury levels are 357 ppb.

NUTRITION FACTS

PER 3-OZ SERVING

82 CALORIES

1.7 G FAT (0.4 G saturated)

58 MG SODIUM

15.7 G PROTEIN

506 MG OMEGA-3S

120 MERCURY LEVELS (PARTS PER BILLION)

19/ Skipjack Tuna

■ Skipjack tuna is smaller than its yellowfin cousin, which helps it to soak up fewer toxins. Even with its smaller size, it still has almost 200 ppb of mercury, so be mindful of the frequency with which you eat it—especially if you purchase bulk-buying mecca Costco's new sustainable (and affordable) skipjack tuna brand. So, what makes tuna sustainable in the first place? It's FAD-free: fish aggregating devices (FADs) are large nets that can kill sharks, rays, and turtles that are caught along with the tuna.

NUTRITION FACTS

PER 3-OZ SERVING

88 CALORIES

0.9 G FAT (0.3 G saturated)

31 MG SODIUM

18.7 G PROTEIN

217 MG OMEGA-3S

198 MERCURY LEVELS (PARTS PER BILLION)

20/ Dungeness Crab

■ Earning their name from a town in Washington where they're found, Dungeness crabs are not a top source of omega-3s per ounce, but when it comes to serving size, a single crab is just under 6 ounces. If you eat the whole thing, you're looking at 28 grams of protein and 500 milligrams of omega-3s per crab. Seafood Watch—one of the most popular sustainable seafood advisory lists—has given the crab a sustainable seafood rating of "Best Choice."

NUTRITION FACTS

PER 3-OZ SERVING

73 CALORIES

0.8 G FAT (0.1 G saturated)

251 MG SODIUM

14.8 G PROTEIN

261 MG OMEGA-3S

120 MERCURY LEVELS (PARTS PER BILLION)

THE LEAST NUTRITIOUS AND/OR MOST DANGEROUS SEAFOOD

★
Tip

Buying frozen fish is a great way to always have a good source of protein in the house. But avoid anything breaded, or with labels like "battered" and "crunchy," which pack on extra calories, fat, and sodium.

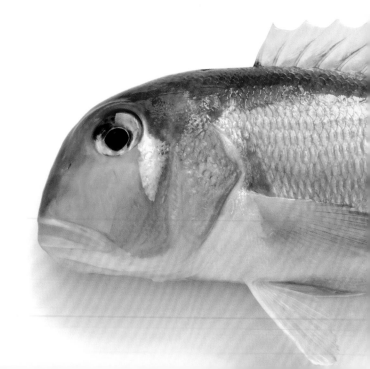

While there's a ton of healthy seafood out there, there's also a boatload of options that don't deserve a spot on your plate. These ten types of seafood are definite don'ts, courtesy of a combination of factors, including their protein and omega-3 content and their mercury levels. And while some aren't so bad—we're looking at you, shrimp—you could still get more bang for your nutritional buck elsewhere.

1/ TILEFISH

Tilefish has the highest mercury level among all varieties of fish, with 883 parts of mercury per billion. And those you find from the Gulf of Mexico? Mercury levels can reach up to 1,445 ppb! That's 45 percent higher than the USDA allowed maximum. Skip this fish!

NUTRITION FACTS
PER 3-OZ SERVING

82 CALORIES

1.96 G FAT (0.4 G saturated)

45 MG SODIUM

14.9 G PROTEIN

365 MG OMEGA-3S

883 MERCURY LEVELS (PARTS PER BILLION)

Not That!

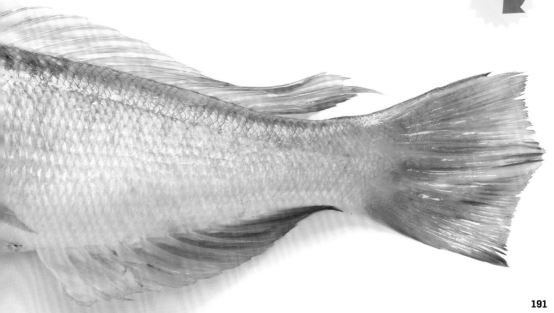

2/ Swordfish

Swordfish contains dangerously high levels of mercury, an element that acts as an endocrine disruptor. An endocrine disruptor is a fake hormone that tricks your body into holding on to fat, burning fewer calories, and reducing levels of leptin—a hormone that regulates appetite. Its high levels of selenium and vitamin D are what make it better for you than some choices—just consume it in moderation.

NUTRITION FACTS

PER 3-OZ SERVING

122 CALORIES

5.7 G FAT (1.4 G saturated)

69 MG SODIUM

16.7 G PROTEIN

641 MG OMEGA-3S

893 MERCURY LEVELS (PARTS PER BILLION)

3/ Tilapia

Deficient in omega-3s, and typically accompanied by an astronomical level of omega-6s, this popular fish is worse for your belly than bacon. Additionally, most tilapia is farm-raised and fed a diet of corn instead of lake plants and algae, making them the turducken of seafood: junk stuffed with junk surrounded by junk.

NUTRITION FACTS

PER 3-OZ SERVING

81 CALORIES

1.4 G FAT (0.5 G saturated)

44 MG SODIUM

17 G PROTEIN

77 MG OMEGA-3S

19 MERCURY LEVELS (PARTS PER BILLION)

4/ Yellowtail

You might see this fish listed on your sushi menu as "hamachi" or "buri." In Tokyo cuisine, "hamachi" is used to describe yellowtail that is farmed. While natural *buri* swim thousands of miles in their lifetimes, hamachi don't get much exercise while being farmed in fish nets, resulting in a noticeable difference in the quality of fish oil, which could account for this tuna's low levels of omega-3s.

NUTRITION FACTS

PER 3-OZ SERVING

93 CALORIES

0.4 G FAT (0.1 G saturated)

38 MG SODIUM

20.7 G PROTEIN

85 MG OMEGA-3S

270 MERCURY LEVELS (PARTS PER BILLION)

5/ Grouper

Popular in Florida, the grouper is a bottom-feeding fish with hearty, but light, meat. This large fish prefers to swallow its prey (including fish, octopi, and crustaceans) whole. Because of its high mercury levels, you'd do best to eat this fish only as often as you vacation.

NUTRITION FACTS

PER 3-OZ SERVING

78 CALORIES

0.9 G FAT (0.2 G saturated)

45 MG SODIUM

16.5 G PROTEIN

210 MG OMEGA-3S

417 MERCURY LEVELS
(PARTS PER BILLION)

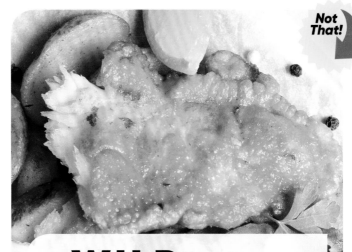

Not That!

6/ WILD PACIFIC COD

If you want to salvage any nutritional value from this fish, please don't bread and fry it for fish sticks. Cod's high protein content and amino acid profile contribute to the fish's satiating properties. In fact, a study in the *European Journal of Clinical Nutrition* found that people ate 11 percent less at dinner after having cod for lunch versus those who ate a beef lunch.

NUTRITION FACTS

PER 3-OZ SERVING

61 CALORIES

0.2 G FAT
(0 G saturated)

93 MG SODIUM

14.9 G PROTEIN

57 MG OMEGA-3S

144 MERCURY LEVELS
(PARTS PER BILLION)

7/ Scallops

Despite being high-protein and low-calorie, these mollusks won't provide you with a ton of omega-3s. However, they're still great for your waistline. One study published in the *Journal of Food Science* found bioactive capsules made from scallop by-products show significant antiobesity effects. Throw tiny bay scallops on top of a salad or eat diver scallops with a lemony farro risotto.

NUTRITION FACTS

PER 3-OZ SERVING

59 CALORIES

0.42 G FAT (0.1 G saturated)

333 MG SODIUM

10.3 G PROTEIN

88 MG OMEGA-3S

40 MERCURY LEVELS (PARTS PER BILLION)

8/ Clams

Steamed, littleneck, cockles, you name it. Clams are a hard-shelled fish with an amazing secret: They are the world's greatest source of vitamin B_{12} (according to the FDA, that is). Cooking the little shells bumps up their vitamin B_{12} levels to 84 micrograms—that's 1,402 percent of your daily recommended value! On the downside, clams are seriously lacking on the omega-3 and protein fronts compared to their peers.

NUTRITION FACTS

PER 3-OZ SERVING

73 CALORIES

0.8 G FAT (0.2 G saturated)

511 MG SODIUM

12.5 G PROTEIN

91 MG OMEGA-3S

28 MERCURY LEVELS (PARTS PER BILLION)

9/ Farmed Catfish

Farmed catfish may be raised in clean, fresh water but they contain significantly fewer valuable omega-3s compared to their wild counterparts. Even though catfish are naturally omnivores, farmed fish are fed unnatural diets of soybeans, corn, and rice.

NUTRITION FACTS

PER 3-OZ SERVING

101 CALORIES

5 G FAT (1.1 G saturated)

83 MG SODIUM

13 G PROTEIN

62 MG OMEGA-3S

12 MERCURY LEVELS (PARTS PER BILLION)

10/ Orange Roughy

This long-living fish is one of the few species that the Natural Resources Defense Council (NRDC) recommends you avoid entirely due to high levels of mercury. The Environmental Defense Fund (EDF) suggests adults limit themselves to only two servings per month, and only one serving per month for children under the age of twelve.

NUTRITION FACTS

PER 3-OZ SERVING

89 CALORIES

0.8 G FAT (0 G saturated)

59 MG SODIUM

19 G PROTEIN

26 MG OMEGA-3S

504 MERCURY LEVELS (PARTS PER BILLION)

Not That!

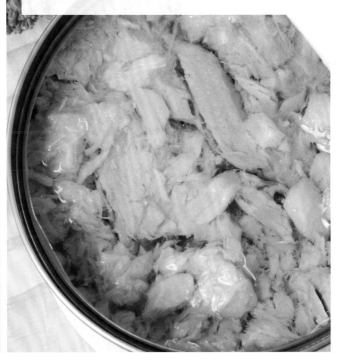

Mercury Matters

Human exposure to mercury primarily comes from seafood consumption—and this exposure can cause adverse neurodevelopmental, cardiovascular, and immunological health effects in sufficient doses. The FDA considers a 1,000 parts per billion (ppb) limit to provide an adequate margin of safety for adult men and women, while environmental advocacy groups like the Natural Resources Defense Council (NRDC) recommend that pregnant women or women planning to become pregnant should avoid eating fish with mercury counts of 500 ppb and above.

CHAPTER 5

THE BEST

FRUITS

YOU CAN HARDLY walk down the produce aisle in your local supermarket without seeing a new "it fruit"—the Ariana Grande of cantaloupes. From sumo oranges to açaí berries, they promise amazing flavor and myriad health benefits at every turn. However, it's not just the new kids on the proverbial block that are worthy of a spot in your cart. And if you're concerned about the high carb counts that frequently give nature's candy a bad rap, you can put those fruit fears to rest: The very same apples and bananas your mom packed in your lunch as a kid are loaded with weight-loss-boosting fiber, meaning their net carbs— a number calculated by subtracting a food's fiber content from its total carbohydrates—are more than low enough to find a spot on any healthy eating plan. They also pack immune-boosting antioxidants and just enough sweetness to keep those candy cravings at bay. So load that fruit bowl to the brim and say hello to a leaner, healthier you.

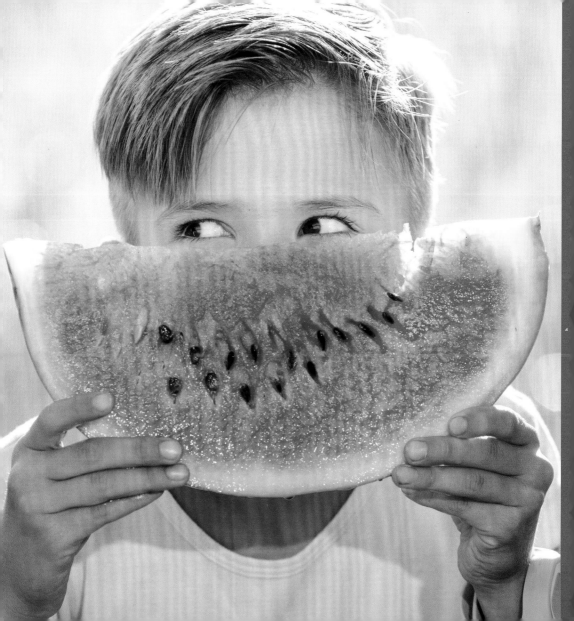

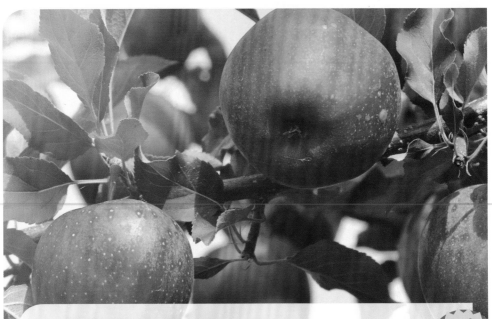

1/ **APPLE**

Eat This! Tip

An apple a day really does keep the doctor away. Just a medium one of these portable powerhouses packs 4 grams of filling soluble fiber—or 17 percent of your daily value (DV)—helping you maintain your digestive health and stabilize your blood sugar, allowing you to silence that voice telling you to hit the vending machine. Better yet, apples are also loaded with the flavonoid pigment quercetin, which has antihistamine and allergy-fighting properties, as well as a hit of vitamin C for much-needed immune support.

Check your local farmers' market for interesting, locally grown varieties, like Pink Lady apples, which boast more antioxidants and flavonoids than any other type.

2/ Avocado

■ The next time someone asks if you want guacamole on that, make sure the answer's a resounding "yes," because avocados are a weight-loss superfood. Delicious, nutrient-rich, full of healthy fats, and just as tasty on a sandwich as in a smoothie, avocados are so versatile they make Meryl Streep look like a one-trick pony. And while they're not exactly light on calories, avocados can still help you slim down—a study published in *Nutrition* reveals that people who ate half an avocado with their meal squashed their snacking impulse for hours afterward.

Eat This! Tip: Try our famous, fiber-packed Zero Belly Green Tea Avocado Smoothie: Toss 1 cup green tea, ½ of a frozen banana, 2 tablespoons fresh lemon juice, ⅛ of an avocado, 1 scoop vanilla plant-based protein powder, and some water into a blender; buzz until smooth.

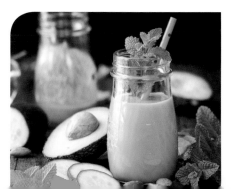

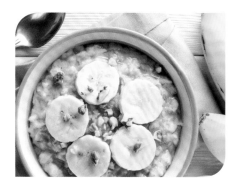

3/ Banana

■ Looking to build lean muscle, shed that spare tire, and wake up feeling refreshed? The answer isn't in a pill—it's in a peel. While bananas aren't super light on carbs, stick to a single 5-inch fruit per day and you'll reap all the benefits of the banana's cravings-crushing fiber and water, filling you up without making your middle mushy. And if you're a regular at the gym, consider bananas your post-workout secret weapon: Their potassium content fights cramps, aids muscle recovery, and even helps you eliminate water retention and bloating, meaning you'll be on track for that "after" picture in no time.

Eat This! Tip: Whether you're using one as the base of your favorite smoothie or the pièce de résistance on your overnight oats, this filling tropical fruit is as delicious as it is versatile—so get ready to go bananas!

4/ **Blackberries**

■ Brimming with fiber, blackberries are antioxidant powerhouses that not only fend off disease, but can help you flatten that belly in a hurry. In just a single cup of blackberries, you'll get a whopping 50 percent of your daily vitamin C, which can help you send your bad cholesterol packing and give your heart health a boost. Blackberries are also loaded with lutein, an antioxidant that can keep your eyes healthy and fend off macular degeneration.

Eat This! Tip: Add them to salads, smoothies, yogurt, and overnight oats, or eat them plain to reap the health benefits and continue dropping pounds.

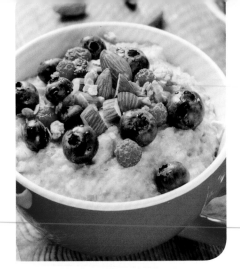

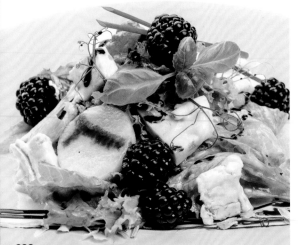

5/ **Blueberries**

■ Packed with more antioxidants than any other North American fruit, blueberries can slash your cancer risk, ward off diabetes, and keep your mind sharp as you age. Not only are they loaded with vitamins A and C and plenty of fiber, keeping your gut healthy and immune system strong, studies show that blueberries can even keep your heart healthy. And don't stress if you can't find fresh ones—blueberries retain most of their antioxidant content when dried or frozen.

Eat This! Tip: Start your day with blueberry benefits: Toss a handful into smoothies or on top of yogurt or over-night oats.

6/CANTALOUPE

Eat This! Tip

Don't let its low carb and calorie counts fool you: Cantaloupe is brimming with essential nutrients. This orange melon has more than 100 percent of your daily vitamin A in every cup, keeping your eyes healthy and your skin clear, and giving your immune system a leg up whenever you snack on a slice.

Ripe cantaloupe is even more delicious when paired with protein-packed cottage cheese. Try combining chopped melon with cucumber, green onion, and cilantro, top the mixture with lime juice and a bit of salt and black pepper, and serve with grilled chicken or fish.

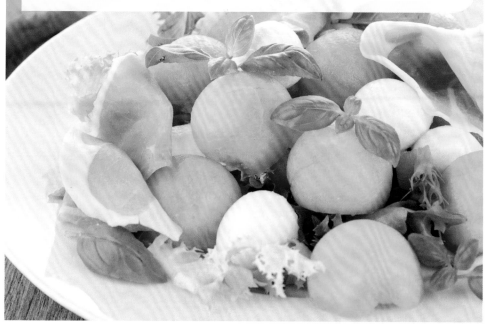

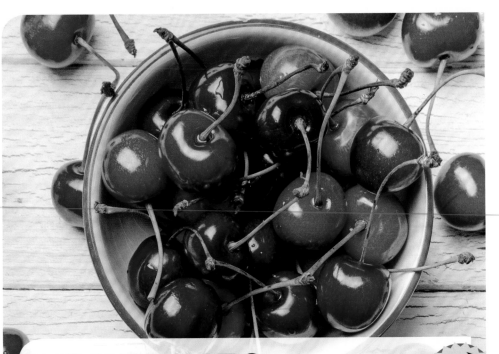

7/CHERRIES

Eat This! Tip

Light on calories—just 87 per cup—but loaded with flavor, these tart treats are a smart addition to any snacker's repertoire. Not only are cherries loaded with immune-boosting vitamin C, a single cup packs 306 milligrams of cramp-fighting potassium—more than you'd get in a small banana.

Nosh on cherries solo as a snack or add them to a bed of arugula or spinach along with some crumbled goat cheese, red onion, and dry-roasted pistachios for a filling side salad. You can even top it off with grilled chicken or fish to make it a meal.

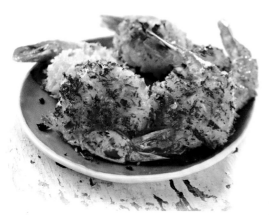

8/ **Coconut**

■ If you're cuckoo for coconuts, keep on cracking. Coconuts aren't just tasty—they're also a great source of medium-chain triglycerides (MCTs), which research has linked to reductions in anxiety symptoms and increases in your body's energy expenditure, per a study published in *Diabetes.* And while they're high in saturated fat, coconuts' wealth of lauric acid makes them a cardio-vascular health superfood, helping to lower high cholesterol.

Eat This! Tip: If you want to add coconut into your regular routine, try replacing cow's milk with coconut milk in your coffee, sip hydrating coconut water post-workout, or stock your freezer with frozen coconut meat to toss into your smoothies when you're in a hurry.

9/ **Figs**

■ These sweet and seedy fruits are more than just a snack cookie filling—in their natural, naked state, they're amazing for your health. They're loaded with potassium, magnesium, bone-strengthening calcium, vitamins A, E, and K, as well as prebiotic fiber, which supports the growth of beneficial gut bacteria and your immune system in the process. Adding one or two figs to your daily menu can help you get healthier while satisfying your sweet tooth.

Eat This! Tip: Try wrapping figs in prosciutto and adding a dollop of goat cheese. This protein-packed salty-and-sweet combo will keep you full for hours, allowing you to crush those cravings for less healthy fare in just a few bites—so don't be afraid to get figgy with it.

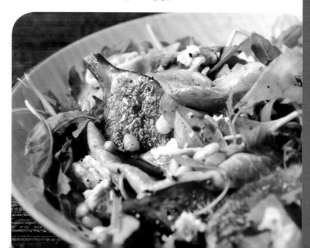

10/ **Guava**

■ Think fruit can't be filling? Think again. Guava packs more protein than any other tropical fruit, with 4 grams per cup, as well as 9 grams of belly-flattening fiber—all for just 112 calories. Guava is also loaded with the cancer-fighting antioxidant lycopene, as well as 600 percent of your daily vitamin C per cup— more than you'd get from seven medium oranges (and without the stomachache).

Eat This! Tip: Whether you're adding it to your fruit salad or eating it solo as a snack, don't be intimidated by the seeds you see when you cut into a guava. They're completely edible, so dig right in.

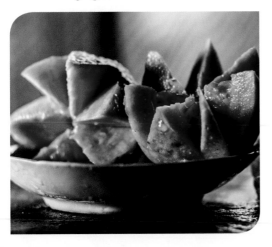

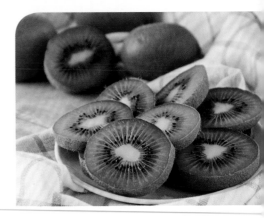

11/ **Kiwi**

■ Good things really do come in small packages—just take the kiwi, for example. Kiwis are full of actinidin, an enzyme that helps your body break down protein, making it easier to digest, while their prebiotic fiber gives the good bacteria in your gut a veritable feast. Research even suggests that a daily serving of kiwifruit can help keep your digestive system running like clockwork, helping you beat bloat and get closer to that six-pack with every bite.

Eat This! Tip: Don't judge a book by its cover—or a fruit by its skin. While many people eat only the kiwifruit's green flesh, its skin is loaded with immune-boosting vitamin C and cholesterol-cutting antioxidants, so after giving your kiwi a good wash, bite into it like you would an apple.

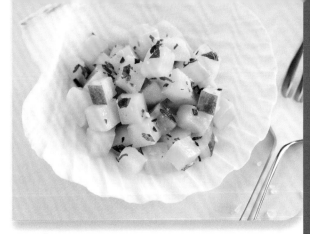

12/ Lemon

■ When life gives you lemons, enjoy them! Lemons top the Centers for Disease Control and Prevention's "powerhouse fruits and vegetables list," beating out every other fruit analyzed—and with good reason. The juice from just half of one of these sunny fruits will load your diet with more than a day's worth of antioxidant vitamin C, shown to significantly slash a person's risk of cardiovascular disease. And for waist-watchers, sour is power: The vitamin C in that lemon can boost your fat-burning ability by as much as 25 percent.

Eat This! Tip: Squeeze a lemon wedge into a glass of hot or cold water to perk you up first thing in the morning, add some fresh lemon juice to olive oil for a bright and fresh salad dressing, or zest the peel to create a flavorful garnish for your favorite pasta or vegetable dish.

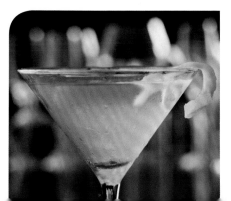

13/ Mango

■ Mangos have so much more going on than meets the eye. The flesh of these tasty fruits is packed with eye-health-protecting vitamin A, heart-healthy B_6, and immune-system-boosting vitamin C. Mangos are also chock-full of antioxidants, like quercetin, isoquercitrin, astragalin, fisetin, gallic acid, and methyl gallate, which have protective effects against leukemia, as well as breast, colon, and prostate cancers. Want to know the easiest way to cut this tricky fruit? Check out these chef tips: eatthis.com/how-to-cut-mango.

Eat This! Tip: When you're making your morning mango smoothie, mix in a scoop of protein powder and a handful of raw oats to load it with filling protein and fiber while slowing your digestion of its sugars.

14/ **PAPAYA**

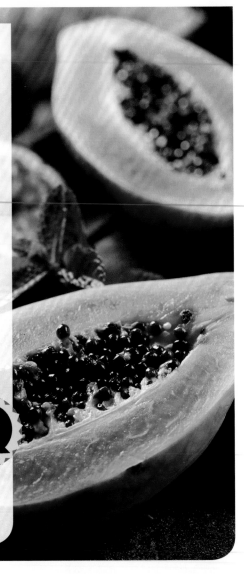

Loaded with vision-strengthening vitamin A and a favorable fiber-to-sugar ratio, papayas are a flavorful, filling, and sweet-tooth-satisfying tropical fruit. The orange-fleshed fruit also packs two enzymes—papain and chymopapain—that have been shown to fight asthma, arthritis, inflammation, and a host of other health issues. For anyone with complexion concerns, papaya is potent medicine too—applied topically, these enzymes are effective acne-fighters, dissolving oil and leaving your skin soft and supple. And save that Botox for another day—a cup of fresh papaya packs 144 percent of your daily value of collagen-strengthening vitamin C, leaving your skin so lineless you might just start getting carded again.

Look for papayas that are mostly yellow and yield slightly to pressure. Papayas are delicious on their own, although their flavor is heightened with a hint of lime juice. Try them in desserts or salads, or just toss some into your favorite smoothie to start the day off right.

Eat This! Tip

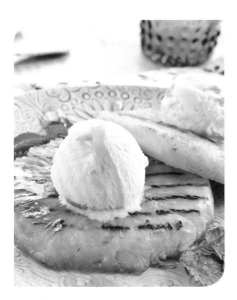

16/ **Pomegranate**

■ Sweet, delicious, and fun to eat, pomegranate would be an enjoyable addition to any diet even if it wasn't so good for you—but make no mistake: It is. Pomegranate seeds, or arils, pack a trifecta of antioxidant polyphenols—tannins, anthocyanins, and ellagic acid— which fend off free radical damage. Pomegranates are also a major source of vitamin C, which keeps your skin glowing and your immune system strong.

Eat This! Tip: Pop the arils as a snack or sprinkle them onto salads, yogurt, or your favorite chicken dishes.

15/ **Pineapple**

■ Move over, coffee—pineapple might just be the best energy-booster out there. A single cup of pineapple packs 76 percent of your daily manganese, a trace element essential for energy production. Pineapple is also loaded with bromelain, an anti-inflammatory enzyme, and the fruit's detoxifying acids can even keep you smelling sweeter, even after a vigorous workout.

Eat This! Tip: Enjoy summer's sweet treat on its own, or with cottage cheese or yogurt. And try tossing some thick-cut slices on the grill for a naturally deliciously caramelized flavor.

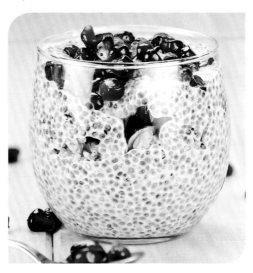

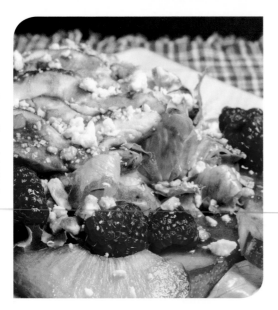

18/ Ruby Red Grapefruit

◼ Eager to shed that spare tire? Start your morning with grapefruit. A study in the *Journal of Medicinal Food* reveals that eating half a grapefruit before meals reduces dangerous visceral (belly) fat—and lowers cholesterol. Participants in the six-week study who added grapefruit to every meal shaved up to an inch off their waistlines, with researchers attributing its fat-burning properties to a potent combo of phytochemicals and vitamin C.

Eat This! Tip: Consider having half a grapefruit before your morning oatmeal or slicing a few segments into a starter salad.

17/ Raspberries

◼ Who knew the road to better health could be so sweet? Raspberries are loaded with anthocyanins, naturally occurring chemicals that boost insulin production, lower blood sugar levels, and fight diabetes. And with just 84 calories, 5 grams of sugar, and tons of fiber in every cup, fruits don't get much more filling—or easy on the waistline—than these.

Eat This! Tip: Enjoy a cup with your morning eggs or make an entrée-size dinner salad by combining the fruit with grilled chicken, mixed greens, goat cheese, and sunflower seeds.

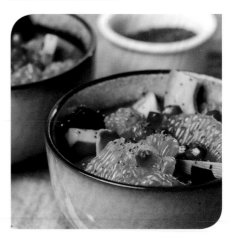

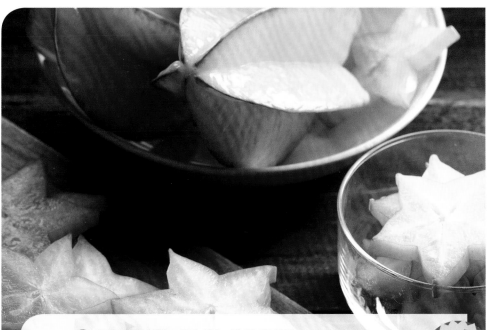

19/STARFRUIT

Eat This! Tip

Looking to make your usual meals a bit more exotic? Look no farther than the starfruit. Tart and slightly sweet, starfruit is sure to become a staple on your menu once you try it. And fruits don't get much more weight-loss-friendly than this one: A medium starfruit has just 28 calories, but also packs 50 percent of your daily vitamin C, which can fight signs of aging, like dry skin and wrinkles, caused by free radical damage.

When thinly sliced into stars, the fruit makes a fun, colorful addition to veggie or fruit salads, and also tastes great laid over seared and broiled chicken breasts.

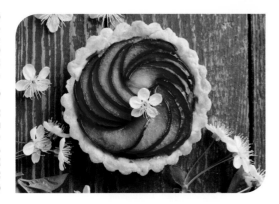

20/ **Stone Fruits**

■ A slimmer you is just a stone's throw away when you eat stone fruits. Studies suggest that stone fruits can ward off metabolic syndrome, a group of belly-fat-related risk factors that increase a person's chances of developing obesity-related diseases including type 2 diabetes. Apricots, peaches, plums, and nectarines pack powerful phenolic compounds that can actually alter your body's fat gene expression. And stone fruits have yet another flat-belly benefit: They've got the lowest fructose content out there, meaning you can snack on them and still slim down easily.

Eat This! Tip: Add tasty stone fruit slices to your morning yogurt or overnight oats, bake into a seasonal pie or tart, and use as an accent to savory dishes (these fruits pair well with chicken, pork, and fish).

21/ **Strawberries**

■ Add some strawberries to your meal plan today—you'll be berry glad you did. Strawberries are loaded with natural chemicals called polyphenols that not only aid weight loss, they actually stop fat from forming. And that fetching crimson hue is more than just eye candy: It comes from antioxidant compounds called anthocyanins, which reduce your risk of heart disease, cancer, cognitive decline, and inflammation. Snacking on strawberries can even lower your levels of the stress hormone cortisol, which triggers belly fat production.

Eat This! Tip: Eat ripened strawberries plain, add them to yogurt, or dip them in melted dark chocolate for a sweet snack.

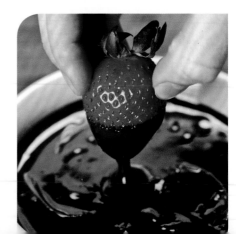

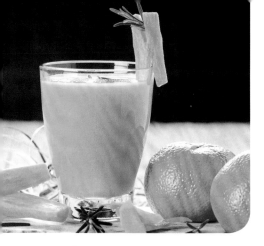

22/ **Tangerine**

■ Also known as mandarin oranges, these sweet citrus fruits pack big nutrition in a small package. A large tangerine has 12.7 grams of sugar, but don't let that scare you—inside those sweet segments are a ton of immune-supporting vitamin C, digestive-health-boosting fiber, and beautifying B_{12}, which promotes hair growth, reduces hair loss, and can even slow the rate at which those lovely locks turn gray.

Eat This! Tip: Nosh on tangerines solo or throw one into your smoothie with some tofu and vanilla plant-based protein powder. The ascorbic acid in tangerines helps the body absorb iron from tofu and the flavors combine to make a grown-up version of a Creamsicle.

23/ **Watermelon**

■ Nothing beats biting into a juicy piece of watermelon on a sweltering summer day. However, it's not just watermelon's sweet flavor that makes it such a summer staple: The fruit gets its rosy hue from lycopene, a carotenoid pigment that can actually protect your skin from sun damage as well as reduce your risk of heart disease. Research even shows that this hydrating fruit can reduce muscle soreness, improve lipid profiles, and lower fat accumulation, making it a top tool in your beach body arsenal.

Eat This! Tip: For a quick, delicious sweet and savory summer salad, toss cubes of watermelon with onion, fresh basil, cilantro, and feta cheese, drizzle with olive oil and balsamic vinegar, and top with some salt and pepper.

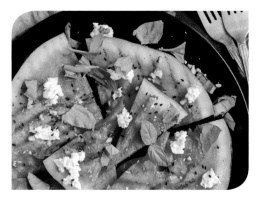

CHAPTER 6

THE BEST

VEGETABLES

OM WAS RIGHT: Most vegetables are extremely healthy for you—and should be at the center of any healthy eating plan. But when it comes to rapid weight loss, some veggies reign supreme. Thanks to their specific nutritional profiles, certain produce-aisle picks can help you trim down by revving your metabolism, turning off belly fat genes, and frying flab—and that's on top of all their other health-boosting benefits.

We've rounded up some of the most powerful veggies to help in your battle of the bulge. Veg out on these fresh picks and discover delicious ways to incorporate them into your diet!

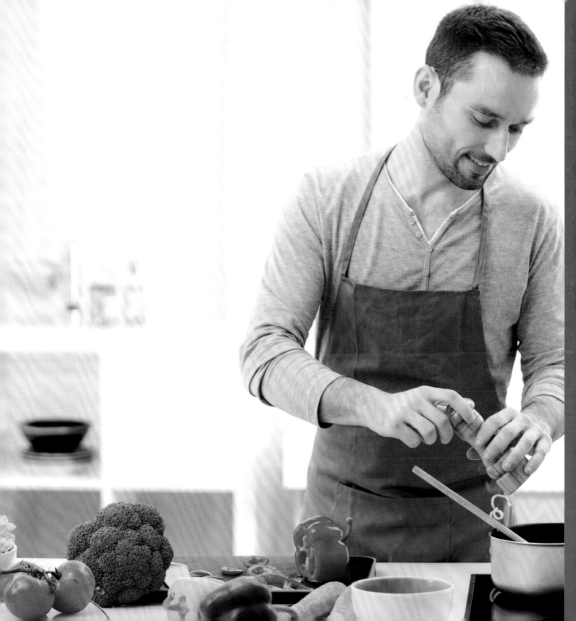

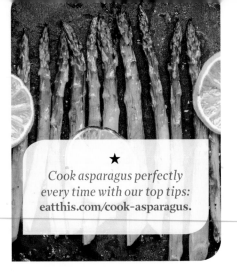

★

*Cook asparagus perfectly
every time with our top tips:*
eatthis.com/cook-asparagus.

1/ **Asparagus**

■ The ultimate spring vegetable, asparagus will help you get that flat belly faster. It's rich in potassium and low in sodium, which helps your body achieve proper electrolyte balance and works to reduce bloating. It's also very low calorie, with only 3 calories per medium spear and just .62 grams carbs. The fiber in asparagus also helps with elimination, further shrinking the appearance of your belly and promoting detoxification.

Eat This! Tip: Roast some spears in the oven with extra-virgin olive oil and dried spices for a simple, yet filling, side dish to serve alongside your favorite seafood or poultry.

2/ **Beets**

■ Feel the beet! A number of studies have shown that consuming the ruby-hued vegetable can improve your athletic performance. According to a recent study, athletes who drank beet juice experienced a 38 percent increase in blood flow to muscles, particularly "fast twitch" muscles that affect bursts of speed and strength. Research has also found that runners who ate baked beets before a 5K race ran 5 percent faster. The secret weapon: nitrates, a natural chemical that increases endurance and lowers blood pressure.

Eat This! Tip: Throw sliced beets into salads or sandwiches for added crunch. You can also reap the health benefits by eating the beet greens, too—toss the bitter leaves in stir-fries or sauté with extra-virgin olive oil and garlic.

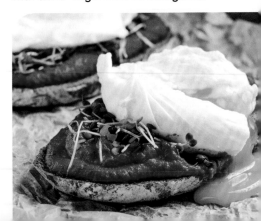

3/BELL PEPPERS

Eat This! Tip

You may have heard that spicy hot peppers can help you scorch calories, but did you know that mild peppers can have the same effect? Thanks to a metabolism-boosting compound, dihydrocapsiate, and their high vitamin-C content, sweet red and green peppers can help you lose weight. A cup of these bell-shaped veggies serves up to three times the day's recommended vitamin C—a nutrient that counteracts stress hormones, which trigger fat storage around the midsection.

Dip slices of bell peppers into hummus for a light snack, add the veggie to omelets and salads, or throw some chicken in a corn tortilla with salsa and slices of avocado, red pepper, and onion for a Tex-Mex-inspired fat-fighting dinner.

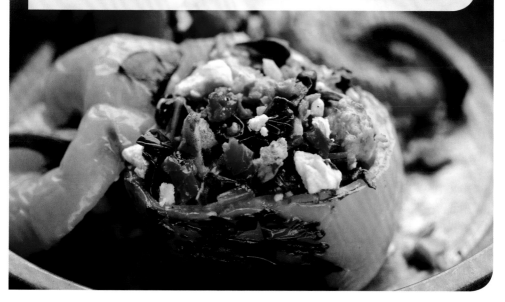

4/ **Broccoli**

■ In addition to warding off prostate, breast, lung, and skin cancers, this cruciferous vegetable can also help you whittle your middle. According to experts, broccoli contains a phytonutrient called sulforaphane that increases testosterone and fights off body fat storage. It's also rich in vitamin C (a mere cup of the stuff can help you hit your daily mark), a nutrient that can lower levels of cortisol during stressful situations, helping those abs take center stage. The only downside? It can make some people with sensitive stomachs a bit gassy. But that's no reason to steer clear of broccoli on a day-to-day basis.

Eat This! Tip: Try simply roasting it with extra-virgin olive oil, black pepper, and Parmesan, or whip up a batch of delicious Broccoli Cheddar Soup. Get the recipe: eatthis.com/broccoli-cheddar.

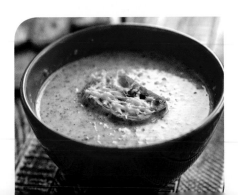

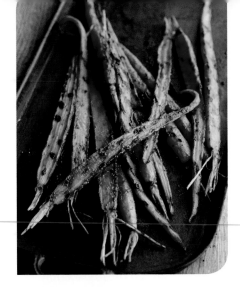

5/ **Carrots**

■ Most red, yellow, or orange vegetables and fruits are spiked with carotenoids—fat-soluble compounds that are associated with a reduction in a wide range of cancers, as well as reduced risk and severity of inflammatory conditions such as asthma and rheumatoid arthritis—but none are as easy to prepare, or have as low a caloric density, as carrots.

Eat This! Tip: Carrots are great for snacking and go well with so many meals—from salads and soups to scooping up hummus instead of using greasy chips to deliciously roasted. Try our simple recipe: eatthis.com/roasted-carrots-recipe

6/ Celery

■ Commonly referred to as a "negative food" (meaning it takes more calories for your body to digest than the food actually contains), celery certainly lives up to the low-cal hype. It has only 6 calories per medium stalk and only 1.19 grams of carbohydrates. Celery is mostly water, so it helps rid your body of any excess water you might be retaining and as a result will reduce puffiness.

Eat This! Tip: Toss the hydrating veggie into a tomato or chicken soup for an added crunch that will easily lower the overall calorie count of your meal. Or munch on celery with almond butter for a filling snack.

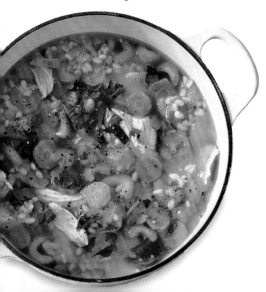

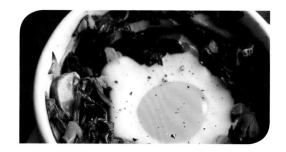

7/ Mushrooms

■ 'Shrooms are high in antioxidants, selenium, and vitamin D, which can play a significant role in muscle building. A study from *Medicine & Science in Sports & Exercise* measured the leg and arm strength of men and women and tested their vitamin D levels; they found that participants with higher levels of D were stronger. A separate analysis found that D supplementation was positively associated with muscle strength. The mightiest mushroom to buy is maitake, a.k.a. hen of the woods (one cup provides three times your daily allowance of D!). Other D-rich varieties: chanterelle, morel, and shiitake.

Eat This! Tip: This super fungus is super versatile in the kitchen—use 'shrooms in salads, soups, and sandwiches, as a homemade pizza topper, or as part of a protein-packed breakfast: eatthis.com/baked-egg-and-spinach.

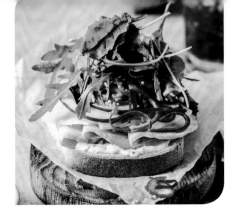

8/ **Onions**

■ Onions are rich in quercetin, a flavonoid that increases blood flow and activates a protein in the body that helps regulate glucose levels, torches stored fat, and keeps new fat cells from forming. Not to mention, onions are basically the unsung hero of cardiovascular health— an important area of wellness for everyone, but especially those who hit the gym hard to accelerate their weight-loss efforts. The culinary staple can help lower cholesterol, ward off hardening of the arteries, and help maintain healthy blood-pressure levels.

Eat This! Tip: Onions are super low-cal and easy to throw into just about anything, from soups, home-made burgers, sandwiches, and tacos to pastas, salads, veggie sides, rice, and omelets.

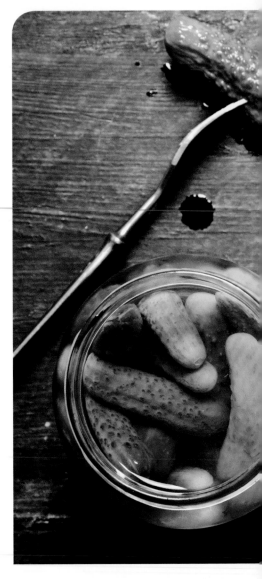

9/PICKLES

Eat This! Tip

Pickles are low-cal, filled with fiber, and covered in vinegar—which is all good news for your waistline. In fact, just one large pickle has 15 calories and 2 grams of belly-filling fiber, so eating three or four can actually leave you feeling pretty satiated for less than 100 calories! Every dieter knows that eating filling snacks are paramount to weight-loss success, but how does the vinegar help the fat-fighting cause? Studies show that acidic foods help increase the rate at which the body burns off carbs by up to 40 percent—and the faster you burn off carbs, the sooner your body starts torching fat.

Add these tangy pickled cucumbers to sandwiches and burgers or munch on them solo to start feeling more confident in your skivvies.

Classic Dill Pickles

Making pickles at home is easier than you may think—and way tastier and healthier. Many store-bought varieties contain harmful additives and artificial dyes. DIY it with our simple recipe!

2 cups water	2 lb pickling cucumbers
1 cup distilled white vinegar	24 sprigs fresh dill weed
2 Tbsp sea salt	4–5 garlic cloves
1–2 Tbsp granulated sugar	

1. Stir water, vinegar, salt, and sugar in a large pot. Bring to a boil, then remove from heat to let cool. Place brine in the fridge until chilled.

2. In the meantime, slice cucumbers into wedges. Stuff cucumber wedges evenly into airtight jars.

3. Divide dill weed and garlic evenly among jars.

4. Divide up brine evenly and pour over cucumbers, until the tops are covered.

5. Cover tightly and shake. Refrigerate for at least 48 hours (up to a week is recommended).

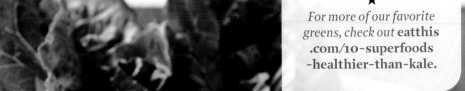

★

For more of our favorite greens, check out **eatthis .com/10-superfoods -healthier-than-kale.**

10/ROMAINE LETTUCE

Eat This! Tip

Romaine lettuce is our salad go-to. The leaves are low calorie, low carb, low in sugar, and high in beneficial nutrients. Romaine has only 15 calories and 1 gram of carbs per cup. It's also a great source of fiber, which will fill you up and keep your BMs regular, and rich in folate, which helps keep energy levels steady and helps to regulate mood.

Use this popular green as a base for salads, as a Bibb substitute in lettuce wraps (try this tasty recipe: **eatthis.com/thai-beef -lettuce-wraps-recipe**), or even tossed into green smoothies.

11/ Spinach

■ It may look pretty unassuming, but Popeye's favorite veggie can actually help take your calorie-burning potential to the next level. How? The green is overflowing with protein (just one cup of the steamed variety has as much protein as a medium hard-boiled egg), a nutrient that aids post-pump muscle recovery and growth. And remember: The more muscle mass you have, the more calories you burn at rest! What's more, the leafy green is also rich in thylakoids, compounds that have been shown to significantly reduce cravings and promote weight loss.

Eat This! Tip: Spinach is undoubtedly one of the most versatile foods out there. Toss it in your morning smoothies, whip up a lunchtime salad or soup, use it in sauces, pasta dishes, dips, and stir-fries, or sauté with garlic, extra-virgin olive oil, and lemon for a healthy and flavorful side dish.

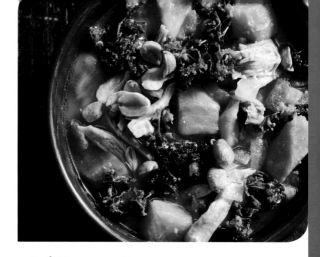

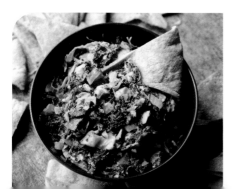

12/ Sweet Potatoes

■ These sweet spuds are one of the cleanest sources of fuel available. High in fiber and carbs (4 grams and 27 grams per serving, respectively), the vibrant tubers have a low glycemic index, meaning they burn slowly, providing a long-term source of energy that helps you power up after a workout and recover your stores of muscle glycogen afterward. The fiber keeps you fuller longer, helping prevent overeating. Bonus: One cup of sweet potato cubes has four times your RDA of vitamin A, which helps your body synthesize protein.

Eat This! Tip: Use the taters in a silky soup, sliced and baked as a base for avocado and eggs, spiralized as a noodle substitute, or tossed in salads.

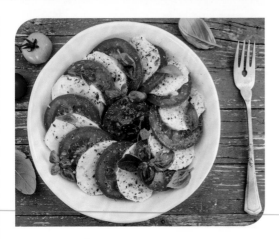

13/ **Tomatoes**

■ There are two things you need to know about tomatoes: Red are the best, because they're packed with more of the antioxidant lycopene, and processed tomatoes are just as potent as fresh ones, because it's easier for the body to absorb the lycopene. Studies show that a diet rich in lycopene can decrease your risk of bladder, lung, prostate, skin, and stomach cancers, as well as reduce the risk of coronary artery disease. Aim for 22 milligrams of lycopene a day, which is about eight red cherry tomatoes or a glass of tomato juice.

Eat This! Tip: There's nothing like a juicy, ripe, fresh summer tomato. Toss in salads or grain bowls, or eat it fresh with extra-virgin olive oil, black pepper, and fragrant herbs.

5 Worst Veggies for Weight Loss

Not all veggie-based dishes and drinks are belly friendly. Be sure to pass on these:

1. Vegetable Tempura → Drenching vegetables in flour and oil is a no-no. No vegetable is healthy enough to stand up to the onslaught of extra calories. For example: One serving of blanched green beans has 22 calories and 0 grams of fat. One serving of tempura green beans has 230 calories and 11 grams of fat. We know, some places make the tempura so light and flaky, it seems like that thin layer of deliciousness can't possible add that many calories. But you can't argue with the math—you're eating ten times as many calories.

2. Vegetable Juice → The juice craze has probably done more for the diet industry than any other trend in recent history. And not because it helped people lose weight, but because it made people pack on pounds and go out searching for weight-loss help. Because not all veggie juices are created equal! For example: One small cup of Kale Orange Power Juice from Jamba Juice has 190 calories and 33 grams of sugar. That's as many calories as a Krispy Kreme glazed doughnut. And the doughnut has 23 fewer grams of sugar, too.

3. Vegetable Dips → Whether it's artichoke or spinach, these dips sound so much better than "green-speckled sour cream dip," but that's really what they are. Nothing sets your night of healthy eating off course like a big bowl of one of these party favorites.

Two tablespoons of Marzetti Dill Veggie Dip gives you 110 calories, almost all of them from fat. And while there are plenty of vegetables pictured on the label, you'll have to supply those yourself. You could eat two tablespoons of Kraft Mayo with Olive Oil straight from the jar and still get less fat and calories than you would from this "veggie" snack.

4. Vegetable Smoothies → Smoothies are like juices on steroids. While they do contain more good-for-you fiber, they usually come with even higher calorie and sugar counts. Bottom line: Drinking your vegetables is the least tasty way to get a sugar high. A small Amazing Greens Smoothie at Jamba Juice is 420 calories and a whopping 54 grams of sugar. That's as many calories as three cans of Coke and as much sugar as four giant Pixie Stix. Nobody wins here.

5. Veggie Chips → We're sorry to break this to you, but veggie chips are just as bad, if not worse, than potato chips. (And in a recent study, potato chips were ranked the worst food for weight gain out of all the foods that exist on the planet!) One serving of Terra Sweet Potato Chips has more calories, fat, and saturated fat than a serving of Cape Cod Potato Chips. Though we like other products from their line, don't assume it's healthier just because the shade of potato is different.

↘ **Whip up delicious, healthy-for-you green smoothies from our Zero Belly Cookbook: eatthis.com/weight-loss-smoothies.**

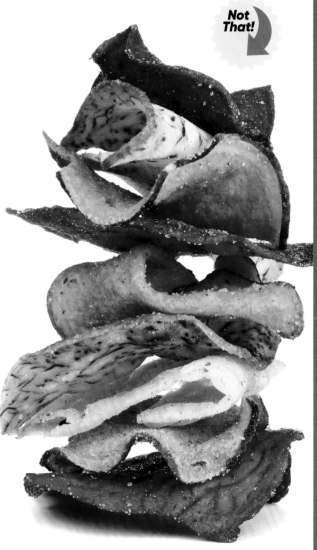

CHAPTER 7

THE BEST (& WORST)

DAIRY

WHILE WHIPPED-CREAM-TOPPED lattes and high-calorie cheeses tend to give dairy a bad reputation among the weight-conscious, it is possible to have your dairy and eat it, too. Better yet, for those allergic, intolerant, or just eager to skip the cow's milk, there are more delicious varieties of dairy alternatives on the market than ever before—ones so good you won't miss the real stuff for a second.

So how can you enjoy your favorite dairy products, maintain your health, and still set your course for that six-pack you've always dreamed of? The answer is simple: moderation and knowing which products to pick. With that in mind, we've rounded up the healthiest, tastiest dairy and dairy alternatives out there, helping you become the master of your own destiny—and the dairy aisle.

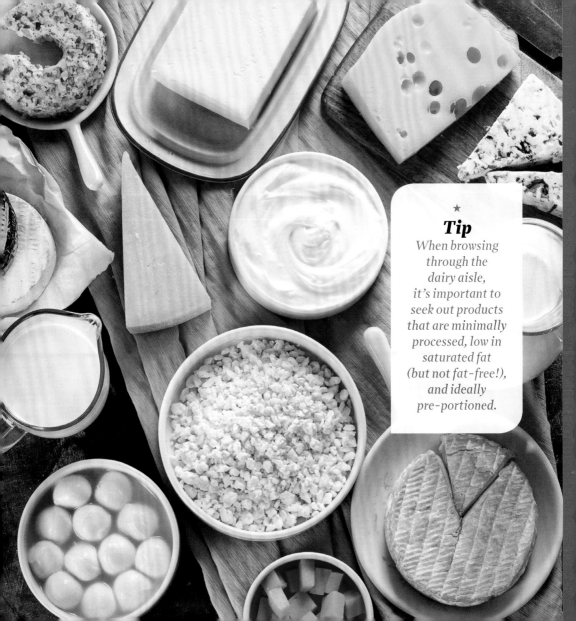

Tip

When browsing through the dairy aisle, it's important to seek out products that are minimally processed, low in saturated fat (but not fat-free!), and ideally pre-portioned.

MILK

Got milk? Sure—but which one is the cream of the crop?

Our grandparents had it easy: The milkman came, dropped off a few quarts, and that was it. Then the shelves of our supermarkets started being lined with 1%, 2%, almond, soy, and even rice varieties, making it harder than ever to determine which milks are the real deal and which are udderly terrible choices.

Still scratching your head? Quiet your confusion with the Eat This—approved guide to milk and milk alternatives.

Drink This!

COW'S MILK

Milk really does do a body good—if you know how to pick the right kind. The two proteins in milk, whey and casein, can help you preserve your lean muscle mass and keep your metabolism revved up even as you shed pounds. Grass-fed milk is the best option—you'll be getting higher levels of healthy omega-3 fatty acids and up to five times more conjugated linoleic acid (CLA) than its corn- and grain-fed counterparts. CLA contains a group of chemicals that provide a wide variety of health benefits, including immune and inflammatory system support, improved bone mass, better blood sugar regulation, reduced body fat, reduced risk of heart attack, and maintenance of lean body mass.

And while that jug of skim may seem like the more weight-loss-friendly option, a little bit of fat in your milk will keep you more satisfied in the long run. Go organic if you can and you'll also sidestep the hormones and antibiotics given to conventionally fed cows.

⤳ Dairy is a common allergen, with about two in three adults having a difficulty in digesting milk, whether it's lactose intolerance or a sensitivity to its casein proteins, which can also cause acne. If dairy doesn't agree with you, read on for alternatives.

Organic Valley Organic Grass-Fed 2% Milk

130 CALORIES

5 G FAT (3 G saturated)

120 MG SODIUM

12 G CARBS (0 G fiber, 11 G sugar)

8 G PROTEIN

30% DV CALCIUM

25% DV VITAMIN D

Kirkland Brand Organic 1% Milk

120 CALORIES

5 G FAT (3 G saturated)

125 MG SODIUM

12 G CARBS (0 G fiber, 12 G sugar)

8 G PROTEIN

25% DV CALCIUM

25% DV VITAMIN D

Not That!

Conventionally produced nonfat milk, brands vary by region

8 FL OZ

90 CALORIES

0 G FAT (0 G saturated)

130 MG SODIUM

13 G CARBS (0 G fiber, 12 G sugar)

8 G PROTEIN

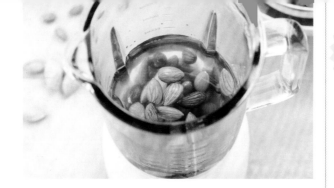

ALMOND MILK

Think almond milk is the creation of modern-day scientists? Think again. Almond milk has actually been around since the Middle Ages. And while almonds are high in vitamin E, manganese, selenium, magnesium, potassium, zinc, iron, fiber, and phosphorous, and boast the highest levels of calcium of any nut, unsweetened almond milk often packs just one-third the calories you'd get in a cup of skim cow's milk. Luckily, those trying to boost their calcium intake have nothing to fear if they go nuts for almond milk: It's typically fortified with calcium, giving it more of the bone-building mineral than traditional dairy milk. And for anyone with trouble digesting dairy, almond milk is a great alternative, putting cereal, lattes, and milk and cookies back on the table without the bloat or discomfort cow's milk can bring.

Drink This!

Blue Diamond Almond Breeze Original Unsweetened
8 FL OZ

30 CALORIES

2.5 G FAT (0 G saturated)

150 MG SODIUM

1 G CARBS (1 G fiber, 0 G sugar)

1 G PROTEIN

45% DV CALCIUM

25% DV VITAMIN D

Not That!

Pacific Organic Unsweetened Original Almond Beverage
8 FL OZ

35 CALORIES

2.5 G FAT (0 G saturated)

190 MG SODIUM

2 G CARBS (0 G fiber, 0 G sugar)

1 G PROTEIN

2% DV CALCIUM

25% DV VITAMIN D

⇘ Choose a milk that doesn't use carrageenan as a thickening and emulsifying agent. Carrageenan is an additive derived from seaweed that has been linked to ulcers, inflammation, and other gastrointestinal problems. Look for brands with no emulsifiers, or those that use sunflower lecithin and gums instead.

Soy Milk

■ Soy is more controversial than Cardi B's tweets. While soy milk is the least processed of all dairy-alternative milks, highest in protein, low in saturated fat, and the most widely available to consumers, soybeans contain high levels of phytic acid, an antinutrient compound that inhibits your body's absorption of essential minerals and may even cause digestive problems.

Since a shocking 94 percent of soybeans in the United States are genetically engineered and research suggests that GMO soybeans have poorer nutritional profiles, it's best to stick to organic, non-GMO brands. And beware flavored varieties, which can be packed with unnecessary sugars.

Drink This
Silk Organic, Non-GMO, Unsweetened Soy Milk
8 FL OZ

80 CALORIES

4 G FAT
(0.5 G saturated)

75 MG SODIUM

4 G CARBS
(2 G fiber, 1 G sugar)

7 G PROTEIN

30% DV CALCIUM

30% DV VITAMIN D

50% DV VITAMIN B_{12}

Drink That!
Soy Dream Enriched Original Organic Soy Milk
8 FL OZ

100 CALORIES

4 G FAT
(0.5 G saturated)

135 MG SODIUM

8 G CARBS
(2 G fiber, 6 G sugar)

7 G PROTEIN

30% DV CALCIUM

25% DV VITAMIN D

50% DV VITAMIN B_{12}

Cashew Milk

■ Made by blending water-soaked cashews with H_2O, this subtly flavored beverage is a good source of fiber, antioxidants, copper (which helps produce and store iron), and magnesium (a mineral needed for proper nerve and muscle function). It can be added to everything from cereals to homemade puddings, but is particularly tasty as an alternative to cream or half-and-half in coffee, thanks to its rich and creamy flavor.

Like almond milk, cashew milk is fairly low in protein and calcium, so if you're replacing cow's milk with this nutty alternative, make sure you're getting plenty of those essential nutrients elsewhere in your diet.

Drink This
Cashew Dream Unsweetened
8 FL OZ

40 CALORIES

3 G FAT
(0.5 G saturated)

120 MG SODIUM

3 G CARBS
(0 G fiber, 0 G sugar)

1 G PROTEIN

30% DV CALCIUM

25% DV VITAMIN D

50% DV VITAMIN B_{12}

Drink That!
So Delicious Unsweetened Cashew Milk Beverage
8 FL OZ

35 CALORIES

3.5 G FAT
(0 G saturated)

85 MG SODIUM

1 G CARB
(0 G fiber, 0 G sugar)

0 G PROTEIN

10% DV CALCIUM

35% DV VITAMIN D

60% DV VITAMIN B_{12}

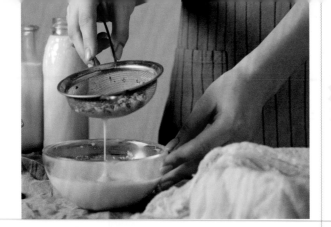

HEMP MILK

This nutty, creamy milk substitute is made from water and cannabis seeds—yes, this is the same plant used to make marijuana. However, hemp milk lacks the psychoactive component of the drug, so don't worry about getting buzzed at breakfast if you pour some in your coffee. Hemp is rich in heart-healthy omega-3 fatty acids and naturally carries ten essential amino acids, making it a good vegan source of protein, and many brands are also fortified with a variety of other good-for-you nutrients like riboflavin and vitamins D_2 and B_{12}. Unlike soy, which can cause digestive issues, hemp doesn't contain belly-bloating complex sugars, and thanks to its subtle flavor, you can easily add hemp milk to everything from baked goods to dishes like mashed potatoes without anyone being the wiser. Downsides: Hemp milk doesn't pack much calcium and it can cost more than other milks at the supermarket.

Drink This!

Living Harvest Tempt Hempmilk Unsweetened Original
8 FL OZ

80 CALORIES

8 G FAT (0.5 G saturated)

125 MG SODIUM

1 G CARBS (0 G fiber, 0 G sugar)

2 G PROTEIN

30% DV CALCIUM

25% DV VITAMIN D

25% DV VITAMIN B_{12}

 Not That!

Pacific Foods Unsweetened Hemp Original
8 FL OZ

70 CALORIES

5 G FAT (0.5 G saturated)

140 MG SODIUM

2 G CARBS (2 G fiber, 0 G sugar)

3 G PROTEIN

30% DV CALCIUM

30% DV VITAMIN D

25% DV VITAMIN B_{12}

Coconut Milk

■ If you're a fan of whole milk or cream, you'll love this naturally sweet milk's texture. Made from fresh grated coconut meat, it has a creamy thickness. Coconut milk is loaded with medium-chain triglycerides (a type of easily digested healthy fat), potassium, and a host of fortified vitamins (some brands even have 50 percent of the day's B_{12}!), making it a healthy way to add a tropical twist to coffees, teas, oatmeal, cereal, and homemade smoothies.

Just don't go coconuts and gulp it by the glass. While the fats in this beverage are the healthy type, moderation is still key—just one cup serves up 20 percent of your daily saturated fat, and some sweetened varieties pack enough sugar to qualify as desserts.

Drink This
Silk Unsweetened Coconut Milk
8 FL OZ

---

45 CALORIES

4 G FAT
(3.5 G saturated)

35 MG SODIUM

<1 G CARBS
(0 G fiber, <1 G sugar)

0 G PROTEIN

45% DV CALCIUM

25% DV VITAMIN D

50% DV VITAMIN B_{12}

Drink That!
So Delicious Unsweetened Coconut Milk Beverage
8 FL OZ

---

45 CALORIES

4.5 G FAT
(4 G saturated)

0 G SODIUM

2 G CARBS
(1 G fiber, 0 G sugar)

0 G PROTEIN

10% DV CALCIUM

30% DV VITAMIN D

50% DV VITAMIN B_{12}

Pea Milk

■ Pea protein–based milk is taking over the health-food scene in a big way. And for good reason: It delivers the same amount of protein as cow's milk, is low in saturated fat, and has 50 percent more calcium than almond milk. And while it's largely legume, it somehow tastes just like real-deal dairy.

⤷ To be clear, we're talking about the variety sold in a carton, not a can, which is extremely calorie-dense and should only be used for cooking.

Drink This
Ripple Original Unsweetened Pea Milk
8 FL OZ

---

75 CALORIES

5 G FAT
(0.5 G saturated)

120 MG SODIUM

0 G CARBS
(0 G fiber, 0 G sugar)

8 G PROTEIN

45% DV CALCIUM

30% DV VITAMIN D

32 MG DHA OMEGA 3'S

Drink That!
Bolthouse Farms Plant Protein Milk Vanilla
8 FL OZ

---

140 CALORIES

5 G FAT
(0.5 G saturated)

120 MG SODIUM

14 G CARBS
(0 G fiber, 12 G sugar)

10 G PROTEIN

35% DV CALCIUM

20% DV VITAMIN D

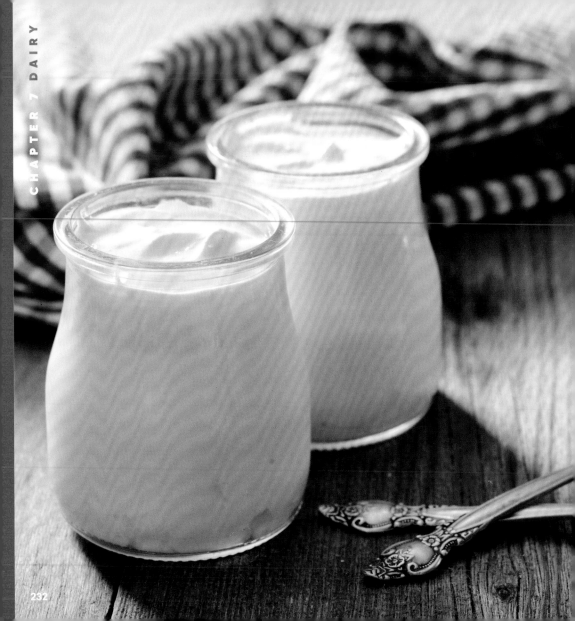

YOGURT

Filled with protein, packed with probiotics, and loaded with bone-building calcium, eating yogurt is one of the easiest ways to aid digestion and get you closer to your health and weight-loss goals. And combined with its versatility, easily subbed for everything from sour cream to the base for sauces, it's easy to see why yogurt is such a dairy dynamo. Even on its own, this protein-packed snack is a near-perfect treat.

But with yogurt becoming such a staple among health-food devotees, the yogurt section of the market has grown and the options have become overwhelming. From Greek to skyr to goat milk 'gurt, find out which yogurts are the best for reaching your health and fitness goals! Here are the ten types you need to know:

⇲ Find more of the best dairy picks for weight loss at eatthis.com/best-dairy-weight-loss.

1/ Traditional Unstrained Yogurt

■ Yogurt is little more than cultured milk thickened with lactic acid–producing cultures, a process that also creates its sour flavor. This kind of yogurt tends to be thinner than Greek or Australian varieties because it hasn't been strained and thus maintains more of its liquid content, making it a great addition to sauces or smoothies.

Maple Hill Creamery Cream on Top Yogurt, Vanilla
PER 6-OZ SERVING

150 CALORIES

7 G FAT (4.5 G saturated)

80 MG SODIUM

15 G CARBS (0 G fiber, 15 G sugar)

6 G PROTEIN

20% DV CALCIUM

2/ Greek Yogurt

🟦 Greeks are the fathers of philosophy and democracy— and some pretty great yogurt, too. Compared to unstrained yogurt, Greek yogurt has twice the protein, less sugar, and fewer carbs. And while there's no FDA standard for what constitutes Greek yogurt, keep an eye out for brands with just two main ingredients: milk and live and active cultures.

Wallaby Organic Aussie Greek Low-Fat Plain

PER 6-OZ SERVING

130 CALORIES

3 G FAT (2 G saturated)

65 MG SODIUM

8 G CARBS (0 G fiber, 5 G sugar)

16 G PROTEIN

20% DV CALCIUM

0% DV VITAMIN D

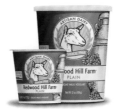

3/ Goat's Milk Yogurt

🟦 For allergy sufferers, this stuff is the GOAT—the greatest of all time. A recent study found that 93 percent of infants allergic to cow's milk were able to drink goat milk with no reaction, making this a great alternative. It also has a smoother, richer, and creamier texture than cow's milk yogurt. There's just one caveat: Its flavor—similar to goat cheese—can turn off some consumers.

Redwood Hill Farm Goat Milk Yogurt, Traditional Plain

PER 6-OZ SERVING

120 CALORIES

6 G FAT (4 G saturated)

70 MG SODIUM

11 G CARBS (0 G fiber, 5 G sugar)

6 G PROTEIN

20% DV CALCIUM

0% DV VITAMIN D

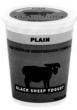

4/ Sheep's Milk Yogurt

🟦 Sheep's milk yogurt is the go-to if you're looking for a similar taste and texture to cow's milk yogurt but don't usually react well to it. This is an excellent source of B vitamins, calcium, and riboflavin, and is perfect for cooking because it doesn't break down like other yogurts do at high temperatures. Just keep an eye on the fat content, which tends to be higher than that of cow's milk.

Old Chatham Black Sheep Yogurt Plain

PER 6-OZ SERVING

140 CALORIES

9 G FAT (5 G saturated)

65 MG SODIUM

7 G CARBS (0 G fiber, 3 G sugar)

10 G PROTEIN

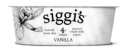

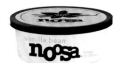

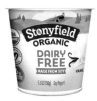

5/ **Skyr**

■ Skyr—a.k.a. Icelandic yogurt—is Greek's biggest competition in the yogurt game. Skyr is Iceland's version of cultured dairy, made with milk and live active cultures, and then strained four times. The thickest in consistency, Icelandic yogurt is something you can really sink your teeth into, and it packs more protein per serving than any other yogurt. While it's traditionally made from skim milk in its native country, it now comes in varieties with 0%, 2%, or 4% (whole).

Siggi's 4% Strained Icelandic-Style Skyr, Vanilla

PER 4.4-OZ SERVING

140 CALORIES

4.5 G FAT (3 G saturated)

55 MG SODIUM

11 G CARBS (0 G fiber, 8 G sugar)

12 G PROTEIN

10% DV CALCIUM

6/**Australian Yoghurt**

■ Australian yoghurt (fancy, right?) isn't strained like the Greek and Icelandic varieties are, so you get a texture closer to traditional yogurt. But because it's typically made with whole milk, it's still rich and delicious. If you don't have much of a sweet tooth, opt for the plain variety, or you're likely to get one sweetened with honey. Flavor-wise, this yogurt is both sweet and tangy, and it just so happens to pack a major portion of muscle-building protein.

Noosa Vanilla

PER 4-OZ SERVING

150 CALORIES

7 G FAT (3 G saturated)

70 MG SODIUM

18 G CARBS (0.5 G fiber, 16 G sugar)

6 G PROTEIN

20% DV CALCIUM

7/**Soy Yogurt**

■ Soy yogurt starts with a soy milk base, which is then combined with live cultures to thicken it up. It's dairy free, low in cholesterol, and a go-to for yogurt lovers staying away from animal protein. The toughest part about this treat: It's hard to find an unsweetened version without any added thickeners, and it's more liquidy than dairy yogurts, making it more difficult to substitute into dishes. The upside: Soy yogurt has been linked to blocking enzymes that impact carbohydrate digestion, which results in a slower rise in blood sugar.

Stonyfield Organic Dairy-Free Vanilla

PER 5.3-OZ SERVING

130 CALORIES

2.5 G FAT (0 G saturated)

40 MG SODIUM

20 G CARBS (<1 G fiber, 18 G sugar)

6 G PROTEIN

Eat This!

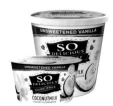

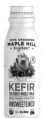

Eat This!

8/ Almond Yogurt

■ Almond yogurt is non-dairy, low in calories, fat, and sodium, but maintains high fiber and calcium contents, making it a great option for those looking to avoid lactose and dairy. It has a similar texture to traditional yogurt—thin and loose—but it's hard to find a brand that doesn't have thickeners and sweeteners even in their plain flavor option. The protein counts are typically lower than dairy-based yogurt, too.

Kite Hill Almond Milk Yogurt, Plain

PER 5.3-OZ SERVING

140 CALORIES

11 G FAT (1 G saturated)

10 MG SODIUM

8 G CARBS (2 G fiber, 5 G sugar)

4 G PROTEIN

9/ Coconut Yogurt

■ To create this yogurt, the healthy-fat-filled white meat of the coconut is pressed with water in order to make coconut milk, which is then combined with live cultures to produce coconut yogurt. As tasty and pleasing as coconut milk might be, coconut yogurt usually lacks in protein and it's difficult to track down a store-bought version without added sugars.

So Delicious Coconutmilk Yogurt Alternative, Unsweetened Vanilla

PER 5.3-OZ SERVING

110 CALORIES

7 G FAT (6 G saturated)

50 MG SODIUM

12 G CARBS (3 G fiber, <1 G sugar)

<1 G PROTEIN

10/ Kefir

■ One of the most under-rated sources of probiotics, kefir is a drinkable yogurt boasting benefits that far outweigh its spoonable counterpart. Kefir is made by combining milk with kefir grains, which are a mix of bacteria and yeast, yielding a drink that contains up to thirty strains of gut-healing bacteria.

Probiotics are essential for maintaining a healthy and flourishing microbiome, which plays a significant role in keeping our digestive systems chugging along.

Maple Hill Organic Whole Milk Kefir, Plain

PER 1-CUP SERVING

180 CALORIES

11 G FAT (7 G saturated)

120 MG SODIUM

11 G CARBS (0 G fiber, 11 G sugar)

9 G PROTEIN

30% DV CALCIUM

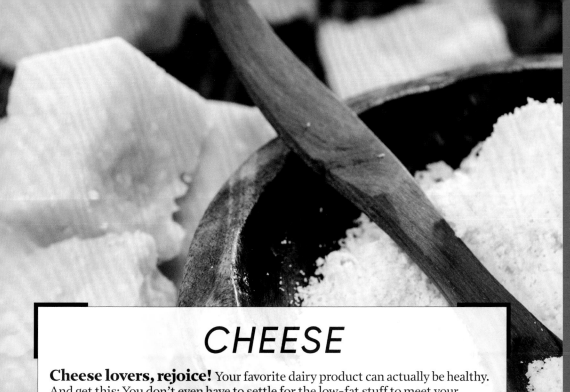

CHEESE

Cheese lovers, rejoice! Your favorite dairy product can actually be healthy. And get this: You don't even have to settle for the low-fat stuff to meet your health goals. With richer flavor than low-fat varieties, full-fat cheeses will satisfy your cravings—and better yet, you'll skip over those unhealthy additives in some low-fat alternatives that are added to make them palatable. Studies have found that consuming full-fat dairy products can even reduce your risk of diabetes.

When you're browsing the cheese aisle, it's a numbers game, but it's not just calorie counts you should be paying attention to: The fewer ingredients, the healthier the cheese. We're talking the bare minimum: dairy, salt, and enzymes. And when it's available for a price that won't break the bank, opt for organic.

For help with your dairy decisions, we've rounded up a list of better-for-you options and some of the worst picks at the store—so say cheese!

Eat This!

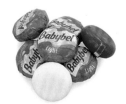

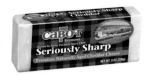

THE BEST CHEESES

AT THE GROCERY STORE

Mini Babybel Light

PER 1 PIECE (21 G)

50 CALORIES

3 G FAT (2 G saturated)

160 MG SODIUM

0 G CARBS (0 G fiber, 0 G sugar)

6 G PROTEIN

■ As far as snacking goes, this cheese wheels its way to number one in our book! "With just 3 grams of fat and 2 grams saturated, this snack has less saturated fats than a Laughing Cow Wedge, and it packs triple the metabolism-boosting protein, with as much as an egg!" says Eat This, Not That! founder Dave Zinczenko. Despite the "light" label, only milk, salt, and enzymes are on the ingredient list, passing our simplicity test with flying colors.

Cabot Vermont Cheese Premium Naturally Aged Cheddar Seriously Sharp

PER 1 OZ (28 G)

110 CALORIES

9 G FAT (6 G saturated)

180 MG SODIUM

<1 G CARBS (0 G fiber, 0 G sugar)

7 G PROTEIN

■ A dietitian go-to with 7 grams of protein, a single portion of this rich cheese will fill you up and satisfy even the most serious savory hankering. This sharp cheese ranks high because it's good quality, natural, and has minimal ingredients—the perfect addition to your next cheese board.

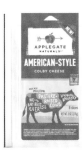

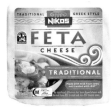

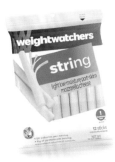

Applegate Naturals American-Style Colby Cheese Slices

PER 1 SLICE (21 G)

80 CALORIES

7 G FAT (4 G saturated)

130 MG SODIUM

0 G CARBS (0 G fiber, 0 G sugar)

5 G PROTEIN

◾ Free of genetically engineered growth hormones such as rBGH (which is banned in other countries around the world because of links to possible increases in cancer), these savory slices will kick sandwiches and burgers up a notch.

Nikos Feta Cheese 8 oz Square

PER 1 OZ

70 CALORIES

4 G FAT (3 G saturated)

340 MG SODIUM

2 G CARBS (0 G fiber, 1 G sugar)

6 G PROTEIN

◾ With a whole lot of flavor and naturally low calorie and fat contents, feta cheese is our go-to salad topper. This brand, unlike most that come already crumbled in a mixture of additives, keeps the ingredient list simple—just dairy, enzymes, and salt. Note: Feta cheese tends to pack a lot of sodium, although choosing a serving of this block versus popular brand Athenos's fat-free feta will save you 90 milligrams of the stuff.

Weight Watchers String Cheese Light Low-Moisture Part-Skim Mozzarella

PER 1 STICK (24 G)

50 CALORIES

2.5 G FAT (1.5 G saturated)

140 MG SODIUM

<1 G CARBS (0 G fiber, 0 G sugar)

6 G PROTEIN

◾ What would a list of cheese be without this fun-to-eat childhood favorite? Great for a school lunch, these grab-and-go snacks are a hit with 6 grams of protein we love and less of the sodium and saturated fats that we don't. For just 1 less gram of protein than your traditional string cheese, this pick has a little more than half the fat and 60 fewer milligrams of sodium.

Not That!

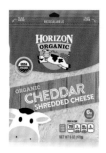

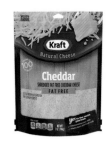

THE WORST CHEESES

AT THE GROCERY STORE

Horizon Shredded Cheddar Cheese

PER ¼ CUP (28 G)

110 CALORIES

9 G FAT (5 G saturated)

180 MG SODIUM

<1 G CARBS (0 G fiber, 0 G sugar)

6 G PROTEIN

Make any dish better with a sprinkle of organic . . . wood chips?! Yes, you heard that right. This company uses cellulose (a.k.a. wood chip powder) to prevent caking in the bag, although they do proudly specify that their cheese isn't bleached with chlorine in the ingredient list (thanks?). Truth is, most shredded, bagged cheeses contain cellulose, so opt for a block of cheese and grate it yourself. Your body will thank you!

Kraft Fat Free Shredded Cheddar Cheese

PER ¼ CUP (28 G)

45 CALORIES

0 G FAT (0 G saturated)

280 MG SODIUM

2 G CARBS (1 G fiber, 0 G sugar)

9 G PROTEIN

Yes, this one uses cornstarch instead of wood chips to prevent caking, but they also use a boatload of artificial color to give their cheese its fluorescent orange color—another shredded cheese fail we want anywhere but our favorite foods.

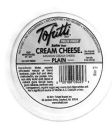

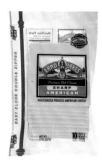

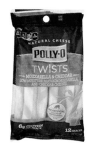

Tofutti Better Than Cream Cheese, Plain

PER 2 TBSP (30 G)

60 CALORIES

5 G FAT (2 G saturated)

120 MG SODIUM

0 G CARBS (0 G fiber, 0 G sugar)

1 G PROTEIN

The ingredient list for this cheese alternative is as long as it is highly processed and bad for your health. A blend of expeller-pressed oils and water, processed gums and cellulose (we'll say it again, wood chips!) are then added to give this imitation mixture its creamy texture. And its nutritional stats are just as bad: It contains only 1 gram of protein and no vitamins or minerals, like calcium, that you'd find in dairy-based cheese.

Land O'Lakes Sharp American Singles

PER 1 SLICE (23 G)

80 CALORIES

7 G FAT (4.5 G saturated)

320 MG SODIUM

1 G CARBS (0 G fiber, 1 G sugar)

5 G PROTEIN

You're going to want to keep a water bottle handy before digging into these dehydrating slices. With ⅓ of the FDA recommended sodium allowance of 2,300 milligrams a day in just one measly thin deli slice, these tip the danger scale for salt and won't even leave you full in the process.

Polly-O Twist Cheese

PER 1 STICK (21 G)

60 CALORIES

4 G FAT (2.5 G saturated)

140 MG SODIUM

0 G CARBS (0 G fiber, 0 G sugar)

6 G PROTEIN

A school lunch favorite because of the satisfying feeling when you successfully separate its two-toned twist, this mozzarella and cheddar string cheese is fine by us in the nutrition department. However, we could do without the added dyes that create its fun colors—and so could you.

⤳ Hungry for more? Check out our guide to the best healthy cheeses at eatthis.com/healthy-cheese-guide.

CHAPTER 8

THE BEST

GRAINS

BEING REFINED IS usually a good thing—unless you're a grain, that is. Unfortunately, research suggests that the vast majority of the grains we're eating on a daily basis are of the refined variety, like white bread, sugary cereals, and those impulse buy pastries practically jumping off the supermarket shelves and into our carts. And it's not just a widening waistline you have to worry about when you load your plate with the refined stuff: They can cause your risk of diabetes and heart disease to skyrocket as well as increase your triglyceride levels, which are linked to everything from heart attacks to strokes. The good news? There's still a silver lining—and one that doesn't involve ditching your favorite carbs for good. Adding healthy, whole grains to your menu can have the opposite effect, flattening your belly, reducing your colon cancer risk, and even fending off trouble with your ticker. So let things get a little unrefined for once—your body will thank you.

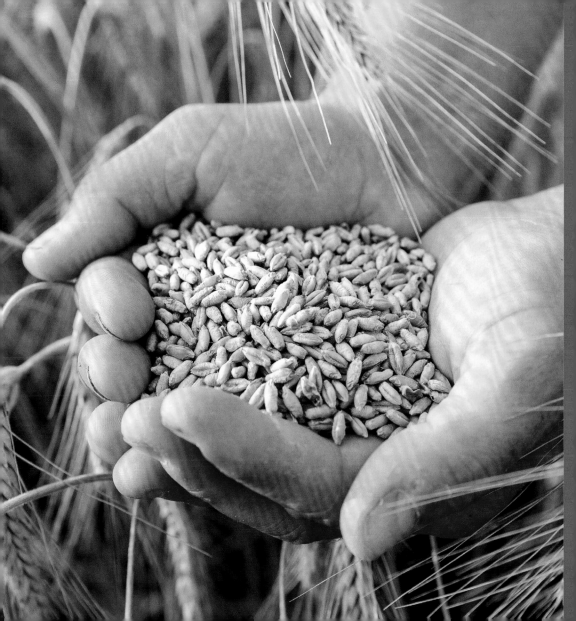

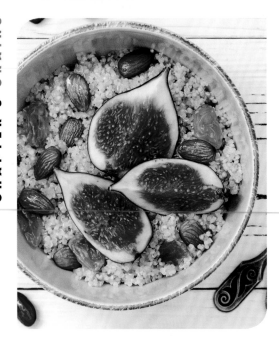

2/ Barley

■ This killer appetite suppressant can help keep your six-pack diet on track all day. Barley boasts belly-filling, mostly soluble fiber that has been linked to lowered cholesterol, decreased blood sugars, and increased satiety, as well as reduced inflammation. And the grain also acts as a bulking agent, which can help push waste through the digestive tract.

Eat This! Tip: Use it as a side dish (replacing rice or quinoa) or make a grain salad with cooked barley, vegetables, and homemade dressing.

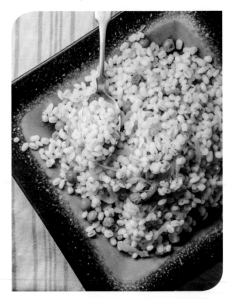

1/ Amaranth

■ Quinoa isn't the only "ancient grain" that comes loaded with health perks. Amaranth, a naturally gluten-free seed, is a good source of digestion-aiding fiber, as well as calcium and bicep-building iron. Amaranth takes on a porridge-like texture when cooked, making it a great alternative breakfast option.

Eat This! Tip: Whip up a batch and be sure to top off your bowl with some tasty, nutrient-packed oatmeal toppings like fresh fruit and nuts.

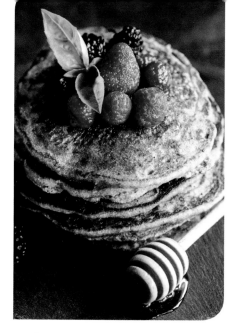

4/ **Bulgur**

■ A whole grain made from cracked wheat, bulgur is another high-fiber staple you should be adding to your diet. It's packed with vitamins and minerals, and known to be great for digestion.

Eat This! Tip: For a delicious side salad, combine bulgur with cucumbers, chickpeas, red onion, and dill and dress with a lemon vinaigrette.

3/ **Buckwheat**

■ Many people living with celiac disease can tolerate this delicious, naturally gluten-free whole grain, along with amaranth and quinoa. And it's one of the best grain-based sources of brain-boosting manganese and magnesium—a wonder mineral that does everything from improve nerve functioning to ease PMS symptoms.

Eat This! Tip: Get your dose of the grain in the AM—use it for buckwheat pancakes or soak overnight for a hearty porridge (similar to overnight oats).

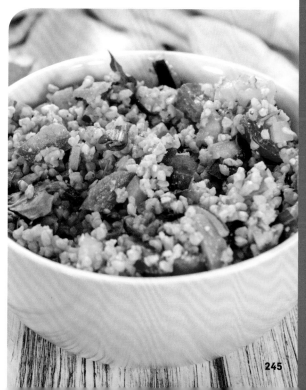

5/ BRAN FLAKES

Eat This! Tip

If you're not a warm porridge person in the morning, fear not: A 1-cup serving of bran flakes can provide you with nearly 6 grams of fiber!

Skip the raisin bran and add in your own fruit to keep sugar counts under control and fiber totals even higher.

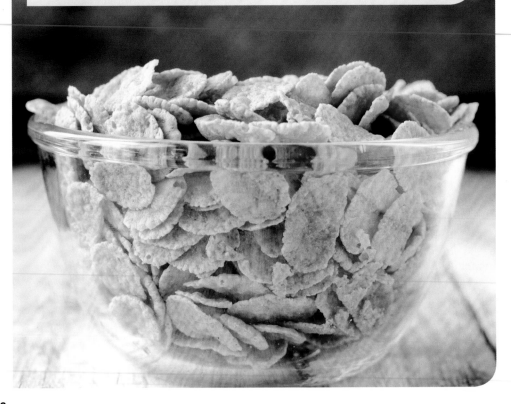

6/ Brown Rice

■ When you choose white rice over its brown cousin, around 75 percent of its nutrients—including nearly all the antioxidants, B vitamins, magnesium, and phosphorus contained in the healthy bran and germ—are left on the milling-room floor. Always opt for brown rice, which also includes brown aromatic varieties like basmati and jasmine.

Eat This! Tip: This versatile grain is one of the simplest foods to make— once you've figured out how to do it. Cook it like a pro with our chef-approved tips: eatthis.com/easiest-way-cook-rice.

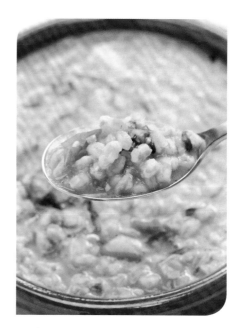

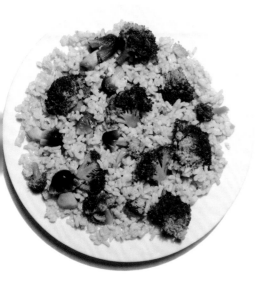

7/ Farro

■ Farro dates back to 17,000 BC, but it wasn't a staple in conventional supermarkets until recently. Brimming with antioxidant vitamins A and E and minerals like magnesium and iron, this Italian wheat grain has a similar taste to brown rice, but with a pleasantly chewier texture and nutty, almost licorice-like flavor. And it packs more protein than quinoa!

Eat This! Tip: Toss this super satiating grain into soups and salads, and swap low-fiber white rice for farro in risotto. Farroto!

247

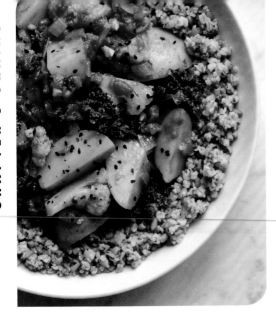

9/ **Kamut**

■ Use this ancient grain in place of quinoa for a punch of protein—nearly 10 grams per 1 cup cooked. Native to the Middle East, Kamut is high in energy-boosting, muscle-protecting minerals like magnesium, potassium, and iron, along with 21 grams of fiber per cup. Bonus: A study published in the *European Journal of Clinical Nutrition* found that eating it reduces cholesterol, blood sugar, and cytokines, which cause inflammation throughout the body.

Eat This! Tip: Toss kamut into salads or enjoy it as a side dish on its own.

8/ **Freekeh**

■ What the heck is freekeh, you ask? This super grain is a staple in Middle Eastern cuisine and boasts a pleasant, nutty flavor and a nutritional profile that rivals quinoa. This nutritious whole grain is low in fat and high in both filling fiber and protein. And once in your stomach, freekeh acts as a prebiotic, stimulating the growth of healthy bacteria that aid digestion. So get your freekeh on!

Eat This! Tip: Combine freekeh with roasted sweet potatoes, succulent pears, and sage for a flavorful side. Or top it with lean protein for a hearty entrée.

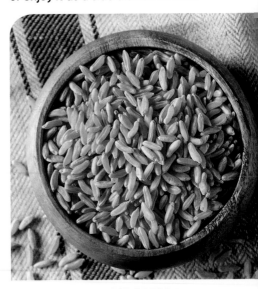

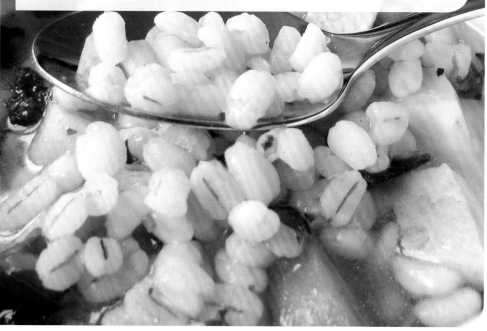

10/ PEARLED BARLEY

Eat This! Tip

The dietary fiber found in pearled barley "helps you extract and remove cholesterol, which is correlated with heart disease," explains Jessica Crandall, a Denver-based RD, certified diabetes educator, and national spokesperson for the Academy of Nutrition and Dietetics.

Incorporate this great grain into soups and stews, or even feature it as a side dish with some added spices.

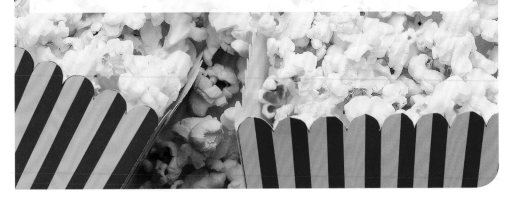

11/ **POPCORN**

Eat This! Tip

When you think of whole grains, chances are this movie theater staple doesn't come to mind—although it should! Since popcorn is considered a whole grain, it's got a healthy helping of fiber, and it's a good source of B vitamins, magnesium, and phosphorus. Whole corn is also thought to increase healthy gut flora, which can ward off diabetes, heart disease, and chronic inflammation.

Be sure to stick to air-popped to avoid unwanted calories or artificial flavors. We recommend these healthy ways to dress up popcorn: **eatthis .com/popcorn-recipes.**

12/ Rolled Oats

■ With 4 grams of fiber per serving, starting your day with a hearty bowl of oatmeal is sure to set you on the right track. A *Nutrition Journal* study found that participants who consumed oatmeal on a regular basis experienced a drop in bad cholesterol (and waist size!) due to their increased fiber intake.

And though oats are loaded with complex carbs, the release of those sugars is slowed by fiber—and because oats also have 10 grams of protein per ½-cup serving, they deliver steady, ab-muscle-friendly energy. Better yet, that fiber is soluble, which lowers the risk of heart disease.

Eat This! Tip: The flaky, thin composition of rolled oats makes them the ideal choice for overnight oats, since they quickly soak up whatever they're saturated in.

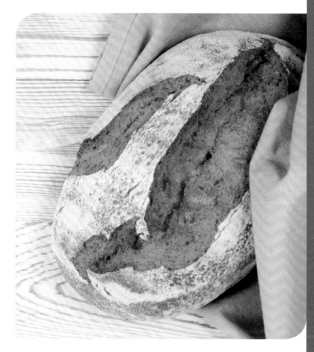

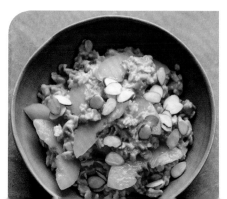

13/ Spelt

■ Yet another grain that's teeming with muscle-building protein— nearly 11 grams per 1-cup serving. Wholesome spelt is a grain related to wheat, but it's packed with more fiber and, obviously, more protein.

Eat This! Tip: Make spelt sourdough! Sub commonly used (and always processed) white flour with wholesome spelt flour in your next sourdough loaf. Find recipe inspo here: **eatthis.com /sourdough-bread-recipe**.

14/ STEEL-CUT OATS

Eat This! Tip

Nicknamed "Irish oats," steel-cut oats contain almost double the amount of fiber that rolled oats do, which is why you should be opting for these instead. These thick, coarse oats are the least processed form of oats and will provide you with the kind of lasting energy we like to see in a good breakfast.

Steel-cut oats are not great for baking due to their rough texture. It's best to eat them in the traditional way—cooking them in water on the stove and then adding a hint of natural sweetness from fruit or honey.

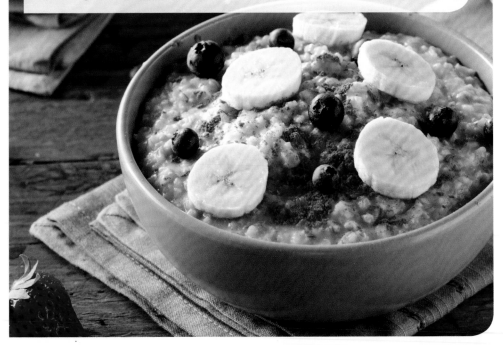

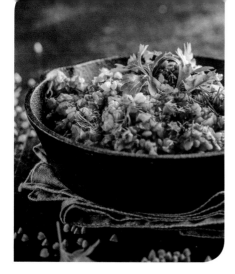

15/ **Teff**

◾ Teff may be the new quinoa, according to Lisa Moskovitz, RD. "It's a more complete amino acid—packed protein than quinoa itself," she says. "That makes it great for anyone who wants to keep calories low and protein high." And the benefits don't stop there. Teff is "also a good source of fiber, in addition to containing 30 percent of your daily value of blood-pumping iron." With more fiber and more protein comes great appetite control.

Eat This! Tip: Trade your morning oatmeal in for a protein-packed teff porridge, or cook it up as a side dish anytime you'd usually go for quinoa or rice.

16/ **Triticale**

◾ While you may have never heard of triticale before, it might just become your go-to grain. This wheat-rye hybrid packs 12 grams of protein per ½ cup and is also rich in brain-boosting iron, bloat-busting potassium, magnesium, and heart-healthy fiber.

Eat This! Tip: Mix triticale with soy sauce, fresh ginger, cloves, shiitake mushrooms, and edamame to make a healthy, Asian-inspired dish. You can also use triticale flour in place of traditional flour in baking.

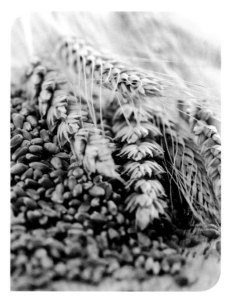

17/ QUINOA

Eat This! Tip

Quinoa is higher in protein than any other grain (8 grams per 1-cup serving), and it packs a hefty dose of heart-healthy unsaturated fats. Plus, it qualifies as a "complete protein," meaning it contains all of the essential amino acids—including the muscle-promoting L-arginine—an impressive feat for a plant-based source. This South American ancient grain is also a great source of fiber, a nutrient that can help you feel fuller, longer.

Try quinoa in the AM (it has twice the protein of most cereals, and fewer carbs), give quinoa bowls a try, or pair a scoop with veggies, beans, or a salad to create a well-balanced meal.

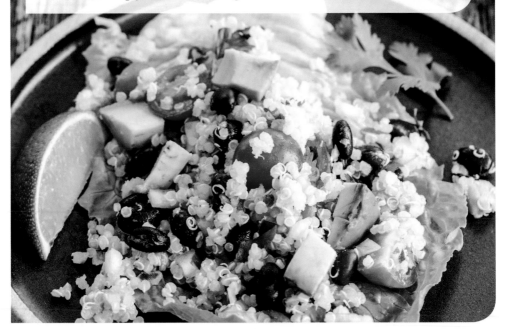

18/ Rye

■ According to research, rye has more nutrients per 100-calorie serving than any other whole grain. It has four times more fiber than standard whole wheat and provides you with nearly 50 percent of your DV of iron. The problem is, most rye bread in grocery stores is made with refined flours. Always look for "whole rye" topping the ingredients list to get the healthy benefits.

Eat This! Tip: Think outside the bread: Whole rye berries can be boiled as a hearty alternative to oatmeal or sprouted and sprinkled into salads. The berries are nutty and slightly sweet, with that unmistakable rye flavor.

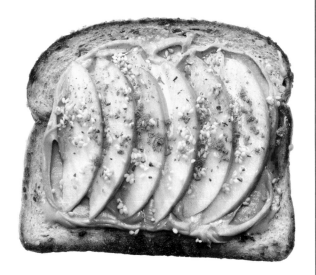

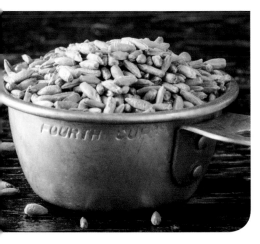

19/ Whole Wheat

■ The word "whole" is crucial here: It means that the endosperm, germ, and bran of the wheat kernel have all been left intact. It can be readily found in bread and pasta products, but don't let the marketers fool you: Terms like "multigrain" and "wheat" just don't cut it. Make sure the label says "100% whole wheat."

Eat This! Tip: When you're shopping for any whole-wheat and whole-grain product, look at the ingredients and make sure the whole grain is at or near the top of the list. And each serving should contain at least 2 or 3 grams of fiber.

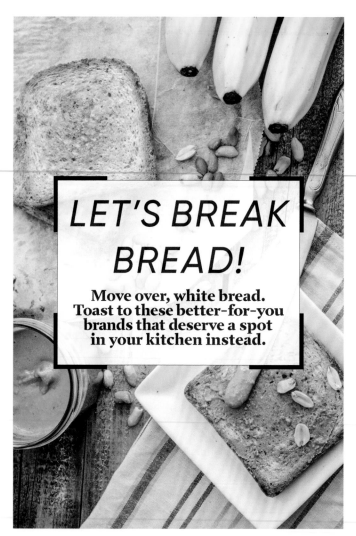

LET'S BREAK BREAD!

Move over, white bread. Toast to these better-for-you brands that deserve a spot in your kitchen instead.

Whole-Grain Bread

■ When scouring the bread aisle, the first ingredient should always read "whole grains"— and it should be devoid of added sugars like high-fructose corn syrup. One slice of a true whole-grain bread can contain around 4 or 5 grams of fiber and upward of 16 grams of inflammation-reducing whole grains. Even better: Some brands double up the fiber content and boast more than 10 grams per slice!

Nature's Own Double Fiber Wheat Bread

PER 1 SLICE

60 CALORIES

0.5 G FAT (0 G saturated)

120 MG SODIUM

13 G CARBS
(5 G fiber, <1 G sugar)

3 G PROTEIN

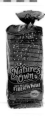

Sprouted Whole-Grain Bread

■ This nutrient-dense bread is loaded with brain-protecting B vitamins. What's more, because it's sprouted, the grains, seeds, and legumes have been pre-digested and divested of their anti-nutrients, giving you an easily digestible bread teeming with even more nutritional benefits.

Ezekiel Bread

■ Made with sprouted grains, wheat, barley, beans, lentils, millet, and spelt, Ezekiel Bread contains 18 amino acids—including all of the nine essential amino acids. That's something most other bread products can't claim. Making this your go-to sandwich base ensures you get at least 8 grams of complete protein every time you sit down to lunch.

Gluten-Free Bread

■ If you don't have a gluten intolerance or sensitivity, you're better off with the high-fiber, nutrient-dense whole-grain bread. That said, if you do want to go gluten-free, stick with Rudi's brand—it's low in calories, sodium, carbs, and sugar while being high where it matters: fiber.

Eat This!

Food For Life 7-Sprouted Grains Bread

PER 1 SLICE

80 CALORIES

0.5 G FAT (0 G saturated)

80 MG SODIUM

15 G CARBS
(3 G fiber, 1 G sugar)

4 G PROTEIN

Ezekiel 4:9 Sprouted Whole Grain Bread

PER 1 SLICE

80 CALORIES

0.5 G FAT (0 G saturated)

75 MG SODIUM

15 G CARBS
(3 G fiber, 0 G sugar)

4 G PROTEIN

Rudi's Gluten-Free Multigrain Bread

PER 1 SLICE

110 CALORIES

4 G FAT (0 G saturated)

180 MG SODIUM

19 G CARBS
(4 G fiber, 3 G sugar)

<1 G PROTEIN

CHAPTER 9

THE BEST (& WORST)

DRINKS

THEY SAY YOU are what you eat, but what you drink can have just as big an impact on your weight-loss goals. While soft drinks, sodas, and sugary coffee concoctions are off-limits (a.k.a. Coolatta non grata), there are plenty of healthy and delicious thirst quenchers to help you stay hydrated, boost your energy, and banish the munchies. Check out our roundup of beverages that belong at the center of any successful weight-loss plan and start sipping your way slim!

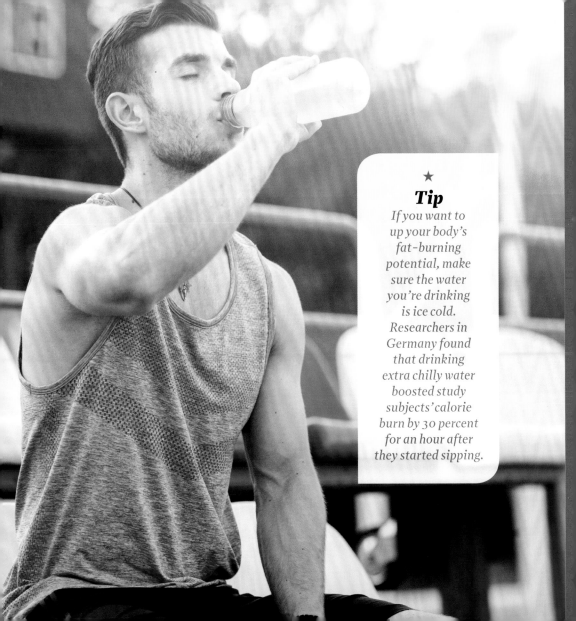

★
Tip
If you want to up your body's fat-burning potential, make sure the water you're drinking is ice cold. Researchers in Germany found that drinking extra chilly water boosted study subjects' calorie burn by 30 percent for an hour after they started sipping.

Drink This!

THE BEST-EVER DRINKS FOR WEIGHT LOSS

Drink to your health with these delicious, slimming beverages.

2/ **Detox Water**

■ Combine plain water with proven fat-burning superfoods to create detox water, and you'll have an elixir that energizes you, fights bloating, and helps you achieve your weight-loss goals. Certain fruits have detox-ifying properties in their flesh and peels; slice them whole into your water to enjoy their nutritional benefits and fresh flavor while easily hitting your water intake quota.

↘ Drink up and de-puff with our list of the 50 Best Detox Waters: eatthis.com /best-detox-water-fat-burning-weight-loss.

1/**WATER**

■ Hands down, the best option for hydration is good ol' H_2O. Since our bodies are made up of about 60 percent water, it's essential that we drink enough to keep our internal organs functioning properly and brains sharp. Drinking water can also fix numerous health issues including headaches, fatigue, bloating, and weight gain. Nature's beverage is calorie-free and cost-free, and will take care of all your hydration needs.

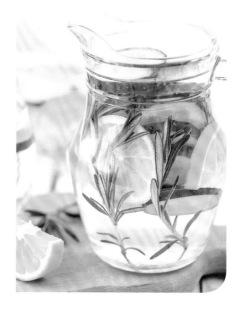

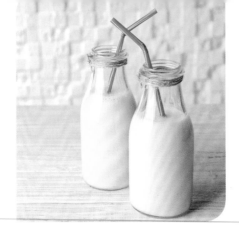

4/ **Cold Brew**

■ When regular brewed coffee is chilled and stored, two things happen: First, it begins to lose whatever nuance of taste it once possessed; second, it starts losing the polyphenols that give coffee its health benefits. The best iced coffee is cold brewed; it takes more time to make, so it's often pricier, but the taste is well worth it. Most notably, it will be less bitter, which means you can get away with adding less sugar. And less sugar = fewer calories.

3/ **Milk**
(2% organic, 100% grass-fed)

■ Moooove over, traditional dairy: Organically raised cows are not subject to the same hormones and antibiotics that conventional cows are, and no antibiotics for them means no antibiotics for you. Grass-fed cows have been shown to have higher levels of healthy omega-3 fatty acids and two to five times more conjugated linoleic acid (CLA), which provides a wide variety of health benefits, including immune system support, improved bone mass, improved blood sugar regulation, reduced body fat, reduced risk of heart attack, maintenance of lean body mass, and anti-inflammatory properties. Go for 2%. Skim is mostly sugar.

⤹ Find info about the best milk and milk alternatives in the Dairy chapter.

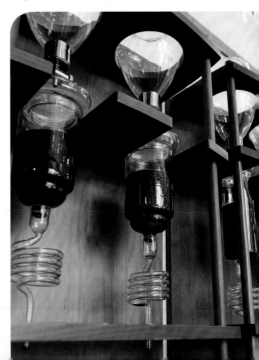

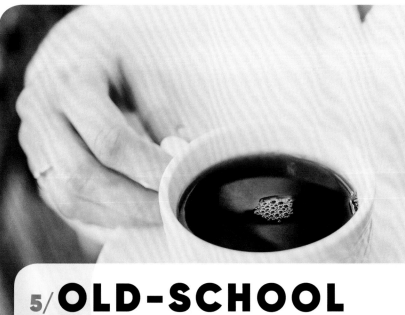

Drink This!

5/OLD-SCHOOL BLACK COFFEE

Drinking that second cup of coffee may do more than get you through the workday—it may also save your life.

At least that's what research published in the journal *Circulation* suggests. To come to this finding, researchers surveyed more than 250,000 Americans over 28 years and asked them questions about their diet and coffee consumption. After analyzing their rates of disease and death over the following twenty years, they found that among nonsmokers, those who drank between three and five cups of java daily were up to 15 percent less likely to die of any cause than those who weren't as friendly with their neighborhood barista.

6/ **Green Tea**

■ Turbocharge your workout's fat-blasting effects by sipping a cup of green tea before hitting the gym. In a recent 12-week study, participants who combined a daily habit of 4 to 5 cups of green tea each day with a 25-minute sweat session lost an average of two more pounds than the non-tea-drinking exercisers. Thank the compounds in green tea called catechins; these flat belly crusaders blast adipose tissue by triggering the release of fat from fat cells (particularly in the belly), and then speeding up the liver's capacity for turning that fat into energy.

Drink This: Lipton, Yogi

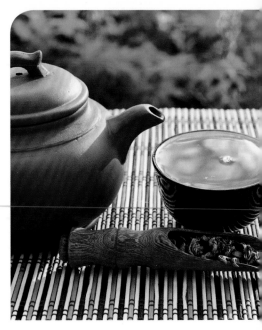

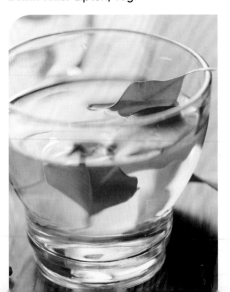

7/ **Oolong Tea**

■ Oolong, a Chinese name for "black dragon," is a light, floral tea that, like green tea, is also packed with catechins, which promote weight loss by boosting your body's ability to metabolize lipids (fat). A study in the *Chinese Journal of Integrative Medicine* found that participants who regularly sipped oolong tea lost six pounds over the course of the six-week time period. That's a pound a week!

Drink This: Bigelow, Stash

8/ Mint Tea

■ Fill a big teacup with soothing peppermint tea and sniff yourself skinny! While certain scents can trigger hunger, others can actually suppress your appetite. Studies have found that people who sniffed peppermint every two hours lost an average of 5 pounds a month. (Although tea is relatively low in caffeine—about 25 percent of what a cup of coffee delivers—decaffeinated varieties are great to have on hand for a soothing bedtime treat.) Consider also adding a few drops of peppermint oil to your pillow or burning a minty candle to fill the room with slimming smells.

Drink This: Tazo, Teavana

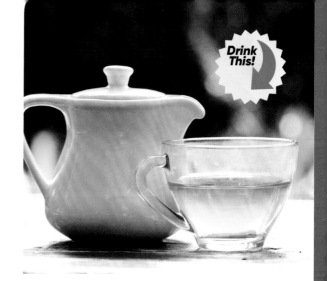

Drink This!

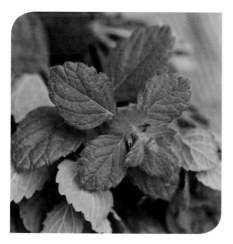

9/ White Tea

■ White tea is dried naturally, often in sunlight, making it the least processed and richest source of antioxidants among the teas out there (as much as three times as many polyphenols as green tea!). A study published in the journal *Nutrition and Metabolism* showed that white tea can simultaneously boost lipolysis (the breakdown of fat) and block adipogenesis (the formation of fat cells) due to high levels of ingredients thought to be active on human fat cells. If there's such a thing as diet tea, this is it.

Drink This: Twinings, The Republic of Tea, Celestial Seasonings Sleepytime

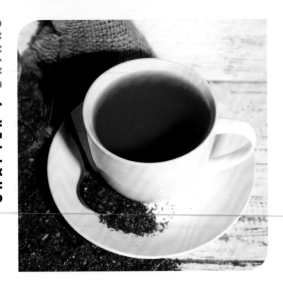

11/ **Black Tea**

■ Researchers found that drinking a cup of black tea per day improves cardiovascular function—and the more cups you drink, the more you benefit! Better cardiovascular function means you can breeze through that 5K you signed up for. And a recent study revealed that drinking 20 ounces of black tea daily causes the body to secrete five times more interferon, a key element of your body's infection-protection arsenal. Just ditch the dairy—adding milk to this tea counteracts these healthy effects.

Drink This: Celestial Seasonings, Republic of Tea, Tazo

⤸ Find even more tasty teas to sip for weight loss: eatthis.com/21-best-teas-for-weight-loss.

10/ **Rooibos Tea**

■ Rooibos tea is made from the leaves of the "red bush" plant, grown exclusively in the small Cederberg region of South Africa, near Cape Town. What makes rooibos particularly good for your belly is a unique and powerful flavonoid called aspalathin. Research shows that this compound can reduce stress hormones that trigger hunger and fat storage and are linked to hypertension, metabolic syndrome, cardiovascular disease, insulin resistance, and type 2 diabetes. Yup, sometimes the kettle can be as effective as the kettlebell.

Drink This: Celestial Seasonings, Harney & Sons

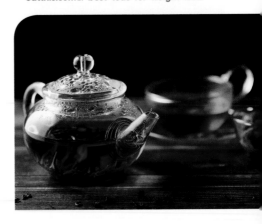

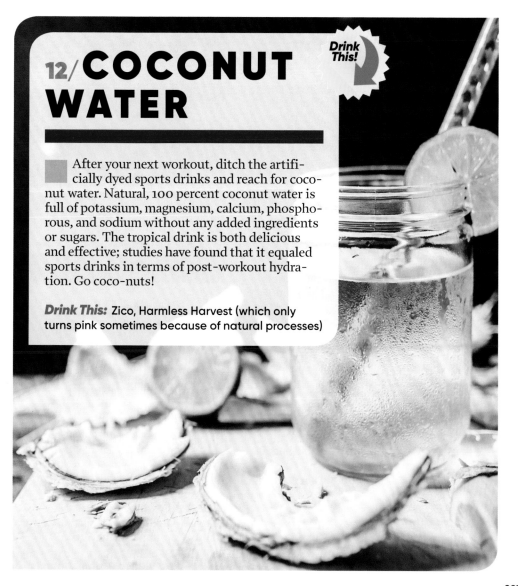

12/ COCONUT WATER

Drink This!

After your next workout, ditch the artificially dyed sports drinks and reach for coconut water. Natural, 100 percent coconut water is full of potassium, magnesium, calcium, phosphorous, and sodium without any added ingredients or sugars. The tropical drink is both delicious and effective; studies have found that it equaled sports drinks in terms of post-workout hydration. Go coco-nuts!

Drink This: Zico, Harmless Harvest (which only turns pink sometimes because of natural processes)

13/ **Watermelon Water**

■ Sipping watermelon water can ease your sore muscles after a gym session. In a study of athletes, researchers found that watermelon juice diminishes post-workout soreness, likely thanks to its high potassium and magnesium content—two electrolytes that aid hydration, muscle relaxation, and restorative sleep. Sure, the sugar count can run a bit high (up to 24 grams in a 16-ounce bottle), but all of the sweet stuff comes from fresh watermelon and lemon juice, which can help replenish depleted glycogen stores after a long workout.

Drink This: WTRMLN WTR

↘ Can't find a bottle near you? Make your own by blending watermelon pieces with a few squeezes of lemon juice and ice.

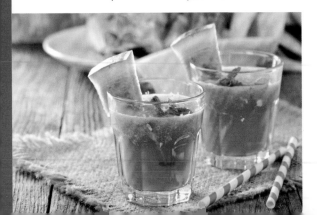

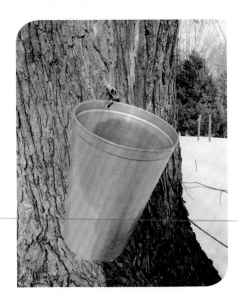

14/ **Maple Water**

■ Before maple tree sap is boiled down to the consistency and sweetness of syrup, it's far thinner and less sugary. And recently, a handful of companies began pasteurizing and bottling the stuff, which they've aptly named maple water. It tastes more or less like water, but is slightly thicker and carries a hint of maple-y sweetness. A 16-ounce bottle has about 6 grams of sugar and provides up to 66 percent of the day's manganese, a nutrient that staves off disease-causing free radicals, joint damage, and inflammation.

Drink This: Vertical Maple Water

15/ Aloe Water

■ When most of us think of aloe, we think of rubbing it all over our sunburned bodies, not drinking it, but it turns out there are benefits to ingesting this skin firmer and fat burner. A great weight-loss secret, aloe vera juice has been a mainstay in Ayurvedic medicine for centuries. The juice helps maintain weight by balancing the digestive system and regulating female hormones; it's also believed to enhance fertility. The only problem? Most aloe drinks are loaded with way too much sugar, which is why we like Aloe Gloe Aloe Water with just 8 grams of the sweet stuff.

Drink This: Aloe Gloe

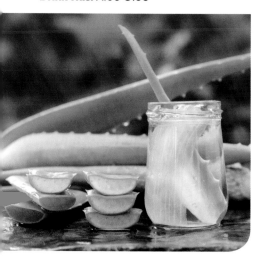

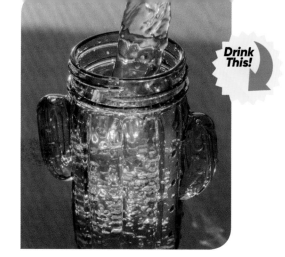

Drink This!

16/ Cactus Water

■ If beautiful, young-looking skin is what you're after, cactus water is the answer. The trendy drink, made from prickly pear cactus extract and its juice, contains betalain—an antioxidant that prevents moisture loss, aiding the appearance of glowing, youthful-looking skin. Aside from its aesthetic benefits, research indicates that consuming prickly pear can lower cholesterol and help diabetics manage their blood glucose. What's more, for a fruit-flavored beverage, it's relatively easy on the waistline: A 16-ounce serving contains just 50 calories and 12 grams of sugar—about half of what you'd find in the same serving of coconut water.

Drink This: Caliwater Cactus Water

SMOOTHIES

You don't have to stick to plain water to reach your weight-loss goals. There's plenty of room for creativity when you make nutritious, delicious smoothies. Need recipe inspo? Our best-selling book *Zero Belly Smoothies* rounds up tons of recipes that combine fat-burning proteins and potent superfoods to slim your waist, rev up your metabolism, soothe your digestive system, and turn off your fat genes forever. Test panelists dropped an impressive 16 pounds in just 14 days! They can make your life easier, too. By blending a smoothie for breakfast, you'll bypass all the extra dishes that typically make your morning meal a chore.

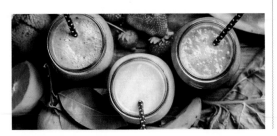

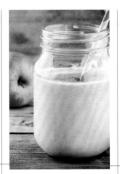

Apple Pi

¼ frozen banana

½ Pink Lady apple with peel, seeded and quartered

½ cup unsweetened almond milk

1 teaspoon flaxseed oil

3.14 dashes of ground cinnamon

1 scoop vanilla plant-based protein powder

   Water to blend (optional but recommended)

273 CALORIES

7.4 G FAT

27 G CARBS
(5.5 G fiber, 15 G sugar)

26 G PROTEIN

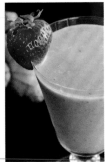

Ginger Man

½ cup frozen strawberries

¼ frozen banana

1 cup unsweetened almond milk

1 tablespoon fresh ginger, peeled and chopped

1 teaspoon ground flaxseed

   Dash of ground pepper

1 scoop plain plant-based protein powder

   Water to blend (optional)

264 CALORIES

5 G FAT

26 G CARBS
(6 G fiber, 11 G sugar)

29 G PROTEIN

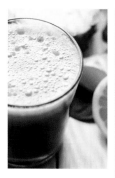

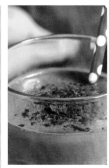

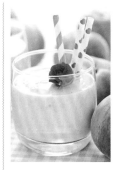

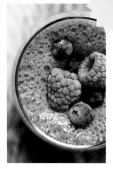

Lemon Kale Protein Detox

½ lemon, peeled and seeded

½ frozen banana

1 cup kale

½ cup unsweetened almond milk

1 scoop plain plant-based protein powder

3 ice cubes

Water to blend (optional)

---

254 CALORIES

---

7 G FAT

---

20 G CARBS
(5 G fiber, 10 G sugar)

---

30 G PROTEIN

Dark Chocolate Banana Nut

½ banana

1 teaspoon dark chocolate morsels (dairy free)

1 cup unsweetened almond milk

⅛ cup chopped walnuts

6 ice cubes

⅓ cup chocolate plant-based protein powder

Water to blend (optional)

---

229 CALORIES

---

11 G FAT

---

26 G CARBS
(7 G fiber, 10 G sugar)

---

28 G PROTEIN

Peachy Keen

1 cup frozen peaches

½ banana

1 cup unsweetened almond milk

1 teaspoon vanilla extract

⅓ cup vanilla plant-based protein powder

½ cup ice cubes

Water to blend (optional)

---

287 CALORIES

---

3 G FAT

---

36 G CARBS
(5 G fiber, 22 G sugar)

---

29 G PROTEIN

Wake Up Call

½ cup frozen mixed berries

Handful of spinach

8 oz unsweetened Silk almond milk

1 scoop plant-based vanilla protein powder

---

230 CALORIES

2.5 G FAT

---

20 G CARBS
(5 G fiber, 7 G sugar)

---

26 G PROTEIN

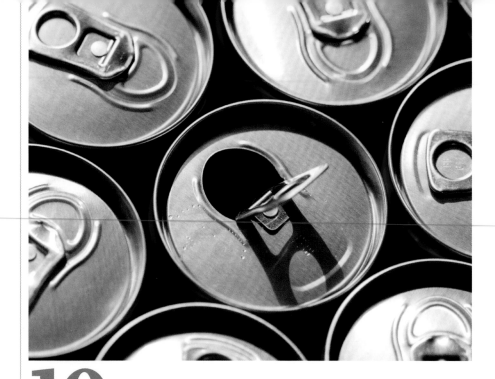

10
Healthy Energy Drinks for a Natural Boost

Energy drinks have gotten a makeover in recent years, and it's about time. Instead of the sugar-laden, waist-widening caffeine bombs you used to pound, the new crop of energizing sips includes sparkling waters with natural fruit flavors and tea-based beverages fueled with B vitamins and brain-boosting adaptogens like L-theanine. They're also canned sans added sugars and have zero artificial sweeteners, flavors, and colors. Some even use cold-pressed vegetable and fruit juices for color and extra nutrients. Check out our favorite healthy energy drinks on the market that will help you tackle your to-do list!

1. MatchaBar Hustle Unsweetened

5 CALORIES

0 G FAT

0 MG SODIUM

1 G CARBS
(1 G fiber, 0 G sugar)

1 G PROTEIN

2. Bai Bubbles Sparkling Antioxidant Infusion

5 CALORIES

0 G FAT

10 MG SODIUM

1 G CARBS
(1 G sugar, 10 G erythritol)

0 G PROTEIN

3. Hiball Sparkling Energy Water

0 CALORIES

0 G FAT

0 G SODIUM

<1 G CARBS
(0 G fiber, 0 G sugar)

0 G PROTEIN

4. Celsius Naturals

10 CALORIES

0 G FAT

5 MG SODIUM

10 G CARBS
(2 G fiber, 0 G sugar)

0 G PROTEIN

5. Zevia Energy

0 CALORIES

0 G FAT

0 MG SODIUM

0 G CARBS
(0 G fiber, 0 G sugar)

0 G PROTEIN

6. RUNA Energy Drinks

0 CALORIES

0 G FAT

0 G SODIUM

1 G CARBS
(0 G fiber, 0 G sugar)

0 G PROTEIN

7. BluePrint Mindful Ma-Tay Tea

45 CALORIES

0 G FAT

0 MG SODIUM

12 G CARBS
(0 G fiber, 8 G sugar)

0 G PROTEIN

8. V8+ Energy

50 CALORIES

0 G FAT

60 MG SODIUM

13 G CARBS
(0 G fiber, 10 G sugar)

0 G PROTEIN

9. Tea Riot

80 CALORIES

0 G FAT

85 MG SODIUM

19 G CARBS
(0 G fiber, 16 G sugar)

0 G PROTEIN

10. Clean Cause Sparkling Energy Water

20 CALORIES

0 G FAT

10 MG SODIUM

5 G CARBS
(0 G fiber, 4 G sugar)

0 G PROTEIN

Not That!

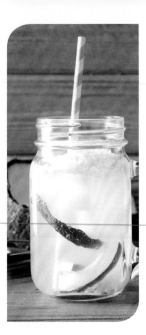

10 POPULAR DRINKS TO AVOID

Liquid calories now account for a whopping 21 percent of our daily calorie intake—more than 400 calories every single day, and more than twice as many as we drank 30 years ago. Simply cutting your drink calories in half could mean shaving off more than 23 pounds in just one year! Avoid these popular, belly-busting drinks to stay lean for life—one sip at a time.

1/ Flavored Coconut Water

Plain coconut water is a wonderful electrolyte replenisher, but once companies throw in added sweeteners and tropical-fruit-flavored syrups (think pineapple coconut water), you often end up drinking more sugar than is in an actual coconut.

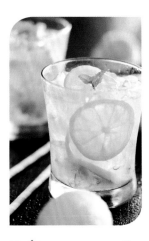

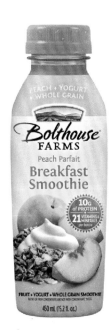

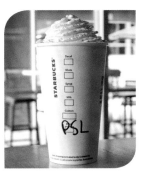

2/ **Lemonade**

While water, sugar, and lemon juice won't make you sick, drinking packaged lemonade in excess could bring on a metabolic condition that will. For example, Minute Maid's version has a whopping 40 grams of sugar in just one 12-ounce can. Craving lemonade? Go homemade! Squeeze fresh lemons, mix the juice with water (or club soda for sparkling lemonade), and add a touch of local honey or agave. For a fun twist to add more flavor, add fresh herbs like mint.

3/ **Drinkable Yogurts**

Probiotics are great for maintaining good gut health, but not when they're tainted with loads of sugar. Take Bolthouse Farms' Peach Parfait Breakfast Smoothie as an example: just one 15.2-fl-oz bottle packs in 360 calories and 45 grams of sugar!

4/ **Pumpkin Spice Lattes**

We know how difficult it can be to resist a classic, comforting PSL, but passing up the pumpkin-flavored bev (or any other seasonal flavor) will do wonders for your waistline. If you order a tall PSL from Starbucks with 2% milk and no whipped cream— a choice that seems slim to most—you're still ingesting 240 calories and 37 grams of sugar. If you really need a caffeine fix, stick to black coffee with a splash of milk and limit your seasonal latte indulgences to once or twice a month.

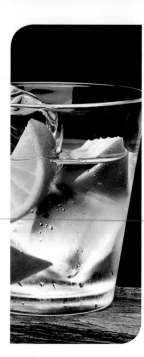

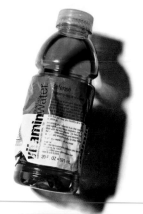

6/ Vitamin-Infused Waters

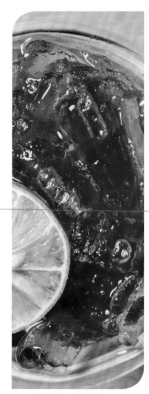

5/ Tonic Water

If you order a gin and tonic at the bar thinking the clear mixer is better for your belly than dark sodas, think again. Just 12 ounces of tonic water can cost you 124 calories and 32 grams of sugar—that's only 7 grams less than soda for the same amount!

While they may have "water" in their name, these bottled beverages are 120 calories each, and every single one of those calories comes from sugar. And it's not just a little bit of sugar, either. There are 32 grams of sugar in a 20-ounce bottle of Vitaminwater, which is 7¾ teaspoons of the sweet stuff. If you want to infuse some flavor and nutrients into your water, ditch the bottled stuff and make a detox water instead.

7/ Fast-Food Iced Tea

Spiked with sugar and caramel coloring, fast-food iced tea is a definite no-go in our book! Our suggestion: Whip up a pitcher of the stuff at home, using natural teas instead.

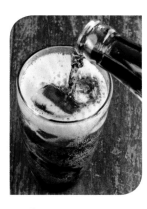

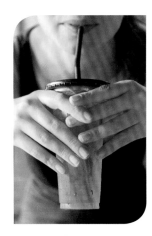

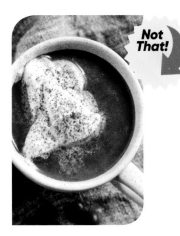

Not That!

8/ Diet Soda

What do artificial colors and fat-causing fake sugars all have in common? They're in your favorite diet fizzy drinks. Nearly all popular diet sodas contain aspartame, an artificial sweetener that was initially developed to aid weight loss and decrease the incidence of metabolic syndrome, but has been found to have the opposite effect. And while they may be largely calorie-free, studies reveal that sugar substitutes can still widen your waistline. Time to kick the soda habit—diet or regular—for good.

9/ Sweet Tea

Word to the wise: If a drink has the word "sweet" in its name, it's probably not going to be great for you. Some bottled sweet teas, like Gold Peak's Sweet Tea, contain 48 grams of sugar (or 96 percent of your daily value of added sugars) in one bottle. Meanwhile, grab a Large Sweet Tea at Sonic, and expect to slurp down 78 grams of the sweet stuff. Your blood sugar will be through the roof after downing that.

10/ Commercial Hot Cocoa

While it's true that packets of hot cocoa aren't great in terms of nutrition, the kind you get from restaurants and coffee joints is far worse. A 16-ounce Starbucks hot chocolate with 2% milk and whipped cream, for example, has half a day's saturated fat, 400 calories, and 43 grams of sugar, which is two and a half times as much as you'll find in the brand's make-at-home packets. Hot coc-no!

CHAPTER 10

COOK THIS, NOT THAT!

IT'S TIME TO stand up for yourself. All the restaurant swaps in the world won't make a difference if you're still putting yourself at the mercy of short-order cooks and corporate food marketers. No matter how smartly you swap one food for another, you can never know for sure that what you're eating is the healthiest possible choice. The only way to do that is to take control, by cooking more at home.

Consider this: Thanks to our restaurant-and-prepared-food culture, the average American woman now eats 1,858 calories a day; the average American man, about 2,697. That's far more than we need to maintain our weight (women should be at or under 1,800, while guys shouldn't top 2,200). And remember, that's to maintain. If you want to lose weight, and you're not signed up for the Boston Marathon, then you need to cut from there.

Does that mean skipping meals? Subsisting only on rice cakes and water? No, but it may mean learning how to wield a spatula. On the following pages, we've created a series of mix-'n'-match recipes that can combine for any number of all-day meal plans. A breakfast-lunch-and-dinner combination from these pages will cost you between 990 and 1,240 calories.

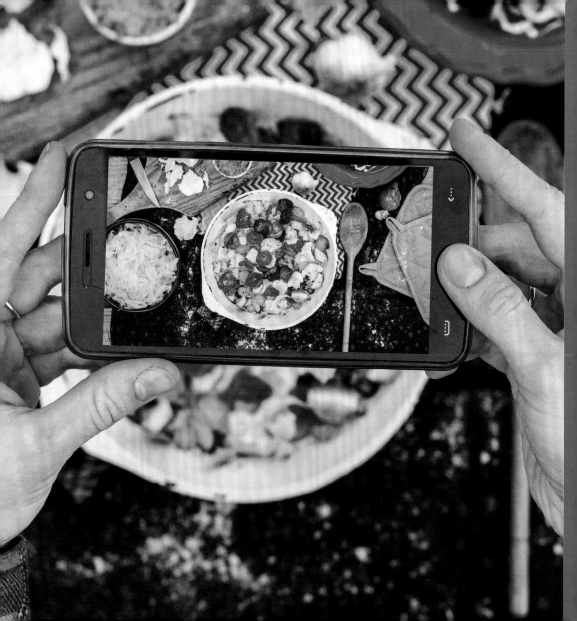

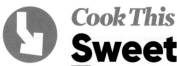

Cook This
Sweet Potato Toasts

HANDS ON: **30 MINUTES** / TOTAL TIME: **30 MINUTES**

YOU'LL NEED

2 medium sweet
   potatoes (16 oz)

ALMOND-CHERRY TOPPINGS

½ cup unsalted almond
   butter

2 cups frozen sweet
   cherries, thawed

   Dash cinnamon

SOUTHWESTERN TOPPINGS

½ cup guacamole

1 cup quartered cherry
   tomatoes

½ cup frozen roasted
   corn, thawed

2 Tbsp snipped fresh
   cilantro

PB&J TOPPINGS

½ cup unsalted peanut
   butter

1 medium banana,
   thinly sliced

3 Tbsp strawberry fruit
   spread

HOW TO MAKE IT

Trim ends of sweet potatoes, leaving skin on. Cut sweet potatoes lengthwise into ¼-inch-thick slices. Discard the short outside slices. Place 4 slices at a time between paper towels. Microwave on high 1 minute. Cool. Place 2 slices, long sides down, in a toaster set for dark toasting. Toast 6 to 8 minutes or until tender, pressing slices back down in the toaster (if they pop up) during toasting. Top as desired.

STORAGE

After microwaving sweet potato slices, cool. Place in an airtight container. Chill up to 3 days.

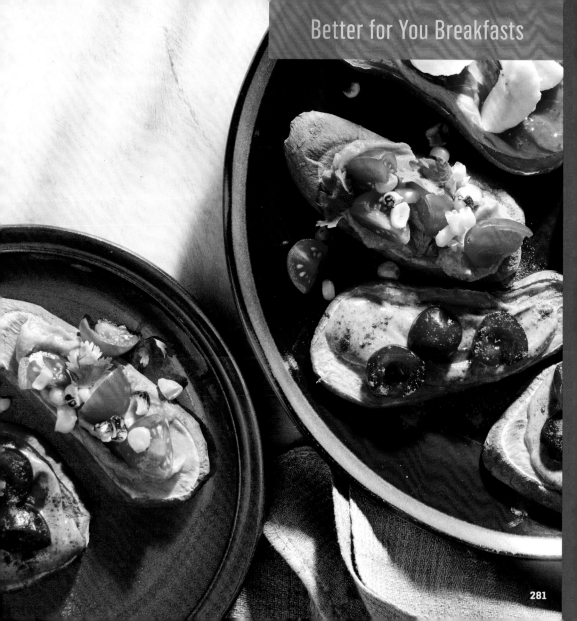

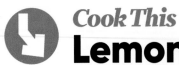

Cook This

Lemon–Poppy Seed Multigrain Pancakes

with Blueberry Compote

HANDS ON: **20 MINUTES** / TOTAL TIME: **30 MINUTES**

YOU'LL NEED

- ¾ cup quick-cooking oats
- ½ cup whole-wheat flour
- ½ cup all-purpose flour
- 1 Tbsp packed brown sugar
- 1 Tbsp baking powder
- 2 tsp poppy seeds
- ½ tsp salt
- 1 Tbsp flaxseed meal
- 3 Tbsp water
- 1 cup fat-free milk
- 1 tsp lemon zest
- 2 Tbsp lemon juice
- 1 Tbsp vegetable oil
  Nonstick cooking spray

BLUEBERRY COMPOTE

- 1½ cups fresh or frozen blueberries
- ½ cup unsweetened applesauce
- ½ cup pure maple syrup

HOW TO MAKE IT

1. In a large bowl, stir together oats, flours, brown sugar, baking powder, poppy seeds, and salt. In another large bowl, combine flaxseed and water; add milk, lemon zest, lemon juice, and oil. Add all at once to flour mixture. Stir just until moistened (the batter should be slightly lumpy).

2. Coat a large nonstick skillet or griddle with cooking spray and place over medium heat. Pour ⅓ cup batter into pan for each pancake, spreading batter if necessary. Cook for 1 to 2 minutes on each side or until pancakes are golden. Turn over when surfaces are bubbly and edges are slightly dry.

3. Meanwhile, in a small saucepan, cook and stir blueberries, applesauce, and maple syrup over high heat until mixture comes to a boil. Reduce heat to medium and cook for 5 minutes. Mash slightly and simmer 3 minutes more or until slightly thickened. Serve over pancakes.

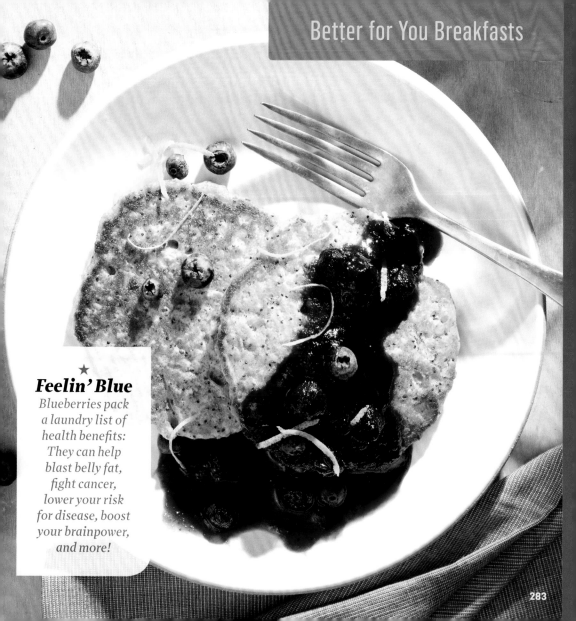

★
Feelin' Blue
Blueberries pack a laundry list of health benefits: They can help blast belly fat, fight cancer, lower your risk for disease, boost your brainpower, and more!

Cook This

Cranberry-Orange Granola

HANDS ON: **15 MINUTES** / TOTAL TIME: **1 HOUR**

YOU'LL NEED

Nonstick cooking spray

2½ cups regular rolled oats

1 cup wheat flakes

⅓ cup whole bran cereal such as Grape-Nuts

⅓ cup coarsely chopped pecans

½ cup orange juice

2 Tbsp pure maple syrup

2 tsp orange zest

½ tsp pumpkin pie spice

½ cup dried cranberries

Fat-free milk, nonfat yogurt, or fresh fruit (optional)

HOW TO MAKE IT

1. Preheat oven to 325°F. Coat a 15 x 10-inch pan with nonstick cooking spray or line with parchment paper; set aside.

2. In a large bowl, stir together oats, wheat flakes, bran cereal, and pecans. In a small saucepan, stir together orange juice, maple syrup, orange zest, and pumpkin pie spice. Cook and stir just until boiling. Remove from heat. Pour over oat mixture; toss just until coated.

3. Spread oat mixture evenly in prepared pan. Bake for 30 to 35 minutes or until oats are lightly browned, stirring twice. Remove from oven and stir in dried cranberries.

4. Immediately turn out onto a large piece of foil; cool completely. Serve with milk or use to make a breakfast parfait with nonfat yogurt and fresh fruit.

STORAGE

Store in an airtight container in the refrigerator for up to 2 weeks or in the freezer for up to 3 months.

NUTRITION FACTS

SERVES 10

Amount per Serving

157 CALORIES

5 G FAT
(1 G saturated)

44 MG SODIUM

4 G FIBER

10 G SUGAR

4 G PROTEIN

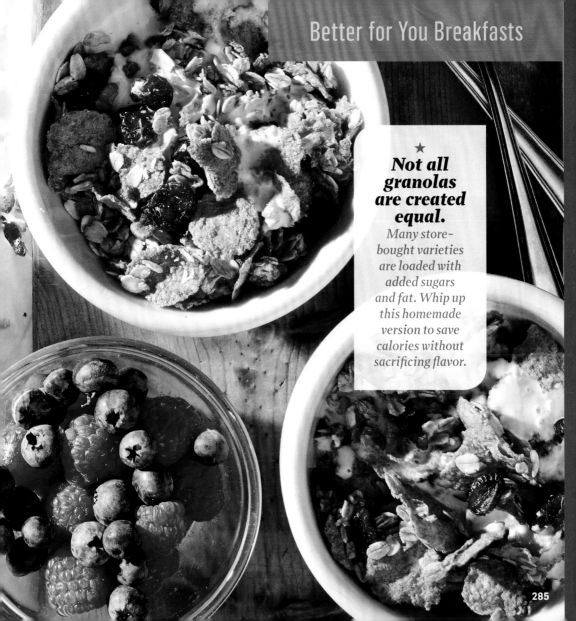

★

Not all granolas are created equal.

Many store-bought varieties are loaded with added sugars and fat. Whip up this homemade version to save calories without sacrificing flavor.

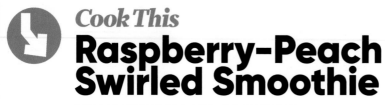

Cook This

Raspberry-Peach Swirled Smoothie

HANDS ON: **15 MINUTES** / TOTAL TIME: **15 MINUTES**

YOU'LL NEED

- ½ cup frozen unsweetened raspberries, thawed
- ⅓ cup orange juice
- 2 5.3-oz cartons nonfat vanilla Greek yogurt
- 1½ cups frozen peach slices
- 1 ripe banana, cut into 2-inch chunks and frozen for at least 2 hours
- 1 Tbsp honey
- ¼ tsp ground ginger
  Fresh raspberries (optional)

HOW TO MAKE IT

1. In a blender, combine raspberries and orange juice. Cover and blend until smooth. Divide between two glasses.

2. Wash out the blender. In the clean blender, combine yogurt, peaches, banana, honey, and ginger. Cover and blend until smooth. Pour over raspberry mixture in glasses. Swirl with a spoon. If desired, top with fresh raspberries. Serve immediately.

NUTRITION FACTS

SERVES 2

Amount per Serving

353 CALORIES

1 G FAT
(0 G saturated)

53 MG SODIUM

7 G FIBER

60 G SUGAR

14 G PROTEIN

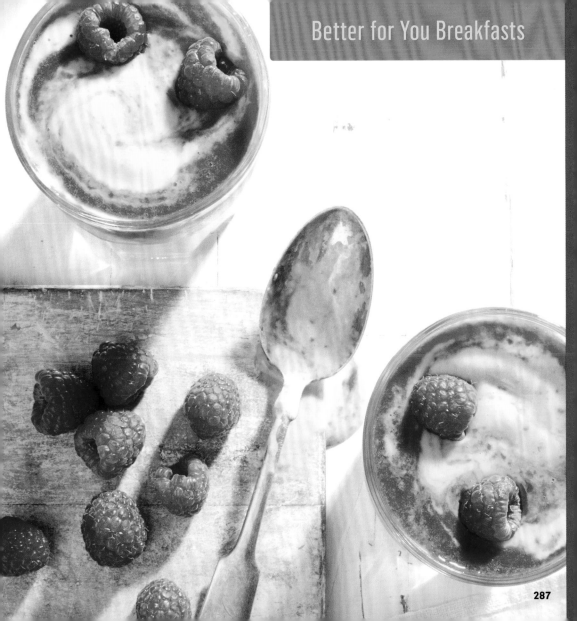

Mango-Ginger Overnight Oats

HANDS ON: **15 MINUTES** / TOTAL TIME: **8 HOURS 15 MINUTES**

YOU'LL NEED

- 2 cups quick-cooking oats
- 1⅓ cups water
- ⅔ cup canned unsweetened light coconut milk
- 2 Tbsp honey
- ½ tsp grated fresh ginger
- 2 cups cubed fresh or frozen mango
- Pomegranate seeds (optional)

HOW TO MAKE IT

1. Place ½ cup oats in each of four pint jars. In a 2-cup measuring cup, combine water, coconut milk, honey, and ginger. Pour over oats in jars. Add ½ cup mango to each jar.

2. Cover; chill overnight or until oats are soft. Top with pomegranate seeds, if desired.

NUTRITION FACTS

SERVES 4

Amount per Serving

264 CALORIES

6 G FAT
(3 G saturated)

38 MG SODIUM

5 G FIBER

20 G SUGAR

6 G PROTEIN

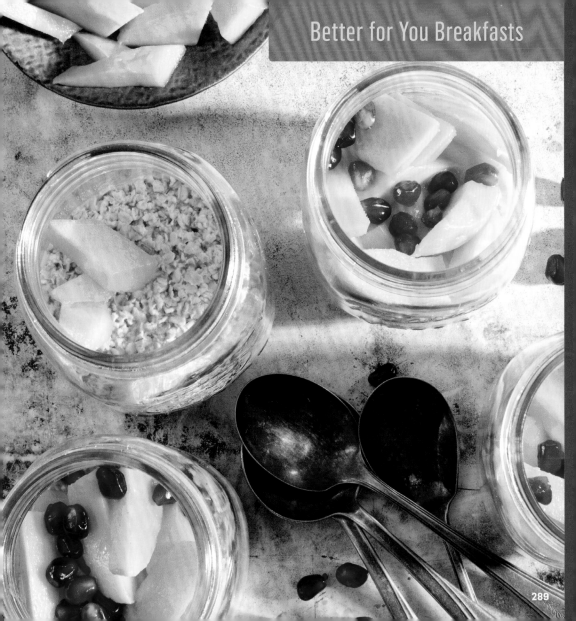

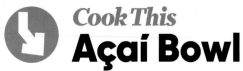

Cook This
Açaí Bowl

HANDS ON: **15 MINUTES** / TOTAL TIME: **15 MINUTES**

YOU'LL NEED

- 1 3.5-oz package frozen açaí pulp
- 2 ripe bananas, cut into 1-inch chunks and frozen at least 2 hours
- 1 Tbsp honey
- 4–5 Tbsp water
- 1 cup fresh or frozen blueberries
- 1 kiwi, peeled and sliced
- 2 Tbsp sliced almonds, toasted
- 2 Tbsp unsweetened coconut, toasted
- 2 Tbsp cocoa nibs

HOW TO MAKE IT

1. In a food processor or high-powered blender, place frozen açaí pulp, frozen banana chunks, and honey. Process until smooth, scraping down sides as needed and adding enough water to make it soft and spoonable.

2. Portion into two bowls. Top with remaining ingredients. Or use your favorite toppings!

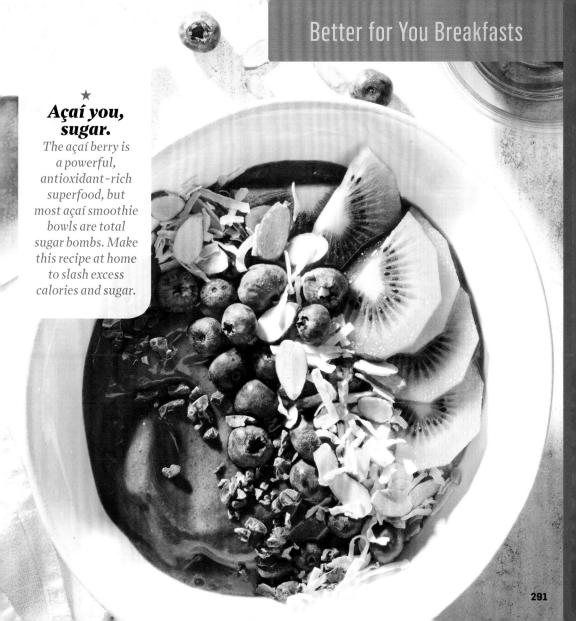

★

Açaí you, sugar.

The açaí berry is a powerful, antioxidant-rich superfood, but most açaí smoothie bowls are total sugar bombs. Make this recipe at home to slash excess calories and sugar.

Cook This

Açaí-Blueberry Smoothie Bowl

TOTAL TIME: **5 MINUTES**

YOU'LL NEED

- 3½ oz frozen pure unsweetened açaí fruit puree
- ½ cup frozen mixed berries
- 10 Tbsp plain whole-milk yogurt, divided
- ¼ cup unsweetened vanilla almond milk
- 2 tsp honey
- 2 Tbsp fresh blueberries
- 1 Tbsp chopped toasted pecans
- ½ tsp chia seeds

HOW TO MAKE IT

In a blender, combine açaí fruit puree, frozen berries, 8 Tbsp of yogurt, almond milk, and honey. Cover and blend until smooth. Pour smoothie into a bowl. Top with remaining 2 Tbsp yogurt, fresh blueberries, pecans, and chia seeds.

NUTRITION FACTS

SERVES 1

Amount per Serving

331 CALORIES

18 G FAT (5 G saturated)

160 MG SODIUM

29 G SUGARS

5 G FIBER

9 G PROTEIN

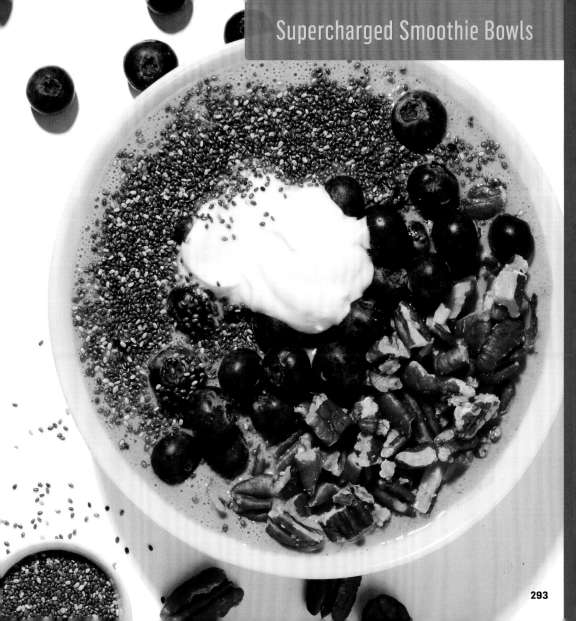

Cook This

Golden Mango Smoothie Bowl

TOTAL TIME: **5 MINUTES**

YOU'LL NEED

- ¾ cup frozen mango chunks
- ½ cup refrigerated unsweetened coconut milk
- ½ tsp ground turmeric
- 1½ tsp honey
- ½ fresh kiwi, peeled and thinly sliced
- ½ cup chopped fresh mango
- 2 Tbsp pomegranate seeds
- 1 Tbsp raw coconut chips, toasted

HOW TO MAKE IT

In a blender, combine frozen mango, coconut milk, turmeric, and honey. Blend until smooth, adding 1 Tbsp water if needed. Pour smoothie into a bowl. Top with kiwi, fresh mango, pomegranate seeds, and coconut.

NUTRITION FACTS

SERVES 1

Amount per Serving

237 CALORIES

5 G FAT
(4 G saturated)

25 MG SODIUM

41 G SUGARS

5 G FIBER

2 G PROTEIN

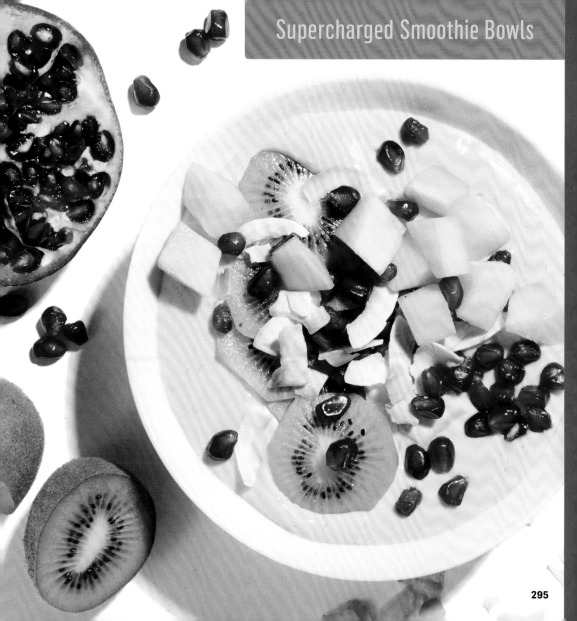

Cook This

Mexican Chocolate Smoothie Bowl

TOTAL TIME: **5 MINUTES**

YOU'LL NEED

- 4 oz silken tofu, drained
- ¾ cup ice cubes
- 2 Tbsp plain low-fat Greek yogurt
- 2 Tbsp dark chocolate almond milk
- 2 tsp pure maple syrup
- ¼ tsp ground cinnamon
- ¼ tsp vanilla
- Pinch salt
- ¼ cup fresh raspberries
- 1 Tbsp roasted unsalted almonds, chopped
- ¼ oz bittersweet chocolate baking bar, chopped

HOW TO MAKE IT

Squeeze tofu between paper towels to remove as much liquid as possible. In a blender, combine tofu, ice cubes, yogurt, almond milk, maple syrup, cinnamon, vanilla, and salt. Blend until smooth. Pour smoothie into a bowl. Top with raspberries, almonds, and chopped chocolate.

NUTRITION FACTS

SERVES 1

Amount per Serving

228 CALORIES

12 G FAT
(2 G saturated)

179 MG SODIUM

14 G SUGARS

4 G FIBER

11 G PROTEIN

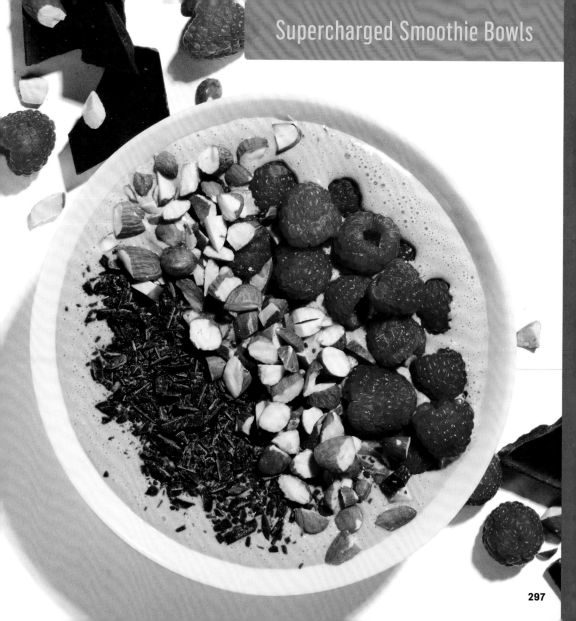

Cook This

Peaches and Green Smoothie Bowl

TOTAL TIME: **5 MINUTES**

YOU'LL NEED

1 cup frozen peach slices

¾ cup chopped kale with stems removed, divided

½ cup unsweetened vanilla almond milk

¼ cup plain low-fat yogurt

2 tsp lemon juice

1 tsp honey

¼ tsp grated fresh ginger

4–5 fresh or frozen peach slices, thawed

2 Tbsp sliced almonds, toasted

HOW TO MAKE IT

In a blender, combine frozen peach slices, ½ cup of kale, almond milk, yogurt, lemon juice, honey, and ginger. Cover and blend until smooth. Pour smoothie into a bowl. Top with fresh peach slices, remaining ¼ cup kale, and almonds.

NUTRITION FACTS

SERVES 1

Amount per Serving

301 CALORIES

9 G FAT
(9 G saturated)

153 MG SODIUM

38 G SUGARS

7 G FIBER

11 G PROTEIN

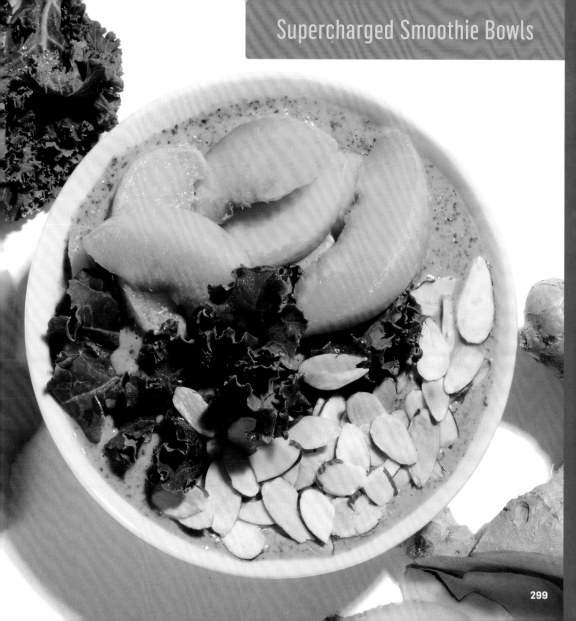

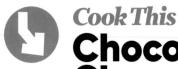

Cook This

Chocolate Covered Cherry Smoothie Bowl

TOTAL TIME: **5 MINUTES**

YOU'LL NEED

- ¾ cup frozen pitted dark sweet cherries
- ¼ small banana, frozen
- ½ cup ice cubes
- ⅓ cup pomegranate-cherry juice
- 1 Tbsp chocolate whey protein powder
- ⅓ cup plain whole-milk yogurt, divided
- 3 fresh dark sweet cherries
- 1 Tbsp raw coconut chips
- 1 tsp cocoa nibs

HOW TO MAKE IT

In a blender, combine frozen cherries, banana, ice cubes, juice, protein powder, and 2 Tbsp of yogurt. Cover and blend until smooth. Pour smoothie into a bowl. Top with remaining yogurt, fresh cherries, coconut, and cocoa nibs.

NUTRITION FACTS

SERVES 1

Amount per Serving

259 CALORIES

7 G FAT
(5 G saturated)

89 MG SODIUM

31 G SUGARS

4 G FIBER

8 G PROTEIN

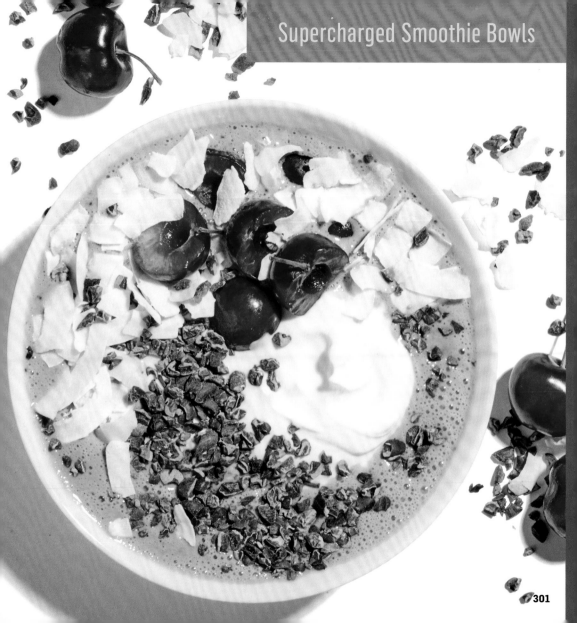

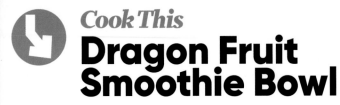

Cook This
Dragon Fruit Smoothie Bowl

TOTAL TIME: **10 MINUTES**

YOU'LL NEED

- 1 cup frozen pineapple chunks
- 1 cup frozen pink dragon fruit flesh
- ½ cup kombucha
- ¼ cup water
- 1 Tbsp vanilla whey protein powder
- ½ cup chopped fresh pineapple
- 4½ tsp raw pepitas
- Fresh mint leaves

HOW TO MAKE IT

In a blender, combine frozen pineapple chunks, dragon fruit, kombucha, water, and protein powder. Cover and blend until smooth. Pour smoothie into a bowl. Top with fresh pineapple, pepitas, and mint.

NUTRITION FACTS

SERVES 1

Amount per Serving

182 CALORIES

4 G FAT
(0 G saturated)

101 MG SODIUM

24 G SUGARS

3 G FIBER

6 G PROTEIN

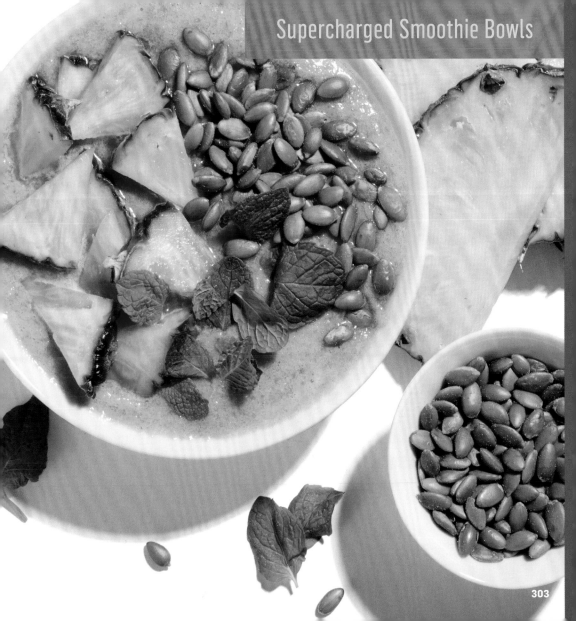

Cook This

Thai Chicken and Rice Casserole

with Peanut Sauce

HANDS ON: **10 MINUTES** / TOTAL TIME: **35 MINUTES**

YOU'LL NEED

Nonstick cooking spray

3 cups cooked brown rice*

2 cups shredded rotisserie chicken

1 16-oz package frozen Asian vegetables, thawed (such as carrots, snap peas, broccoli, and corn)

¾ cup reduced-sodium chicken broth

¼ cup unsalted peanut butter

3 Tbsp lime juice

2 Tbsp reduced-sodium soy sauce

2 tsp pure maple syrup

½ tsp ground ginger

¼ tsp crushed red pepper

OPTIONAL GARNISHES:

Shredded carrot

Thinly sliced fresh jalapeño peppers

Chopped fresh cilantro

Sliced green onions

Chopped unsalted peanuts

Lime wedges

HOW TO MAKE IT

1. Preheat oven to 350°F. Coat a 3-quart baking dish with cooking spray. In a large bowl, combine rice, chicken, and frozen vegetables.

2. In a small saucepan, whisk together the next seven ingredients (through crushed red pepper). Cook and stir over medium heat until mixture is just simmering and peanut butter is melted and smooth. Stir into rice mixture. Pour into prepared baking dish. Bake 20 to 25 minutes or until lightly browned. Top with shredded carrot, jalapeño slices, cilantro, green onions, peanuts, and/or lime wedges, if desired.

NUTRITION FACTS

SERVES 6

Amount per Serving

364 CALORIES

11 G FAT
(2 G saturated)

584 MG SODIUM

4 G FIBER

8 G SUGAR

27 G PROTEIN

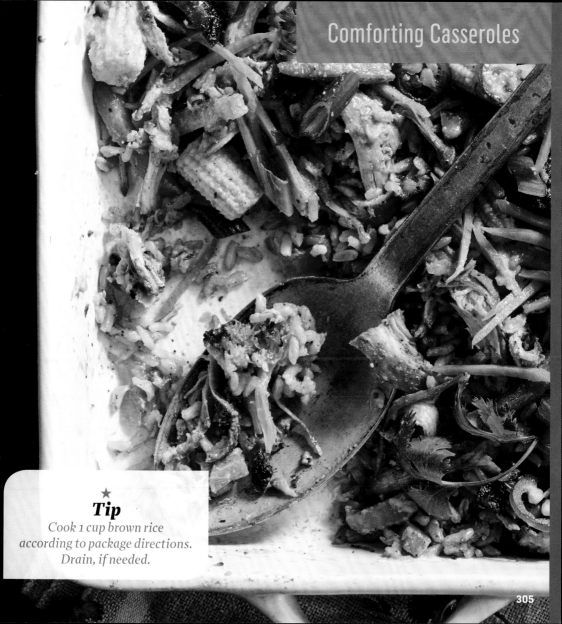

★
Tip
*Cook 1 cup brown rice
according to package directions.
Drain, if needed.*

Cook This
Combo Pizza Casserole

HANDS ON: **20 MINUTES** / TOTAL TIME: **1 HOUR**

YOU'LL NEED

Nonstick cooking spray

1 Tbsp olive oil

8 oz sliced fresh button mushrooms (3 cups)

1 medium onion, chopped

1 medium green bell pepper, chopped

2 tsp minced garlic

3 cups sliced, stemmed fresh kale

1 12-oz package fully cooked Italian-flavor chicken sausage, sliced ½ inch thick

2 15-oz cans no-salt-added cannellini beans, rinsed and drained

1 14.5-oz can no-salt-added fire-roasted diced tomatoes, undrained

1 cup lower-sodium marinara sauce

1 tsp dried oregano, crushed

1 cup shredded part-skim mozzarella cheese (4 oz)

12 whole-grain melba toasts, crumbled (¾ cup)

2 Tbsp sliced pitted ripe black olives

Crushed red pepper

Chopped fresh basil and/or oregano (optional)

HOW TO MAKE IT

1. Preheat oven to 350°F. Coat a 13 x 9-inch baking dish or six 12- to 14-ounce individual casserole dishes with cooking spray; set aside.

2. In a very large skillet, heat oil over medium heat. Add mushrooms, onion, bell pepper, and garlic. Cook, stirring occasionally, 3 to 5 minutes or until vegetables are nearly tender. Stir in kale and chicken sausage. Cook and stir 5 minutes more or until kale has started to wilt.

3. Remove from heat and stir in beans, diced tomatoes, marinara, and dried oregano. Pour into prepared baking dish(es).

4. Bake 20 to 25 minutes or until starting to bubble around the edges. Sprinkle with cheese, melba toast, and black olives. Bake about 10 minutes more or until cheese is melted. Let stand 5 minutes before serving. Top with crushed red pepper and fresh basil and/or oregano, if desired.

NUTRITION FACTS

SERVES 6

Amount per Serving

363 CALORIES

12 G FAT
(3 G saturated)

688 MG SODIUM

9 G FIBER

9 G SUGAR

25 G PROTEIN

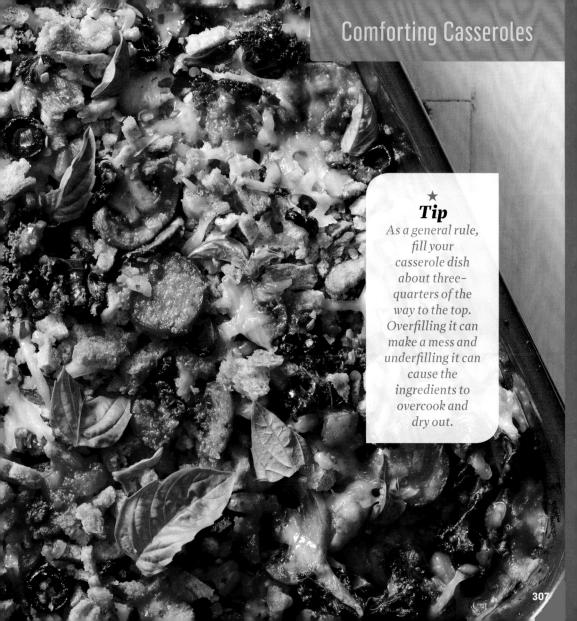

★
Tip

As a general rule, fill your casserole dish about three-quarters of the way to the top. Overfilling it can make a mess and underfilling it can cause the ingredients to overcook and dry out.

Cook This
Cauliflower Macaroni and Cheese

HANDS ON: **20 MINUTES** / TOTAL TIME: **1 HOUR 20 MINUTES**

YOU'LL NEED

Nonstick cooking spray

1 10- to 12-oz package fresh riced cauliflower

10 oz reduced-fat cheddar cheese, shredded (2½ cups)

8 oz dry multigrain high-protein elbow macaroni (2 cups)

2 cups milk (2%)

1 14.5-oz can reduced-sodium chicken or vegetable broth

1 Tbsp cornstarch

1 tsp onion powder

1 tsp dry mustard

½ tsp black pepper

⅛ tsp salt

Dash cayenne pepper

3 Tbsp grated Parmesan cheese

3 Tbsp whole-wheat panko bread crumbs

2 Tbsps snipped fresh parsley

HOW TO MAKE IT

1. Preheat oven to 350°F. Coat a 13 x 9-inch baking dish with cooking spray. Place riced cauliflower, cheddar cheese, and macaroni in baking dish. Toss lightly to combine. In a large bowl, whisk together the next eight ingredients (through cayenne pepper). Pour over cauliflower mixture; cover with foil.

2. Bake 30 minutes. Stir, re-cover, and bake 20 minutes more. In a small bowl, combine Parmesan, panko, and parsley. Remove foil and sprinkle topping over casserole. Bake 10 to 15 minutes or until topping is browned in places and macaroni is tender. Let stand at room temperature 5 minutes before serving.

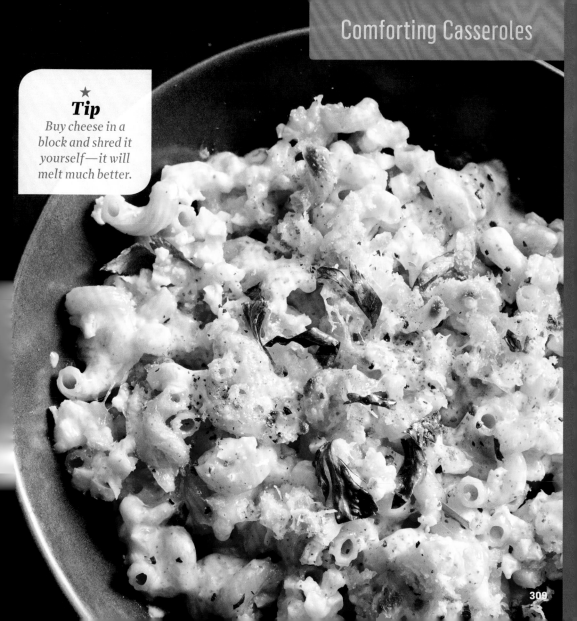

> ★
> **Tip**
> *Buy cheese in a block and shred it yourself—it will melt much better.*

Cook This
African Chicken Peanut Stew

HANDS ON: 20 MINUTES /
SLOW COOK: 7 TO 8 HOURS (LOW) OR 3½ TO 4 HOURS (HIGH) PLUS 30 MINUTES (HIGH)

YOU'LL NEED

- 3 lb bone-in chicken thighs, skinned
- 1 lb sweet potatoes, peeled and cut into ¾-inch chunks
- ½ cup chopped onion
- 3 cups unsalted chicken broth
- ⅓ cup creamy peanut butter
- 2 Tbsp no-salt-added tomato paste
- 2 tsp minced garlic
- 1 tsp grated fresh ginger
- 1 tsp ground cumin
- 1 tsp salt
- ¼ tsp black pepper
- ⅛ tsp cayenne pepper
- 3 cups coarsely chopped stemmed fresh kale

- 1 14.5-oz can no-salt-added diced tomatoes, drained
- ¼ cup coarsely chopped salted dry-roasted peanuts
  Lime wedges (optional)

HOW TO MAKE IT

1. In a 5- to 6-quart slow cooker, combine chicken, sweet potatoes, and onion.

2. In a large bowl, whisk together 1 cup of the broth and the next eight ingredients (through cayenne pepper). Whisk in remaining broth. Pour broth mixture over chicken mixture in cooker. Cover and cook on low 6 to 7 hours or high 3 to 3½ hours or until chicken is done (175°F).

3. Using tongs, transfer chicken to a cutting board. Remove and discard bones. Coarsely shred chicken. If using low heat, raise to high. Return chicken to cooker and add kale and diced tomatoes. Cover and cook 30 minutes more. Top with peanuts before serving. Serve with lime wedges, if desired.

NUTRITION FACTS

SERVES 6

Amount per Serving

338 CALORIES

15 G FAT
(3 G saturated)

632 MG SODIUM

6 G FIBER

8 G SUGAR

29 G PROTEIN

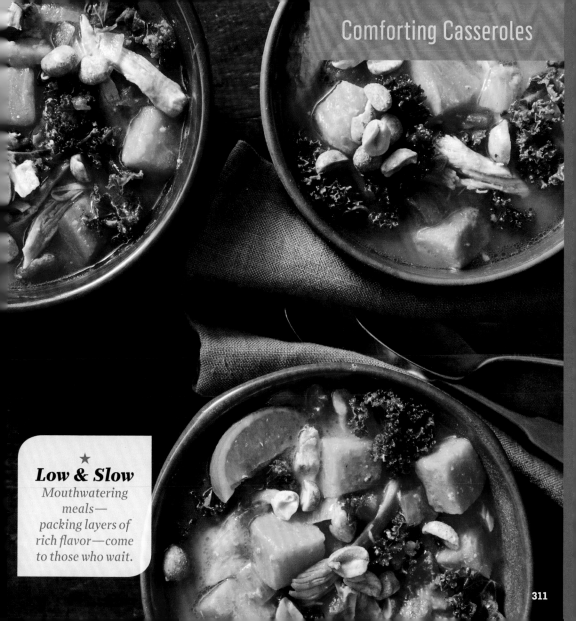

★ Low & Slow
Mouthwatering meals—packing layers of rich flavor—come to those who wait.

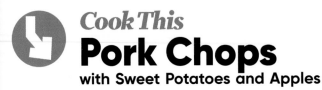

Cook This
Pork Chops
with Sweet Potatoes and Apples

HANDS ON: **20 MINUTES** / TOTAL TIME: **1 HOUR**

YOU'LL NEED

Nonstick cooking spray

2 Tbsp olive oil

2 medium sweet potatoes, peeled and cut into ½-inch chunks (4 cups)

½ cup chopped onion

3 red cooking apples, cored and coarsely chopped

6 boneless pork top loin chops, cut ½ inch thick (about 1½ lb total)

½ tsp salt

½ tsp black pepper

3 Tbsp apple cider or juice

3 Tbsp pure maple syrup

1 Tbsp coarse ground mustard

1 tsp chopped fresh thyme

¼ tsp ground cinnamon

HOW TO MAKE IT

1. Preheat oven to 350°F. Coat a 13 x 9-inch baking dish with cooking spray.

2. In a very large skillet, heat 1 tablespoon of the oil over medium heat. Add sweet potatoes and onion; cook 4 minutes, stirring occasionally. Add apples and cook 4 minutes more (vegetables will not be tender at this point). Spoon vegetable mixture into prepared baking dish.

3. In the same skillet heat remaining 1 table-spoon oil over medium-high heat. Add pork chops and cook about 4 minutes or until lightly browned on one side. Place pork chops on top of vegetable mixture, browned-side up. Season pork chops with ¼ teaspoon each salt and pepper.

4. In the same skillet combine apple cider, maple syrup, mustard, thyme, cinnamon, and the remaining ¼ teaspoon each salt and pepper. Bring just to a boil. Pour over pork chops and vegetables. Cover with foil.

5. Bake about 30 minutes or until sweet potatoes are tender and pork chops just slightly pink in the center (145°F).

NUTRITION FACTS

SERVES 6

Amount per Serving

345 CALORIES

8 G FAT
(2 G saturated)

405 MG SODIUM

5 G FIBER

20 G SUGAR

29 G PROTEIN

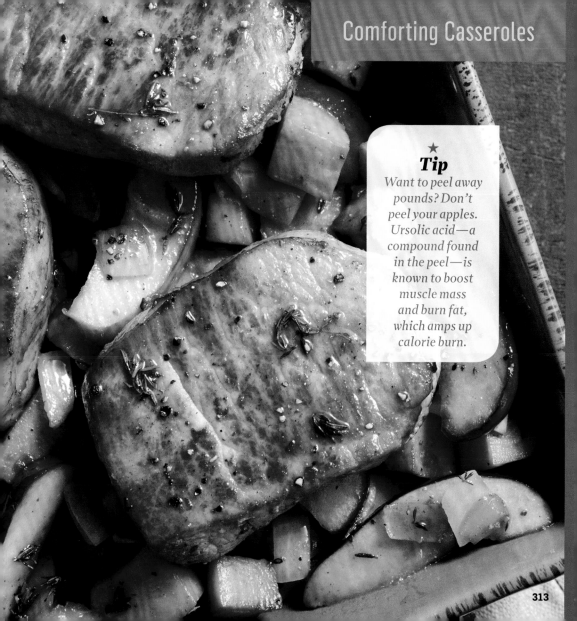

★
Tip

Want to peel away pounds? Don't peel your apples. Ursolic acid—a compound found in the peel—is known to boost muscle mass and burn fat, which amps up calorie burn.

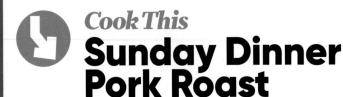

Cook This
Sunday Dinner Pork Roast
with Vegetables

HANDS ON: **20 MINUTES** / SLOW COOK: **7 TO 8 HOURS (LOW) OR 3½ TO 4 HOURS (HIGH)**

YOU'LL NEED

1 8-oz can no-salt-added tomato sauce

3 Tbsp honey

1 Tbsp chili powder

1 tsp onion powder

1 tsp dry mustard

1 tsp paprika

¾ tsp salt

½ tsp garlic powder

½ tsp black pepper

1 2½- to 3-lb boneless pork sirloin roast

1½ lb small round red potatoes, quartered

1½ lb multicolor carrots, halved lengthwise

1 medium red onion, cut into ½-inch-thick wedges

HOW TO MAKE IT

1. In a small bowl, stir together tomato sauce, honey, chili powder, onion powder, dry mustard, paprika, ½ teaspoon of the salt, the garlic powder, and ¼ teaspoon of the pepper. Set aside.

2. Heat a large nonstick skillet over medium-high head. Add pork roast and cook 8 minutes or until browned on all sides. Cool slightly and brush half of the tomato-honey mixture on all sides of pork.

3. In a 5- to 6-quart slow cooker, combine potatoes, carrots, and onion. Sprinkle vegetable mixture with remaining ¼ teaspoon salt and black pepper. Place pork on top of vegetables in cooker. Drizzle remaining tomato-honey mixture over pork. Cover and cook on low 7 to 8 hours or high 3½ to 4 hours or until center of pork roast reaches 145°F.

4. Transfer pork from cooker to a cutting board. Let stand 3 minutes. Slice pork and serve with vegetables.

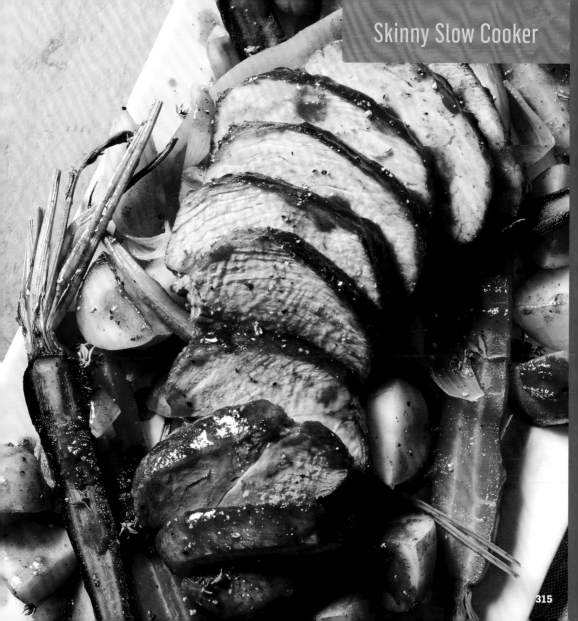

Cook This
Caribbean Beef Stew

HANDS ON: 15 MINUTES /
SLOW COOK: 7 TO 8 HOURS (LOW) OR 3½ TO 4 HOURS (HIGH) PLUS 30 MINUTES (HIGH)

YOU'LL NEED

Nonstick cooking spray

1 lb beef stew meat

12 oz sweet potatoes, peeled and cut into 1-inch chunks (2 cups)

1 10-oz can no-salt-added diced tomatoes with green chilies, such as Rotel brand

½ cup chopped onion

½ cup sliced celery

1 cup reduced-sodium beef broth

3 Tbsp no-salt-added tomato paste

2 Tbsp packed brown sugar

2 tsp minced garlic

2 tsp grated fresh ginger

½ tsp salt

½ tsp ground allspice

¼ tsp black pepper

⅛ tsp ground cinnamon

½ cup frozen green peas

HOW TO MAKE IT

1. Coat a large skillet with cooking spray. Heat skillet over medium-high heat. Add beef and cook 6 minutes or until browned on all sides.

2. In a 3½- or 4-quart slow cooker, combine beef and the next four ingredients (through celery). In a small bowl, whisk together broth and the next eight ingredients (through cinnamon). Pour over meat mixture in cooker. Cover and cook on low 7 to 8 hours or high 3½ to 4 hours.

3. If using low heat, raise to high. Stir in peas. Cover and cook 30 minutes more.

NUTRITION FACTS

SERVES 4

Amount per Serving

303 CALORIES

5 G FAT
(2 G saturated)

575 MG SODIUM

6 G FIBER

15 G SUGAR

29 G PROTEIN

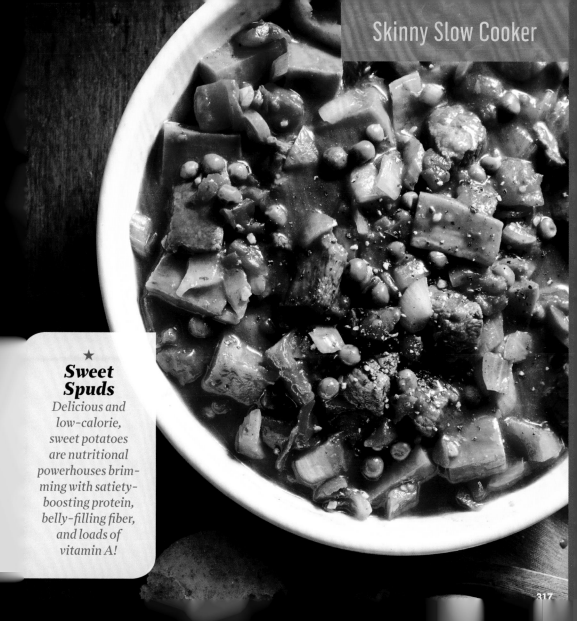

★
Sweet Spuds

Delicious and low-calorie, sweet potatoes are nutritional powerhouses brimming with satiety-boosting protein, belly-filling fiber, and loads of vitamin A!

Cook This

Chipotle-Orange Carnitas Tacos

HANDS ON: **25 MINUTES** / SLOW COOK: **8 TO 10 HOURS (LOW) OR 4 TO 5 HOURS (HIGH)**

YOU'LL NEED

- 1 2½- to 3-lb boneless pork shoulder roast, trimmed of fat and cut into 3-inch chunks
- ½ cup chopped onion
- ½ cup orange juice
- 1 Tbsp ground cumin
- 1 Tbsp finely chopped canned chipotle pepper in adobo sauce
- 1 tsp dried oregano, crushed
- ¾ tsp salt
- ¼ tsp black pepper
- ½ tsp orange zest
- 2 tsp red wine vinegar
- 18 6-inch corn tortillas, warmed
- 1 cup shredded red cabbage
- ½ cup matchstick-sliced radishes
- ½ cup crumbled queso fresco
- ½ cup chopped fresh cilantro
  Orange Crema (optional)*

HOW TO MAKE IT

1. In a 3½- or 4-quart slow cooker, combine pork and onion. In a small bowl, whisk together orange juice, cumin, chipotle, oregano, salt, and black pepper. Pour over pork mixture in cooker.

2. Cover and cook on low 8 to 10 hours or high 4 to 5 hours. Remove meat from cooker. Shred meat using two forks. Stir in orange zest, vinegar, and enough cooking liquid to moisten meat.

3. Serve meat in tortillas with cabbage, radishes, cheese, and cilantro. If desired, top each taco with 2 teaspoons Orange Crema.*

✶ NOTE

In a small bowl, combine ¾ cup plain fat-free Greek yogurt and ½ teaspoon orange zest. Stir in 2 to 3 tablespoons fat-free milk to reach drizzling consistency. Yields about ¾ cup.

NUTRITION FACTS

SERVES 3

Amount per Serving

372 CALORIES

12 G FAT
(4 G saturated)

482 MG SODIUM

6 G FIBER

6 G SUGAR

30 G PROTEIN

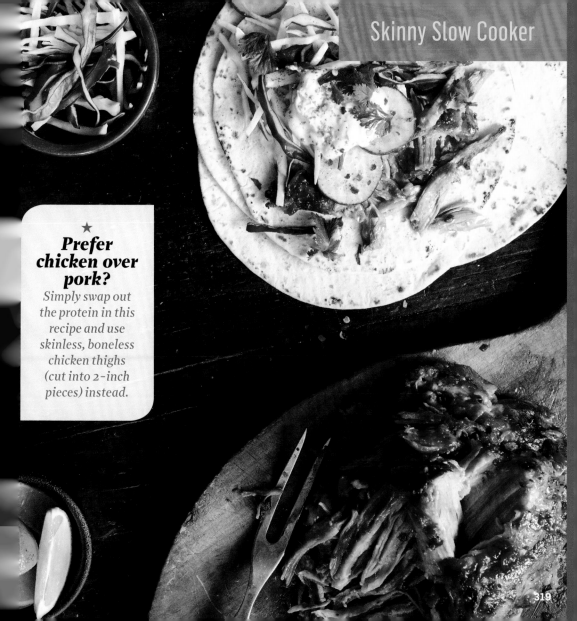

★
Prefer chicken over pork?

Simply swap out the protein in this recipe and use skinless, boneless chicken thighs (cut into 2-inch pieces) instead.

Cook This
Korean Beef and Carrots
with Snap Peas

HANDS ON: **15 MINUTES** /
SLOW COOK: **7 TO 8 HOURS (LOW) OR 3½ TO 4 HOURS (HIGH) PLUS 15 MINUTES (HIGH)**

YOU'LL NEED

- 1 lb beef stew meat
- ¼ tsp black pepper
- ⅛ tsp salt
- 2 tsp olive oil
- 1 8-oz package sliced fresh button mushrooms
- 2 cups frozen pearl onions
- 3 Tbsp reduced-sodium soy sauce
- 1 Tbsp packed brown sugar
- 1 Tbsp lime juice
- 2 tsp minced garlic
- ¼ tsp crushed red pepper
- 2 cups packaged julienne-cut carrots
- 1 8-oz package fresh snap peas
- 2 cups hot cooked quinoa
  Chopped fresh cilantro and/or sriracha sauce (optional)

HOW TO MAKE IT

1. Season beef with black pepper and salt. In a large skillet, heat oil over medium-high heat. Add beef and cook 5 minutes or until browned on all sides.

2. In a 3½- or 4-quart slow cooker, combine the browned meat, mushrooms, and pearl onions. In a small bowl, whisk together soy sauce, brown sugar, lime juice, garlic, and crushed red pepper. Pour over meat mixture in cooker. Cover and cook on low 7 to 8 hours or high 3½ to 4 hours.

3. If using low heat, raise to high. Stir in carrots and snap peas. Cover and cook 15 minutes more. Serve over quinoa. If desired, sprinkle with cilantro and/or drizzle with sriracha.

NUTRITION FACTS

SERVES 4

Amount per Serving

390 CALORIES

10 G FAT
(3 G saturated)

641 MG SODIUM

7 G FIBER

15 G SUGAR

34 G PROTEIN

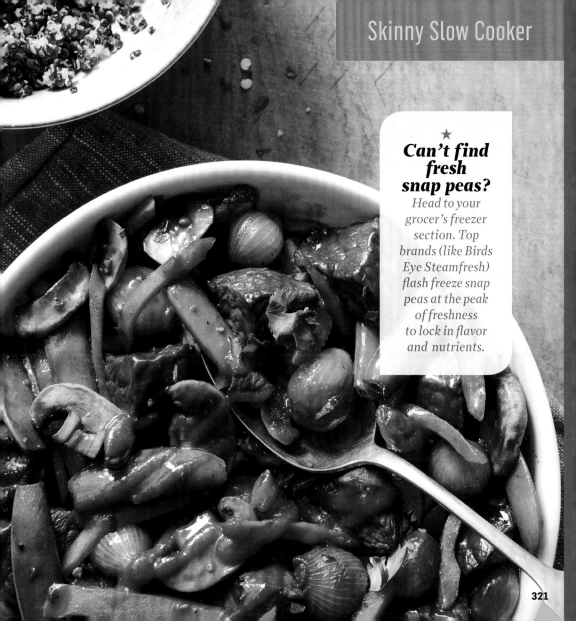

★
Can't find fresh snap peas?

Head to your grocer's freezer section. Top brands (like Birds Eye Steamfresh) flash freeze snap peas at the peak of freshness to lock in flavor and nutrients.

Cook This
Louisiana-Style Red Beans and Rice

HANDS ON: **10 MINUTES** / SLOW COOK: **8 HOURS (LOW) OR 4 HOURS (HIGH) PLUS 1 HOUR (HIGH)**

YOU'LL NEED

- 1 cup dried small red beans
- 2½ cups unsalted chicken broth
- ½ cup chopped onion
- ½ cup chopped celery
- ½ cup chopped green bell pepper
- 1 bay leaf
- 2 tsp minced garlic
- 1 tsp dried thyme, crushed
- ¼ tsp cayenne pepper
- 2 8.8-oz pouches cooked whole-grain brown rice
- 1 12-oz package fully cooked andouille-style chicken sausage links, sliced ½ inch thick
- ½ tsp salt
- ¼ tsp black pepper
- Sliced green onions

HOW TO MAKE IT

1. Rinse beans. In a large pot, combine beans and 4 cups water. Bring to boiling; reduce heat. Simmer, uncovered, for 10 minutes. Remove from heat. Cover and let stand 60 minutes. Drain and rinse beans.

2. In a 4- to 5-quart slow cooker, combine beans and the next eight ingredients (through cayenne pepper). Cover and cook on low 8 hours or high 4 hours.

3. If using low heat, raise to high. Stir in rice, sausage, salt, and black pepper. Cover and cook 1 hour more. Remove and discard bay leaf. Top with green onions before serving.

NUTRITION FACTS

SERVES 6

Amount per Serving

329 CALORIES

7 G FAT
(1 G saturated)

547 MG SODIUM

8 G FIBER

2 G SUGAR

21 G PROTEIN

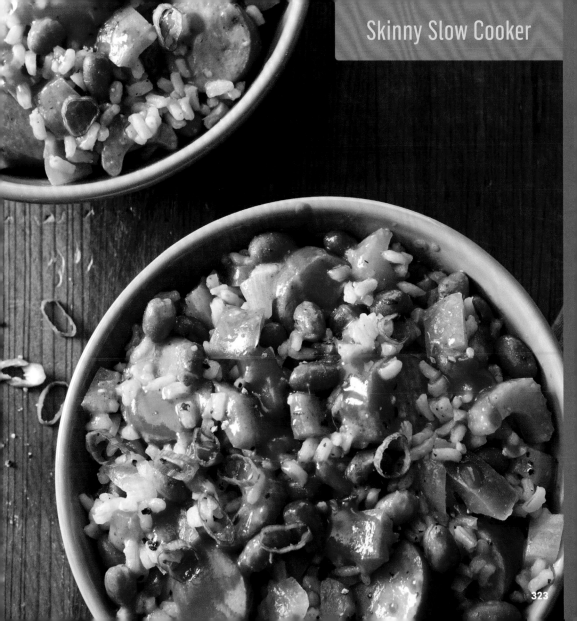

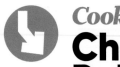

Cook This
Cherry-Coffee Rubbed Pork
with Smashed Parmesan Potatoes

HANDS ON: **20 MINUTES** / TOTAL TIME: **1 HOUR 15 MINUTES**

YOU'LL NEED

- 8 small red potatoes (1½ to 2 inches in diameter) (about 8 oz)
- 2 Tbsp butter, melted
- 1 Tbsp olive oil
- 1 1-lb pork tenderloin
- 1 Tbsp water
- ½ tsp instant espresso coffee powder
- ¼ cup cherry preserves (large pieces snipped)
- ½ tsp black pepper
- ½ tsp paprika
- ¼ tsp salt
- ¼ tsp garlic powder
- ¼ tsp onion powder
- ¼ tsp dry mustard
- 8 oz fresh broccolini or small broccoli florets, trimmed
- 2 Tbsp freshly grated Parmesan cheese
- 2 tsp chopped fresh thyme

HOW TO MAKE IT

1. Preheat oven to 425°F. Line a 15 x 10-inch baking pan with foil. Prick potatoes with a fork and place on one-half of the prepared baking pan. Bake 25 minutes.

2. Holding a folded dish towel, gently press down on one potato at a time to flatten to about ½-inch thickness. In a small bowl, stir together butter and oil. Brush half of the butter mixture onto both sides of the smashed potatoes.

3. Place pork on the other half of the pan. In a small bowl, stir together the water and espresso powder until dissolved. Stir in preserves, ¼ teaspoon of the pepper, and the next five ingredients (through dry mustard). Brush over the pork. Bake 15 minutes. Add broccolini to the pan and brush with remaining butter mixture. Turn the potatoes. Bake 15 to 20 minutes more or until pork is done (145°F), potatoes are golden and crisp, and broccolini is tender, adding Parmesan, thyme, and remaining pepper to potatoes the last 5 minutes of baking time.

4. Remove pork from pan to a cutting board and tent with foil. Let stand 10 minutes before carving.

NUTRITION FACTS

SERVES 4

Amount per Serving

331 CALORIES

12 G FAT
(5 G saturated)

320 MG SODIUM

3 G FIBER

11 G SUGAR

27 G PROTEIN

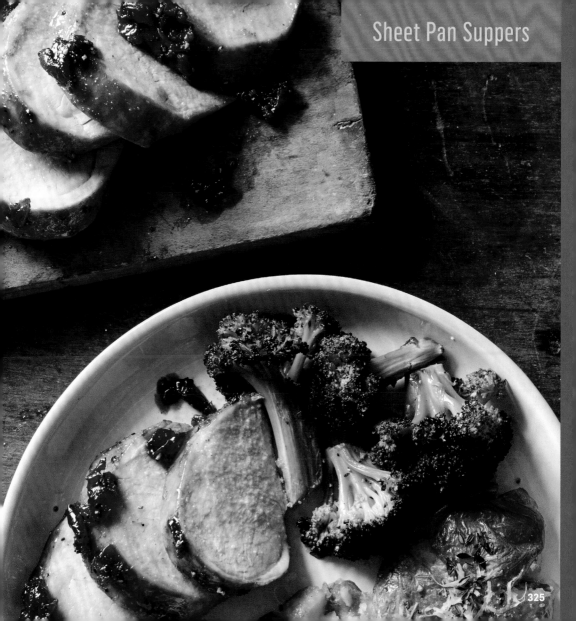

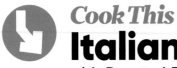

Cook This

Italian Turkey Burgers
with Roasted Brussels Sprouts

HANDS ON: **20 MINUTES** / TOTAL TIME: **40 MINUTES**

YOU'LL NEED

Nonstick cooking spray

1 egg, lightly beaten

3 Tbsp freshly grated Parmesan cheese

3 Tbsp fine dry whole-wheat bread crumbs

1 tsp Italian seasoning, crushed

½ tsp black pepper

1 lb 93% lean ground turkey

12 oz Brussels sprouts, trimmed and halved

1 Tbsp balsamic vinegar

1 Tbsp olive oil

⅛ tsp salt

½ cup lower-calorie pasta sauce, such as Prego brand

⅓ cup shredded part-skim mozzarella cheese

4 reduced-calorie wheat hamburger buns, split and toasted

1 cup fresh arugula

HOW TO MAKE IT

1. Preheat oven to 425°F. Coat a 15 x 10-inch baking pan with cooking spray.

2. In a large bowl, stir together egg, Parmesan, bread crumbs, ½ teaspoon of the Italian seasoning, and ¼ teaspoon of the pepper. Add turkey and stir just to combine (do not overmix). Form into four ¾-inch-thick patties. Place on one-half of the prepared baking pan.

3. Place Brussels sprouts on the other half of the pan. Drizzle with vinegar and oil; sprinkle with salt and the remaining ½ teaspoon Italian seasoning and ¼ teaspoon pepper. Toss to coat.

4. Bake 10 minutes. Turn turkey burgers and top with pasta sauce and mozzarella. Bake about 10 minutes more or until burgers are cooked through (165°F), cheese is melted, and Brussels sprouts are browned and tender.

5. Place burgers on buns and top with arugula. Serve with Brussels sprouts.

NUTRITION FACTS

SERVES 4

Amount per Serving

401 CALORIES

17 G FAT
(6 G saturated)

635 MG SODIUM

10 G FIBER

8 G SUGAR

35 G PROTEIN

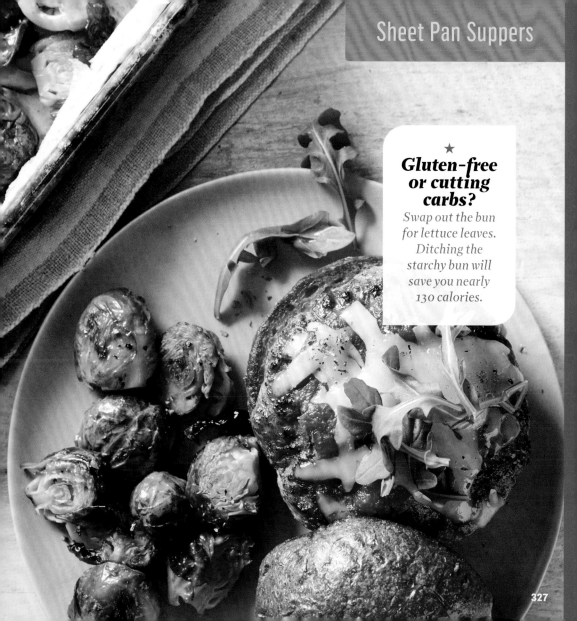

★
Gluten-free or cutting carbs?

Swap out the bun for lettuce leaves. Ditching the starchy bun will save you nearly 130 calories.

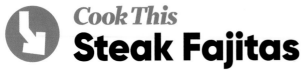

Cook This
Steak Fajitas

HANDS ON: **25 MINUTES** / TOTAL TIME: **45 MINUTES**

YOU'LL NEED

2 red, yellow, orange, and/or green bell peppers, sliced (2 cups)

1 cup sliced red onion

4 tsp vegetable oil

½ tsp salt

½ tsp black pepper

1 Tbsp chili powder

2 tsp ground cumin

½ tsp dried oregano, crushed

12 oz beef flank steak

8 6-inch white corn tortillas, warmed

1 avocado, halved, seeded, peeled, and thinly sliced

Lime wedges, plain fat-free Greek yogurt, and/or crumbled cotija cheese (optional)

HOW TO MAKE IT

1. Preheat broiler. In a medium bowl, combine the bell peppers, onion, 2 teaspoons of the oil, ¼ teaspoon of the salt, and ¼ teaspoon of the black pepper; set aside.

2. In a small bowl, combine chili powder, cumin, oregano, and remaining 2 teaspoons oil, ¼ teaspoon salt, and ¼ teaspoon black pepper. Trim fat from steak. Using a sharp knife, score a diamond pattern in both sides of steak. Using your hands, rub spice mixture onto both sides of steak. Place steak in a 15 x 10-inch baking pan.

3. Broil steak 4 to 6 inches from the heat 6 minutes. Turn steak and add bell peppers and onion to the pan around the steak. Broil 5 to 7 minutes more or until vegetables are lightly charred and steak reaches desired doneness (145°F for medium).

4. Transfer steak to a cutting board and cover loosely with foil; let stand 5 minutes. Toss pepper mixture with pan juices. Thinly bias-slice steak across the grain. Serve steak and pepper mixture in the tortillas and top with avocado. If desired, serve with lime wedges, yogurt, and/or cheese.

NUTRITION FACTS

SERVES 4

Amount per Serving

312 CALORIES

16 G FAT
(3 G saturated)

396 MG SODIUM

6 G FIBER

3 G SUGAR

21 G PROTEIN

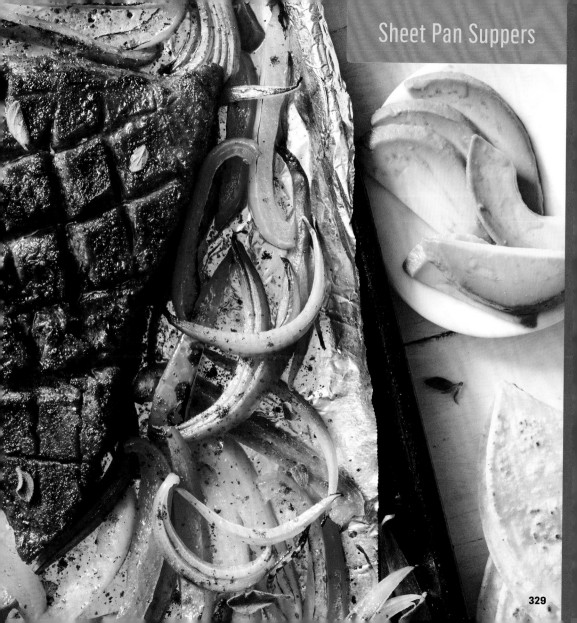

Cook This
Orange Shrimp Dinner

HANDS ON: **25 MINUTES** / TOTAL TIME: **40 MINUTES**

YOU'LL NEED

- 2 oranges
- 3 Tbsp Asian sweet chili sauce
- 1 Tbsp reduced-sodium soy sauce
- 2 cloves garlic, minced
- ½ tsp grated fresh ginger
- ¼ tsp crushed red pepper
- 1 lb fresh or frozen jumbo shrimp, thawed, peeled, and deveined
- 4 heads baby bok choy, halved lengthwise
- 2 cups sugar snap peas
- ½ cup bias-sliced carrots
- 1 Tbsp canola oil
- ¼ tsp salt
- ¼ tsp black pepper
- Toasted sesame seeds

HOW TO MAKE IT

1. Preheat oven to 425°F. Line a 15 x 10-inch baking pan with foil. Remove ¼ teaspoon zest and squeeze 1 tablespoon juice from one of the oranges. Cut the second orange into wedges; set aside.

2. In a large bowl, whisk together the orange zest, orange juice, and the next five ingredients (through crushed red pepper). Add shrimp and toss to coat; set aside.

3. Arrange bok choy (cut-side up), snap peas, and carrots in the prepared baking pan. Brush with oil and sprinkle with salt and pepper.

4. Roast, uncovered, 10 minutes. Add shrimp on top of vegetables. Roast 5 minutes more or until bok choy halves are lightly charred and shrimp is opaque. Remove from oven. Divide among four serving plates. Sprinkle with sesame seeds and serve with orange wedges.

NUTRITION FACTS

SERVES 4

Amount per Serving

196 CALORIES

4 G FAT
(0 G saturated)

655 MG SODIUM

3 G FIBER

13 G SUGAR

23 G PROTEIN

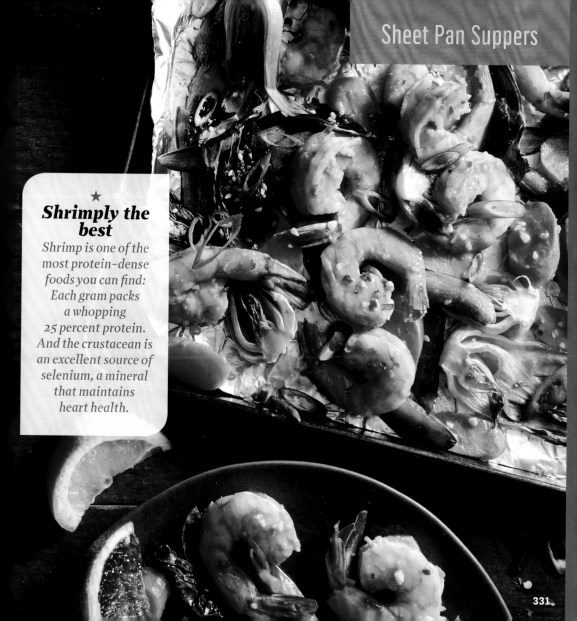

★

Shrimply the best

Shrimp is one of the most protein-dense foods you can find: Each gram packs a whopping 25 percent protein. And the crustacean is an excellent source of selenium, a mineral that maintains heart health.

Cook This

Oven-Fried Chicken

with Curried Vegetables

HANDS ON: **15 MINUTES** / TOTAL TIME: **35 MINUTES**

YOU'LL NEED

- 5 tsp olive oil
- 2 tsp stone-ground mustard
- 2 tsp curry powder
- ½ tsp salt
- 2 cups cauliflower florets
- 1 medium red onion, cut into ½-inch-thick wedges
- 8 oz russet potatoes, peeled and cut into ¾-inch chunks (1 cup)
- 2 eggs, lightly beaten
- ⅓ cup all-purpose flour
- ⅓ cup panko bread crumbs
- 4 6-oz skinless, boneless chicken breast halves
- ¼ cup plain fat-free Greek yogurt (optional)
- 2 Tbsp chopped fresh cilantro (optional)
- 2–3 tsp water (optional)

HOW TO MAKE IT

1. Preheat oven to 425°F. Line a large rimmed baking sheet with foil.

2. In a large bowl, whisk together 4 teaspoons of the olive oil, the mustard, 1 teaspoon of the curry powder, and ¼ teaspoon of the salt. Add cauliflower, onion, and potatoes. Toss to coat. Spread in an even layer on one-half of the prepared baking sheet.

3. Place eggs in a shallow dish. Place flour in a second shallow dish. In a third shallow dish, combine panko and the remaining 1 teaspoon olive oil, 1 teaspoon curry powder, and ¼ teaspoon salt. Dip chicken in flour, then egg, then panko mixture to coat. Place chicken on the other half of the baking sheet.

4. Bake 20 to 25 minutes or until chicken is no longer pink (165°F) and vegetables are tender and browned.

5. Meanwhile, if desired, in a small bowl, stir together yogurt, cilantro, and the water. If needed, add additional water to reach desired consistency. Drizzle over chicken.

NUTRITION FACTS

SERVES 4

Amount per Serving

394 CALORIES

12 G FAT
(2 G saturated)

478 MG SODIUM

4 G FIBER

4 G SUGAR

44 G PROTEIN

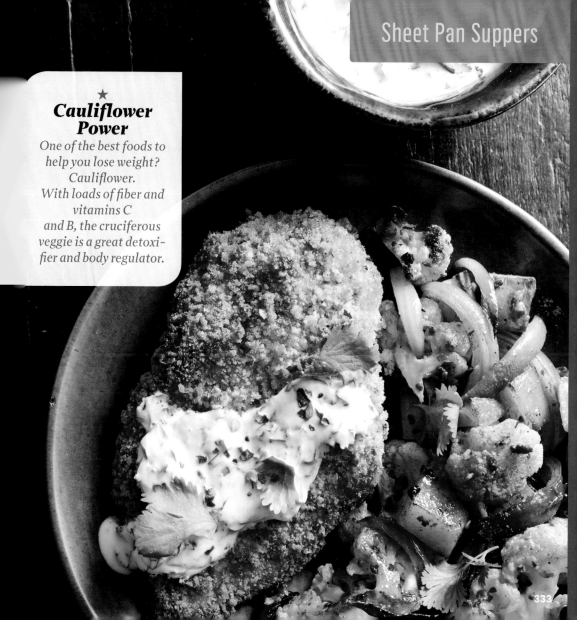

★ Cauliflower Power

One of the best foods to help you lose weight? Cauliflower. With loads of fiber and vitamins C and B, the cruciferous veggie is a great detoxifier and body regulator.

Cook This

Sweet and Spicy Glazed Salmon

with Roasted Green Beans, Cherry Tomatoes, and Yellow Squash

HANDS ON: **15 MINUTES** / TOTAL TIME: **40 MINUTES**

YOU'LL NEED

Nonstick cooking spray

2 cups cherry tomatoes

8 oz fresh green beans, trimmed

1 medium yellow squash, halved lengthwise and cut into ½-inch-thick slices

2 Tbsp olive oil

¼ tsp salt

¼ tsp black pepper

1 Tbsp pure maple syrup

1 Tbsp reduced-sodium soy sauce

2 cloves garlic, minced

⅛ tsp cayenne pepper

1 1-lb fresh skinless salmon fillet

HOW TO MAKE IT

1. Preheat oven to 425°F. Line a 15 x 10-inch baking pan with foil. Coat foil with cooking spray.

2. Place tomatoes, green beans, and squash in the prepared baking pan. Drizzle with oil and sprinkle with salt and pepper. Stir to coat. Arrange in an even layer in the pan. Roast 10 minutes.

3. Meanwhile, in a small bowl, whisk together maple syrup, soy sauce, garlic, and cayenne pepper.

4. Push vegetables to one side of the baking pan. Place salmon on other side of pan. Brush with the maple syrup mixture. Roast 10 to 15 minutes more or until fish flakes easily (145°F) and vegetables are tender.

NUTRITION FACTS

SERVES 4

Amount per Serving

281 CALORIES

14 G FAT
(2 G saturated)

342 MG SODIUM

3 G FIBER

8 G SUGAR

25 G PROTEIN

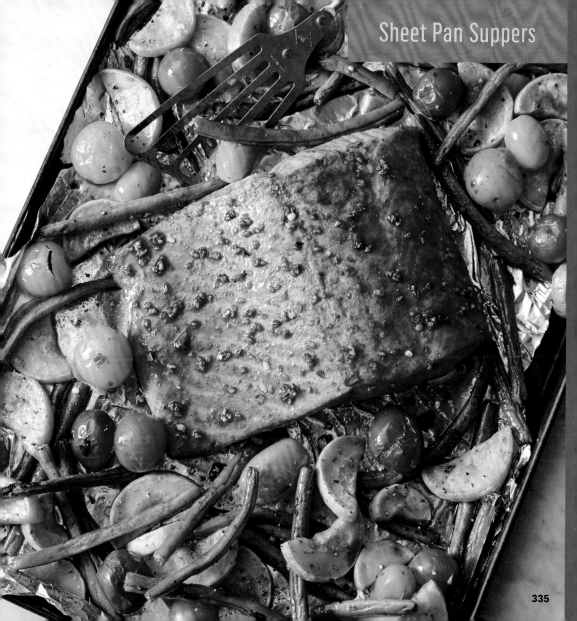

Cook This
Roasted Beet Salad with Barley

HANDS ON: **25 MINUTES** / TOTAL TIME: **25 MINUTES PLUS CHILLING**

YOU'LL NEED

- 6 Tbsp buttermilk
- 3 Tbsp light mayonnaise
- 3 Tbsp chopped fresh chives or green onions
- 1½ tsp lemon juice
- ¼ tsp salt
- ⅛ tsp black pepper
- 2 8-oz packages refrigerated cooked whole baby beets, drained and cut into bite-size pieces
- 1 5-oz package baby arugula
- 4 hard-cooked eggs, halved and sliced
- 1 cup cooked barley or farro
- 2 oz goat cheese, crumbled
- ¼ cup chopped walnuts, toasted

HOW TO MAKE IT

In a small bowl, combine buttermilk, mayonnaise, chives, lemon juice, salt, and pepper. Whisk until smooth. Divide beets among four pint jars. Top with arugula, dressing, eggs, barley, goat cheese, and walnuts. Cover and chill up to 3 days.

NUTRITION FACTS

SERVES 4

Amount per Serving

302 CALORIES

16 G FAT
(5 G saturated)

454 MG SODIUM

5 G FIBER

15 G SUGAR

14 G PROTEIN

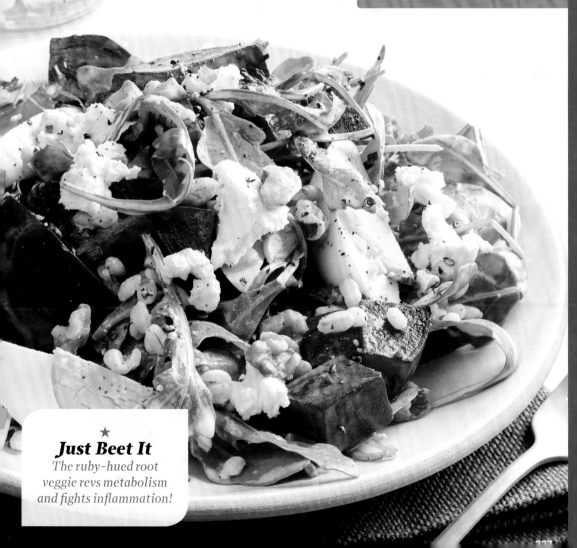

★
Just Beet It
The ruby-hued root veggie revs metabolism and fights inflammation!

Cook This
Clean Bean, Pink, and Green Salad

HANDS ON: **20 MINUTES** / TOTAL TIME: **30 MINUTES PLUS CHILLING**

YOU'LL NEED

- 2 4-oz salmon fillets
- ¼ tsp salt, plus more to taste
- ⅛ tsp black pepper, plus more to taste
- 3–4 Tbsp water
- 2 Tbsp tahini
- 2–3 tsp lemon juice
- 4 tsp olive oil
- ¼ tsp garlic powder
- 10 cups chopped kale
  Dash kosher salt
- 1 grapefruit
- ½ cup canned no-salt-added garbanzo beans, rinsed and drained
- 1 avocado
  Black or white sesame seeds (optional)

HOW TO MAKE IT

1. Preheat oven to 450°F. Line a small rimmed baking sheet with foil and coat with nonstick cooking spray. Place salmon fillets on prepared baking sheet. Pat dry. Season with salt and pepper to taste. Bake 8 to 10 minutes or until salmon flakes easily with a fork.

2. Meanwhile, in a small bowl, combine water, tahini, lemon juice, 1 tsp oil, garlic powder, ¼ tsp salt, and ⅛ tsp pepper.

3. In a large bowl, rub kale with the remaining 3 tsp oil and kosher salt. Divide prepared kale among four pint jars.

4. Cut off a slice from both ends of the grapefruit. Cut away the peel and the white part of the rind (the pith), working from top to bottom. Working over a bowl to collect juice, hold the grapefruit in one hand; tip the grapefruit to its side and cut into the center between one section and the membrane. Cut along the other side of the section next to the membrane to free the section. Set sections and juice aside.

5. Top kale with salmon and garbanzo beans. Top with grapefruit sections.

6. Peel, seed, and chop avocado. Place pieces in bowl with grapefruit juice. Toss to coat. Divide avocado among pint jars. Drizzle with dressing. Cover and chill up to 3 days. Garnish with sesame seeds, if desired.

NUTRITION FACTS

SERVES 4

Amount per Serving

369 CALORIES

20 G FAT
(3 G saturated)

347 MG SODIUM

11 G FIBER

8 G SUGAR

24 G PROTEIN

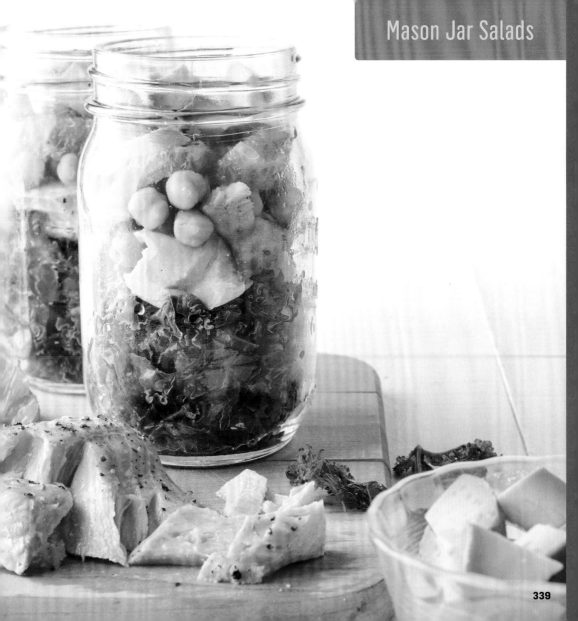

Cook This
Butternut Squash Pasta Salad

HANDS ON: **15 MINUTES** / TOTAL TIME: **35 MINUTES PLUS CHILLING**

YOU'LL NEED

Nonstick cooking spray

1 12-oz package purchased butternut squash cubes (2½ cups)

1 Tbsp olive oil

½ tsp smoked paprika

¼ tsp salt

¼ tsp black pepper

6 oz multigrain or whole-wheat bow tie, penne, or elbow pasta

2 Tbsp apple cider vinegar

1 Tbsp olive oil

1 Tbsp pure maple syrup

1 tsp Dijon-style mustard

¼ tsp salt

1 medium red apple, cored and sliced or chopped

¼ cup dried cherries or cranberries

4 cups spring mix greens

¼ cup pine nuts, toasted

HOW TO MAKE IT

1. Preheat oven to 400°F. Line a shallow baking pan with foil; coat foil with cooking spray. Add butternut squash, olive oil, paprika, salt, and ⅛ tsp pepper to pan; toss to coat. Roast squash 20 minutes or until tender, stirring once.

2. Meanwhile, cook pasta according to package directions. Drain.

3. In a large bowl, whisk together vinegar, oil, maple syrup, mustard, salt, and the remaining ⅛ tsp pepper until smooth. Remove 1 tsp dressing to a small bowl; add apple and toss to coat. Add hot cooked pasta and dried cherries to remaining dressing; toss to coat. Divide greens among four pint jars. Top with pasta mixture, apple, roasted butternut squash, and pine nuts. Cover and chill up to 3 days.

NUTRITION FACTS

SERVES 4

Amount per Serving

387 CALORIES

14 G FAT
(2 G saturated)

334 MG SODIUM

7 G FIBER

17 G SUGAR

9 G PROTEIN

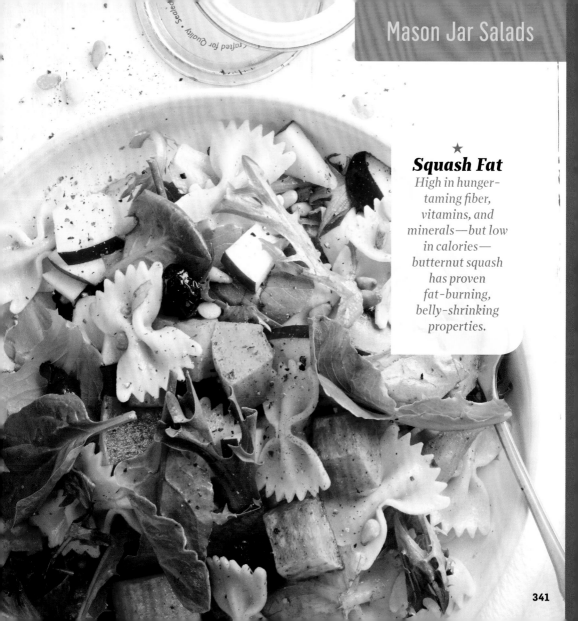

★
Squash Fat
High in hunger-taming fiber, vitamins, and minerals—but low in calories—butternut squash has proven fat-burning, belly-shrinking properties.

Cook This

Cinnamon–Roasted Sweet Potato Salad

with Wild Rice

HANDS ON: **20 MINUTES** / TOTAL TIME: **40 MINUTES PLUS CHILLING**

YOU'LL NEED

Nonstick cooking spray

12 oz sweet potato, scrubbed and cut into ½-inch pieces

1 medium red or yellow onion, sliced into wedges

4 Tbsp olive oil

1 tsp salt

½ tsp black pepper

¼ tsp ground cinnamon

2 Tbsp rice wine vinegar

1 Tbsp curry powder

2 tsp honey

2 cups cooked wild rice

4 oz cooked chicken, shredded

¼ cup golden or regular raisins

2 medium carrots, shaved

¼ cup snipped fresh cilantro

HOW TO MAKE IT

1. Preheat oven to 400°F. Line a rimmed baking sheet with foil and coat with cooking spray. In a medium bowl, combine sweet potato, onion, 1 Tbsp oil, ½ tsp salt, ¼ tsp pepper, and cinnamon; toss to coat. Transfer potato mixture to prepared baking sheet. Roast about 20 minutes or until tender.

2. Meanwhile, in a small bowl, combine remaining 3 Tbsp oil, vinegar, curry powder, honey, the remaining ½ tsp salt, and the remaining ¼ tsp pepper. Whisk until smooth.

3. Divide rice among four pint jars. Top with roasted potatoes, chicken, raisins, and carrots. Drizzle with dressing and top with cilantro. Cover and chill up to 3 days.

NUTRITION FACTS

SERVES 4

Amount per Serving

403 CALORIES

16 G FAT
(3 G saturated)

695 MG SODIUM

7 G FIBER

16 G SUGAR

14 G PROTEIN

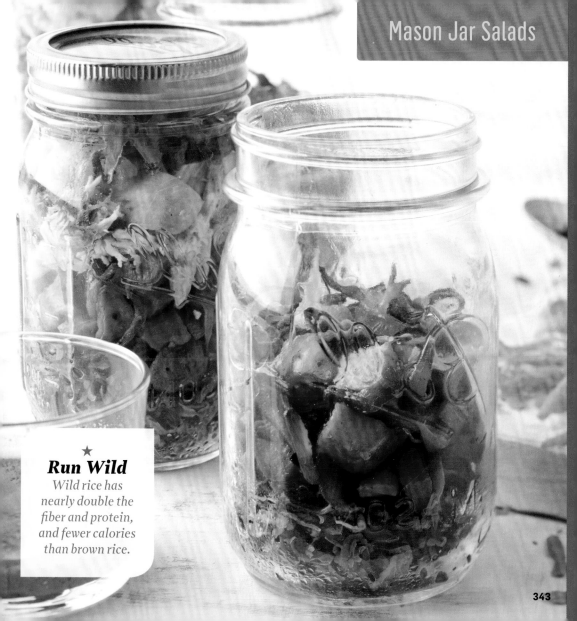

★
Run Wild
Wild rice has nearly double the fiber and protein, and fewer calories than brown rice.

Cook This

Spinach-Pomegranate Salad with Roasted Turkey

HANDS ON: **15 MINUTES** / TOTAL TIME: **15 MINUTES PLUS CHILLING**

YOU'LL NEED

- 2 Cara Cara oranges
- ¼ cup olive oil
- 1 small shallot, finely chopped
- 1 tsp snipped fresh thyme
- ½ tsp Dijon-style mustard
- ¼ tsp salt
- ⅛ tsp black pepper
- 8 cups baby spinach leaves
- 8 oz leftover roasted turkey breast, sliced or shredded
- ¼ cup pomegranate seeds
- ¼ cup chopped pecans, toasted
- ¼ cup shredded Parmesan cheese

HOW TO MAKE IT

1. Using a paring knife, cut off a thin slice from both ends of one of the oranges. Place a flat end of the fruit on a cutting board and cut away the peel and white part of the rind (the pith), working from top to bottom.

2. Working over a glass measuring cup, hold the orange in one hand; tip the fruit to its side and cut into the center between one section and the membrane. Cut along the other side of the section next to the membrane to free the section. Continue with the remaining fruit sections and repeat with remaining orange. Squeeze enough juice from the membranes to

equal ¼ cup. Set sections aside.

3. To the orange juice add oil, shallot, thyme, mustard, salt, and pepper. Whisk to combine.

4. Divide spinach among four pint jars. Top with turkey, reserved orange sections, and pomegranate seeds. Cover and chill up to 3 days. Before serving, drizzle each salad with about 2 Tbsp of the dressing and sprinkle with 1 Tbsp each pecans and Parmesan.

NUTRITION FACTS

SERVES 4

Amount per Serving

337 CALORIES

22 G FAT
(4 G saturated)

340 MG SODIUM

4 G FIBER

8 G SUGAR

21 G PROTEIN

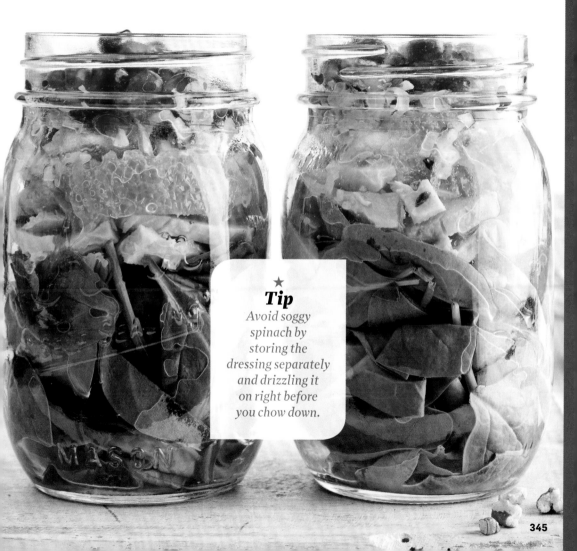

★
Tip
Avoid soggy spinach by storing the dressing separately and drizzling it on right before you chow down.

Cook This

Mexican Quinoa and Chicken Salad

HANDS ON: **30 MINUTES** / TOTAL TIME: **30 MINUTES PLUS CHILLING**

YOU'LL NEED

- 8 oz skinless, boneless chicken breast, cooked and shredded
- 3 Tbsp refrigerated salsa
- 2 cups cooked quinoa
- 1 cup chopped tomato
- ¾ cup canned no-salt-added black beans, rinsed and drained
- ¾ cup frozen roasted corn, thawed
- 1 small red onion, thinly sliced (½ cup)
- 1 avocado, halved, seeded, peeled, and chopped
- 2 Tbsp lime juice
- 2 Tbsp olive oil
- 1 clove garlic, minced
- 2 Tbsp snipped fresh cilantro
- ½ tsp salt
- ¼ tsp black pepper

HOW TO MAKE IT

1. In a small bowl, combine chicken and salsa.

2. Divide quinoa among four pint jars. Layer with tomato, black beans, corn, chicken mixture, onion, and avocado, pressing ingredients down as you fill, if necessary.

3. In another small bowl, combine lime juice, oil, garlic, cilantro, salt, and pepper. Whisk until smooth. Spoon dressing over layers in jars. Cover and chill up to 3 days. Shake jars before serving.

NUTRITION FACTS

SERVES 4

Amount per Serving

413 CALORIES

19 G FAT
(3 G saturated)

375 MG SODIUM

9 G FIBER

5 G SUGAR

21 G PROTEIN

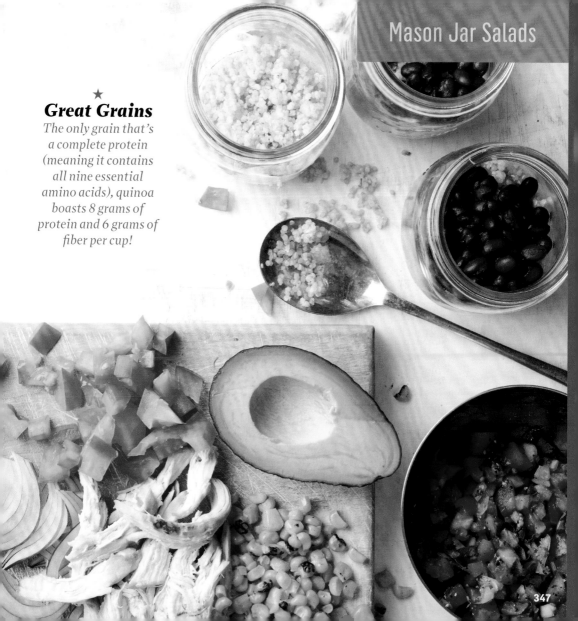

★
Great Grains

The only grain that's a complete protein (meaning it contains all nine essential amino acids), quinoa boasts 8 grams of protein and 6 grams of fiber per cup!

Cook This
Loaded Sweet Potato Skins

HANDS ON: **20 MINUTES** / TOTAL TIME: **1 HOUR 20 MINUTES**

YOU'LL NEED

4 baked sweet potatoes (6 to 8 oz each)

2 tsp canola oil

1 tsp chili powder

Several drops hot pepper sauce

1 cup shredded sharp white cheddar cheese

6 slices lower-sodium, less-fat bacon, crisp-cooked and crumbled

Ranch Drizzle (recipe follows)

Chopped fresh chives

HOW TO MAKE IT

1. Preheat oven to 425°F. Cut baked sweet potatoes in half lengthwise. Scoop out the inside of each potato half, leaving a ¼-inch shell. (Cover and chill the scooped-out potato flesh for another use.)

2. Line a large rimmed baking sheet with foil. In a small bowl, stir together oil, chili powder, and hot pepper sauce. Arrange potato skins cut-sides up on prepared pan. Brush insides of skins with oil mixture. Sprinkle with cheese and bacon.

3. Bake for about 10 minutes or until cheese is melted and potatoes are heated through. Drizzle potato skins with Ranch Drizzle and sprinkle with chives.

RANCH DRIZZLE

In a small bowl, stir together ⅓ cup light sour cream, 3 Tbsp light mayonnaise, 1 to 2 Tbsp fat-free milk, 1 small clove garlic (minced), and ⅛ tsp each dry mustard and onion powder, adding enough milk to make a drizzling consistency.

★ TIPS FOR BAKED POTATOES

1. Preheat oven to 425°F. Scrub potatoes thoroughly with a brush; pat dry. Prick potatoes with a fork. Bake for 40 to 60 minutes or until tender.

2. If desired, use half sweet potatoes and half russet potatoes. Use white cheddar cheese on the sweet potatoes and yellow cheddar cheese on the russet potatoes.

NUTRITION FACTS

SERVES 4

Amount per Serving

305 CALORIES

18 G FAT
(8 G saturated)

469 MG SODIUM

3 G FIBER

5 G SUGAR

13 G PROTEIN

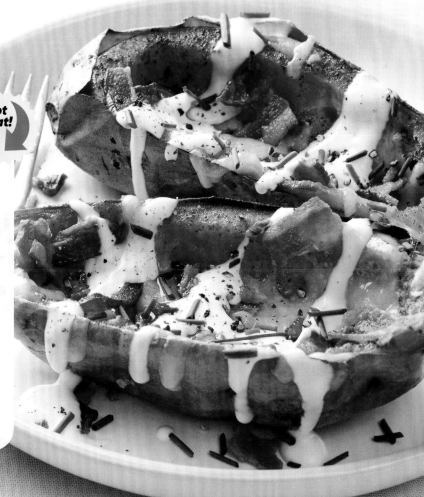

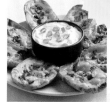

Not That!

T.G.I. Friday's Loaded Potato Skins

1,620 CALORIES

91 G FAT (33 G saturated)

1,910 MG SODIUM

24 G FIBER

9 G SUGAR

51 G PROTEIN

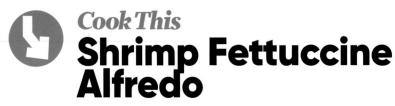

Cook This
Shrimp Fettuccine Alfredo

HANDS ON: **20 MINUTES** / TOTAL TIME: **30 MINUTES**

YOU'LL NEED

- 8 oz fresh or frozen peeled, deveined medium shrimp
- 6 oz dry whole-grain fettuccine
- 8 oz fresh asparagus spears, trimmed and cut into 1-inch pieces
- 1 tsp butter
- ¼ cup finely chopped onion
- 2 cloves garlic, minced
- ½ cup light sour cream
- 3 Tbsp all-purpose flour
- 1½ cups fat-free half-and-half
- ½ cup reduced-sodium chicken broth
- ¼ tsp salt
- ¼ tsp ground white pepper
- ½ cup finely shredded Parmesan cheese

HOW TO MAKE IT

1. Thaw shrimp, if frozen. Cut shrimp in half lengthwise. In a Dutch oven, cook fettuccine according to package directions; add shrimp and asparagus for the last 2 minutes of cooking. Drain well. Return to saucepan; cover and keep warm.

2. In a large skillet, melt butter over medium heat. Add onion and garlic; cook for about 3 minutes or until onion is tender.

3. Meanwhile, in a large bowl, whisk together sour cream and flour. Gradually whisk in half-and-half and broth. Add salt and pepper.

4. Stir half-and-half mixture into onion in skillet. Cook and stir over medium heat just until bubbly; cook and stir for 2 minutes more. Stir in Parmesan until melted. Pour sauce over pasta mixture in Dutch oven; toss to coat.

★ TIP

Slicing shrimp in half lengthwise doubles the number of shrimp pieces without adding any calories!

NUTRITION FACTS

SERVES 4

Amount per Serving

367 CALORIES

10 G FAT
(5 G saturated)

589 MG SODIUM

6 G FIBER

7 G SUGAR

26 G PROTEIN

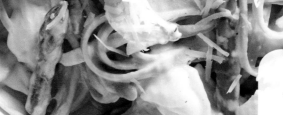

Not That!

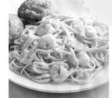

Red Lobster Shrimp Linguini Alfredo

1,170 CALORIES

56 G FAT (23 G saturated)

2,700 MG SODIUM

9 G FIBER

5 G SUGAR

50 G PROTEIN

★
Alfred-no
The restaurant version contains an entire day's worth of fat and sodium! We fixed that.

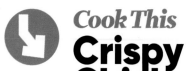

Cook This
Crispy Parmesan Chicken Bites

HANDS ON: **15 MINUTES** / TOTAL TIME: **30 MINUTES**

YOU'LL NEED

- 1¼ lb skinless, boneless chicken breast halves
- 2 egg whites
- ⅔ cup grated Parmesan or Romano cheese (4 oz)
- ⅔ cup whole-wheat panko bread crumbs
- ¼ tsp onion powder
- ¼ tsp black pepper
- Nonstick cooking spray

HOW TO MAKE IT

1. Preheat oven to 425°F. Line a large rimmed baking sheet with parchment paper. Cut chicken into 24 equal pieces (about 1½ inches).

2. In a small bowl, whisk egg whites until frothy. In a shallow dish, combine Parmesan, panko, onion powder, and pepper.

3. Add chicken to egg whites; toss to coat. Transfer chicken, a few pieces at a time, to cheese mixture; turn to coat. (If necessary, press lightly to adhere.) Arrange chicken on prepared baking sheet, leaving 1 to 2 inches of space between pieces. Lightly coat chicken with cooking spray.

4. Bake for about 15 minutes or until chicken is cooked through (165°F) and coating is lightly browned, turning once halfway through baking time.

★ TIP FOR SUGGESTED SAUCES

Serve with low-sodium BARBECUE sauce.

Or homemade HONEY MUSTARD (Stir together ¼ cup light mayo and 2 Tbsp honey mustard.)

Or LIGHT RANCH (Stir together ⅓ cup fat-free plain Greek yogurt and 2 tsp ranch dry salad dressing mix.)

NUTRITION FACTS

SERVES 4

Amount per Serving

284 CALORIES

8 G FAT
(3 G saturated)

349 MG SODIUM

1 G FIBER

0 G SUGAR

40 G PROTEIN

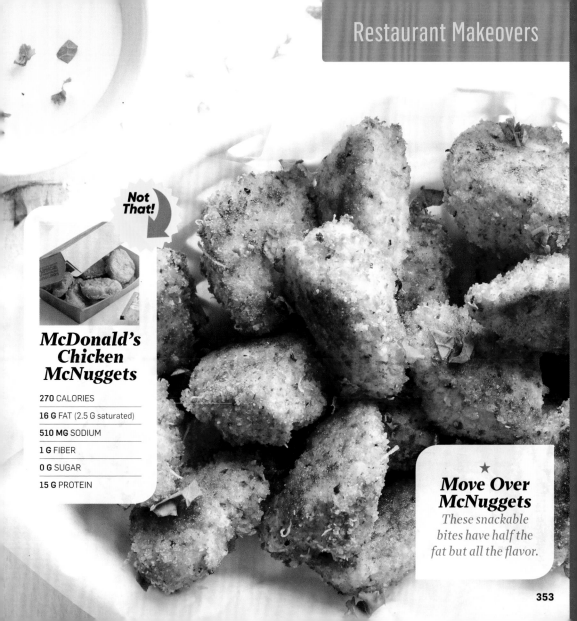

Not That!

McDonald's Chicken McNuggets

270 CALORIES

16 G FAT (2.5 G saturated)

510 MG SODIUM

1 G FIBER

0 G SUGAR

15 G PROTEIN

★
Move Over McNuggets
These snackable bites have half the fat but all the flavor.

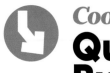

Cook This

Quick Carnitas Burrito Wraps

HANDS ON: **40 MINUTES** / TOTAL TIME: **40 MINUTES**

YOU'LL NEED

- 1 Tbsp olive oil
- 12 oz pork tenderloin, trimmed and cut into bite-size strips
- ½ cup thin strips red bell pepper
- ½ cup thin wedges red onion
- ⅔ cup canned no-salt-added black beans or pinto beans, rinsed and drained
- 4 8-inch whole-wheat flour tortillas
- ¾ cup shredded Monterey Jack cheese (plain or with jalapeño peppers)
- Nonstick cooking spray
- ½ cup fresh tomato salsa
- Fresh cilantro leaves

HOW TO MAKE IT

1. In a large nonstick skillet, heat oil over medium-high heat. Cook and stir pork, bell pepper, and onion in hot oil for about 5 minutes or until pork is no longer pink. Remove from heat. Stir in beans.

2. Place tortillas between paper towels. Microwave on high for 20 to 40 seconds or until warm. Using a slotted spoon, spoon pork mixture onto tortillas just below centers. Top with cheese. Fold bottom edge of each tortilla up and over filling. Fold in opposite sides; roll them up from the bottom. Lightly coat outsides of wraps with cooking spray.

3. Preheat an indoor grill or panini press according to manufacturer's directions. Place wraps, half at a time if necessary, in grill. Close lid and grill for 4 to 6 minutes or until tortillas are toasted and filling is heated through. (Or use a skillet or grill pan to heat wraps. Place wraps in a preheated skillet; place a large skillet on top of wraps. You may need to add a few unopened cans of food to skillet for extra weight. Cook 2 to 3 minutes or until golden brown on bottoms. Carefully remove top skillet [it may be hot]. Turn wraps. Replace skillet and weights; cook 2 to 3 minutes more or until wraps are golden.) Top with salsa and cilantro.

NUTRITION FACTS

SERVES 4

Amount per Serving

377 CALORIES

15 G FAT
(6 G saturated)

552 MG SODIUM

6 G FIBER

5 G SUGAR

27 G PROTEIN

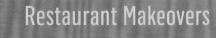

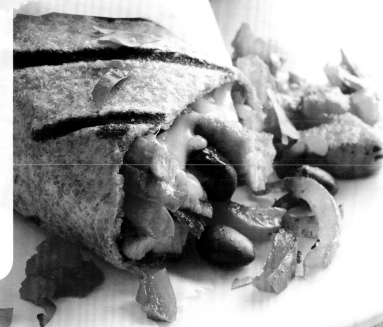

Not That!

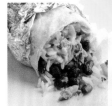

Chipotle Carnitas Burrito with Queso

1,320 CALORIES

60 G FAT (17 G saturated)

2,500 MG SODIUM

22.5 G FIBER

10 G SUGAR

55 G PROTEIN

Cook This
Bacon Cheeseburger Stack

HANDS ON: **20 MINUTES** / TOTAL TIME: **24 MINUTES**

YOU'LL NEED

- 1 egg, lightly beaten
- ¼ cup quick-cooking rolled oats
- ⅛ tsp plus a dash cayenne pepper
- 1 lb ground turkey breast
- 3 Tbsp light mayonnaise
- 2 tsp dill pickle relish
- 1 tsp ketchup
- ¼ tsp dry mustard
- 4 slices thinly sliced sharp cheddar cheese, halved
- 4 light whole-wheat hamburger buns, toasted
- ¼ cup chopped bell or hot cherry peppers
- 4 slices lower-sodium, less-fat bacon, halved and crisp-cooked
- 4 leaves lettuce (optional)
- 4 slices tomato (optional)

HOW TO MAKE IT

1. In a large bowl, combine egg, oats, and ⅛ tsp cayenne pepper. Add turkey; mix well. Shape turkey mixture into eight 3½-inch-diameter patties.

2. For sauce, in a small bowl, stir together mayonnaise, pickle relish, ketchup, dry mustard, and the dash of cayenne pepper.

3. Grill burgers on a greased grill rack directly over medium heat, covered, for 4 to 5 minutes or until done (160°F), turning once and adding a half slice of cheese to each burger the last 1 minute of cooking.

4. To assemble burgers, spread sauce over cut sides of bun tops. Stack two burgers in buns with chopped peppers, bacon, and, if desired, lettuce and tomato.

★ TIP

To toast hamburger buns, grill them cut-side down over medium heat for 30 to 60 seconds or until toasted.

NUTRITION FACTS

SERVES 4

Amount per Serving

407 CALORIES

17 G FAT
(7 G saturated)

707 MG SODIUM

7 G FIBER

3 G SUGAR

43 G PROTEIN

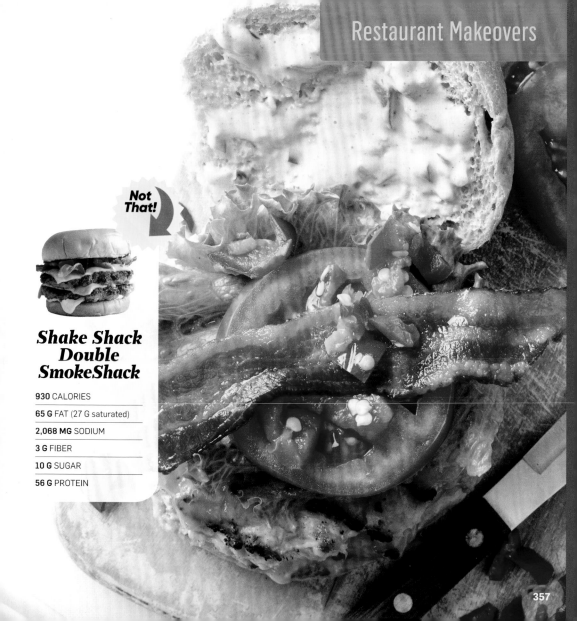

Not That!

Shake Shack Double SmokeShack

930 CALORIES

65 G FAT (27 G saturated)

2,068 MG SODIUM

3 G FIBER

10 G SUGAR

56 G PROTEIN

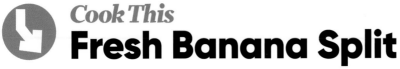

Cook This
Fresh Banana Split

HANDS ON: **15 MINUTES** / TOTAL TIME: **15 MINUTES**

YOU'LL NEED

1 small banana, peeled and halved lengthwise

3 ¼-cup scoops vanilla, chocolate, and/or strawberry light or low-fat ice cream

1 Tbsp chocolate-flavored syrup

⅓ cup chopped fresh strawberries, lightly mashed

⅓ cup chopped fresh pineapple, lightly mashed

2 Tbsp pressurized whipped dessert topping

1 Tbsp sliced almonds, toasted

2 fresh sweet cherries, pitted (optional)

HOW TO MAKE IT

Place banana halves along sides of an individual oblong serving dish. Top with ice cream scoops. Top one scoop with chocolate syrup, one scoop with strawberries, and one scoop with pineapple. Add 1 Tbsp of dessert topping between each scoop of ice cream. Sprinkle almonds over top. If desired, add cherries to whipped topping.

★ TIP

If desired, chop and mash pineapple and strawberries up to 8 hours ahead of time. Cover and store in the refrigerator until ready to serve.

NUTRITION FACTS

SERVES 1

Amount per Serving

393 CALORIES

10 G FAT
(4 G saturated)

74 MG SODIUM

6 G FIBER

50 G SUGAR

8 G PROTEIN

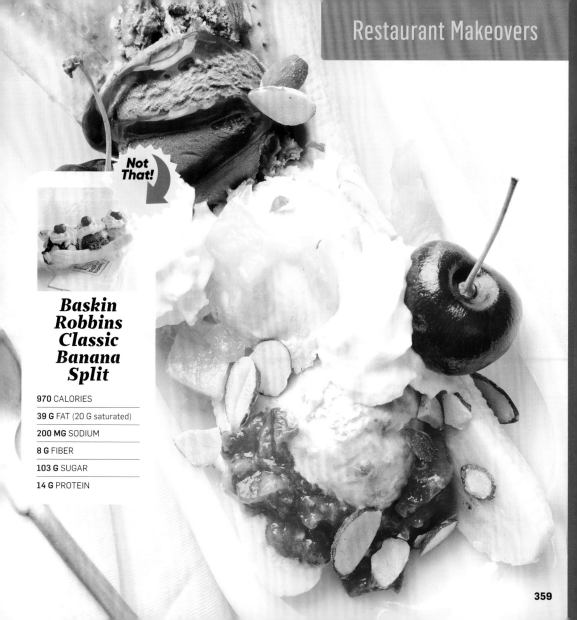

Not That!

Baskin Robbins Classic Banana Split

970 CALORIES

39 G FAT (20 G saturated)

200 MG SODIUM

8 G FIBER

103 G SUGAR

14 G PROTEIN

T